JAMIE'S
30
MINUTE
MEALS

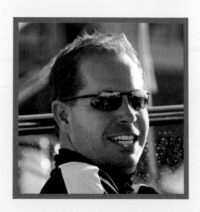

SIMON LAURENCE KINDER
7 April 1962 – 16 May 2010

I dedicate this book to Simon Kinder, a dear friend of mine who has sadly passed away. He was the Managing Director of Magimix UK and one of the very best and most loved figures in the food industry. He was certainly one of my favourite people to be around, and his passion for food and friendship was always appreciated. He'll be sorely missed by me and my team, as well as all of his staff at Magimix. Our love goes out to his wonderful children, Max and Katya, their mother, Monica, and to all of his family.

He would have loved this book because we use food processors and liquidizers left, right and centre to make it speedy. Bless him.

THE MEALS

BROCCOLI ORECCHIETTE   courgette & bocconcini salad, prosciutto & melon salad   24

PREGNANT JOOLS'S PASTA   crunchy chicory & watercress salad, little frangipane tarts   30

CAULIFLOWER MACARONI   chicory salad with insane dressing, lovely stewed fruit   34

TRAPANI-STYLE RIGATONI   griddled chicory salad, rocket & Parmesan salad, limoncello kinda trifle   40

WONKY SUMMER PASTA   herby salad, pear drop tartlets   44

SUMMER VEG LASAGNE   Tuscan tomato salad, quick mango frozen yoghurt in baby cornets   48

SPAGHETTI ALLA PUTTANESCA   crunchy salad, garlic bread, silky chocolate ganache   54

CHEAT'S PIZZA   3 delish salads, squashed cherries & vanilla mascarpone cream   58

OOZY MUSHROOM RISOTTO   spinach salad, quick lemon & raspberry cheesecake   64

SPINACH & FETA FILO PIE   cucumber salad, tomato salad, coated ice cream   70

TOMATO SOUP   chunky croutons, crunchy veg and guacamole, sticky prune sponge puddings   76

CURRY ROGAN JOSH   fluffy rice, carrot salad, poppadoms, flatbread   80

GREEN CURRY   crispy chicken, kimchee slaw, rice noodles   86

CHICKEN PIE   French-style peas, sweet carrot smash, berries, shortbread & Chantilly cream   90

MUSTARD CHICKEN   quick dauphinoise, greens, Black Forest affogato   96

TRAY-BAKED CHICKEN   squashed potatoes, creamed spinach, strawberry slushie   102

KILLER JERK CHICKEN   rice & beans, refreshing chopped salad, chargrilled corn   106

CHICKEN SKEWERS   amazing Satay sauce, fiery noodle salad, fruit & mint sugar   110

STUFFED CYPRIOT CHICKEN   pan-fried asparagus & vine tomatoes, cabbage salad, St Clement's drink, vanilla ice cream float   116

PIRI PIRI CHICKEN   dressed potatoes, rocket salad, quick Portuguese tarts   120

DUCK SALAD   giant croutons, cheat's rice pudding with stewed fruit   126

THAI RED PRAWN CURRY   jasmine rice, cucumber salad, papaya platter   130

GRILLED SARDINES   crispy halloumi, watercress salad & figs, thick chocolate mousse   134

TASTY CRUSTED COD   my mashy peas, tartare sauce, warm garden salad   140

SWEDISH-STYLE FISHCAKES   roasted baby new potatoes, sprout salad, fresh zingy salsa   146

JAMIE'S 30 MINUTE MEALS

JAMIE OLIVER

Photography by
DAVID LOFTUS

MICHAEL JOSEPH
an imprint of PENGUIN BOOKS

MICHAEL JOSEPH

Published by the Penguin Group
Penguin Books Ltd, 80 Strand, London WC2R 0RL, England
Penguin Group (USA) Inc., 375 Hudson Street, New York, New York 10014, USA
Penguin Group (Canada), 90 Eglinton Avenue East, Suite 700, Toronto, Ontario, Canada M4P 2Y3
(a division of Pearson Penguin Canada Inc.)
Penguin Ireland, 25 St Stephen's Green, Dublin 2, Ireland (a division of Penguin Books Ltd)
Penguin Group (Australia), 250 Camberwell Road, Camberwell, Victoria 3124, Australia
(a division of Pearson Australia Group Pty Ltd)
Penguin Books India Pvt Ltd, 11 Community Centre, Panchsheel Park, New Delhi – 110 017, India
Penguin Group (NZ), 67 Apollo Drive, Rosedale, North Shore 0632, New Zealand
(a division of Pearson New Zealand Ltd)
Penguin Books (South Africa) (Pty) Ltd, 24 Sturdee Avenue, Rosebank, Johannesburg 2196, South Africa

Penguin Books Ltd, Registered Offices: 80 Strand, London WC2R 0RL, England

www.penguin.com

First published 2010
1

Printed in Germany by Mohn media
Colour reproduction by Altaimage Ltd

A CIP catalogue record for this book is available from the British Library

ISBN: 978–0–718–15477–6

jamieoliver.com

STICKY PAN-FRIED SCALLOPS   sweet chilli rice, dressed greens, quick brownies   150

SERIOUSLY GOOD FISH TAGINE   fennel & lemon salad, couscous, orange & mint tea   154

SMOKED SALMON   potato salad, beets & cottage cheese, rye bread & homemade butter   160

SMOKY HADDOCK CORN CHOWDER   spiced tiger prawns, rainbow salad, raspberry & elderflower slushie   164

FISH TRAY-BAKE   Jersey Royals, salsa verde, simple spinach salad, cheat's banoffee pie   168

BLOODY MARY MUSSELS   herby salad, gorgeous rhubarb millefeuille   174

SEA BASS & CRISPY PANCETTA   sweet potato mash, Asian greens, 1-minute berry ice cream, sparkling lemon ginger drink   180

ASIAN-STYLE SALMON   noodle broth, beansprout salad, lychee dessert   186

CRISPY SALMON   jazzed-up rice, baby courgette salad, gorgeous guacamole, berry spritzer   190

ROAST BEEF   baby yorkies, little carrots, crispy potatoes, super-quick gravy   194

STEAK SARNIE   crispy new potatoes, cheesy mushrooms, beetroot salad   200

RIB-EYE STIR-FRY   dan dan noodles, chilled hibiscus tea   204

SUPER-FAST BEEF HASH   jacket potatoes, goddess salad, lovely butter beans & bacon   210

STEAK INDIAN-STYLE   spinach & paneer salad, naan breads, mango dessert   216

MEATBALL SANDWICH   pickled cabbage, chopped salad, banana ice cream   220

LIVER & BACON   onion gravy, smashed potato, dressed greens, meringues   226

STUFFED FOCACCIA   prosciutto, celeriac remoulade, dressed mozzarella, fresh lemon & lime granita   230

SEARED PORK FILLET & CATHERINE WHEEL SAUSAGE   meaty mushroom sauce, celeriac smash, garlicky beans   236

PORK CHOPS & CRISPY CRACKLING   crushed potatoes, minty cabbage, peaches 'n' custard   240

KINDA SAUSAGE CASSOULET   warm broccoli salad, berry & custard ripple   244

BRITISH PICNIC   sausage rolls, mackerel pâté, lovely asparagus, crunch salad, Pimm's Eton mess   250

CATHERINE WHEEL SAUSAGE   horseradish mash, apple salad, sage & leek gravy, stuffed apples   256

TAPAS FEAST   tortilla, glazed chorizo, manchego cheese, cured meats & honey, stuffed peppers, rolled anchovies   260

MOROCCAN LAMB CHOPS   flatbreads, herby couscous, stuffed peppers, pomegranate drink   264

SPRING LAMB   vegetable platter, mint sauce, Chianti gravy, chocolate fondue   268

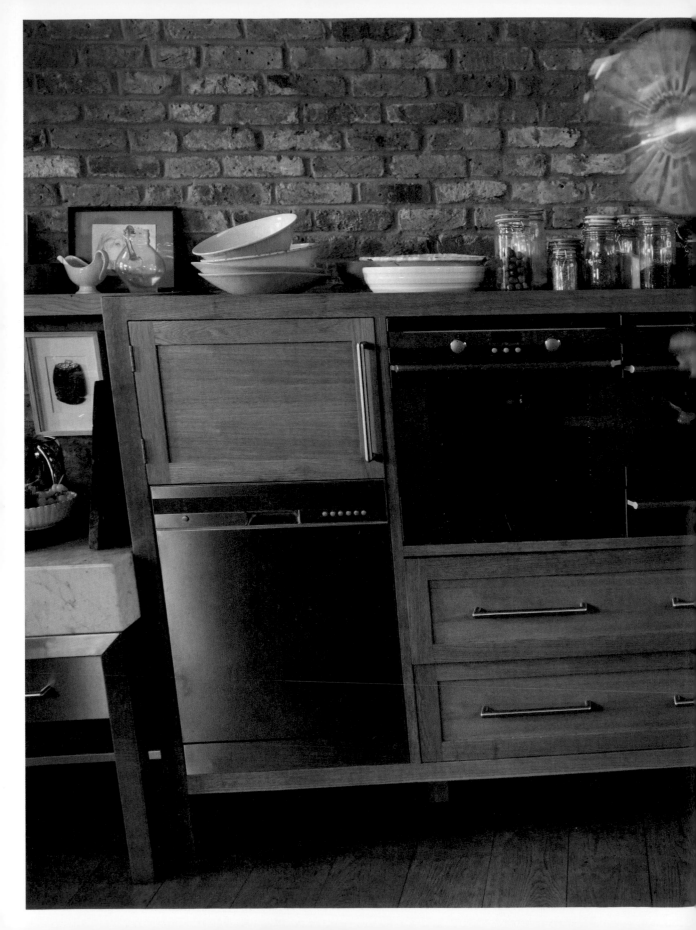

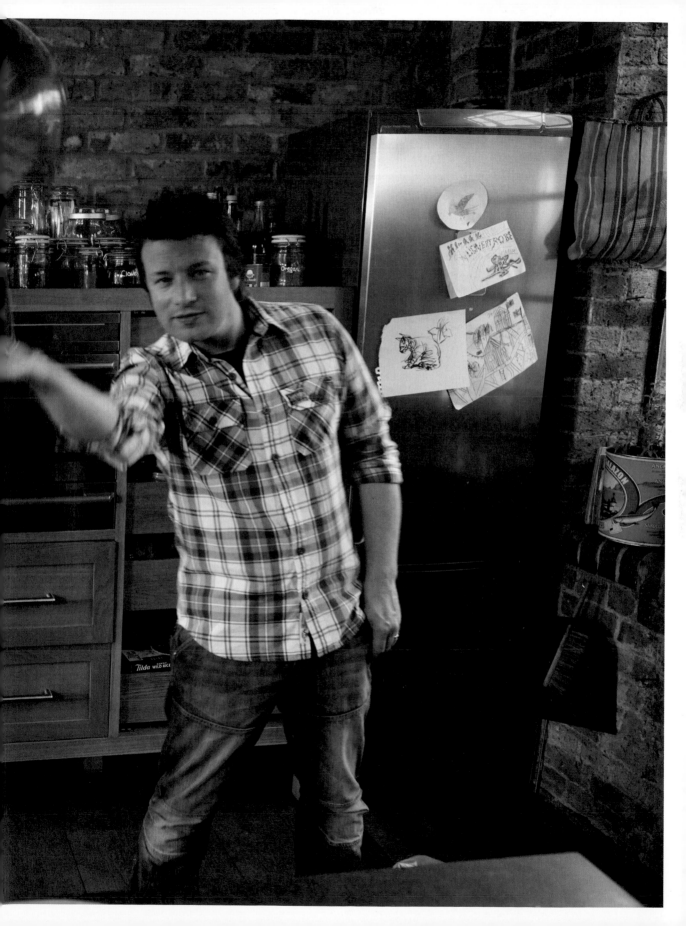

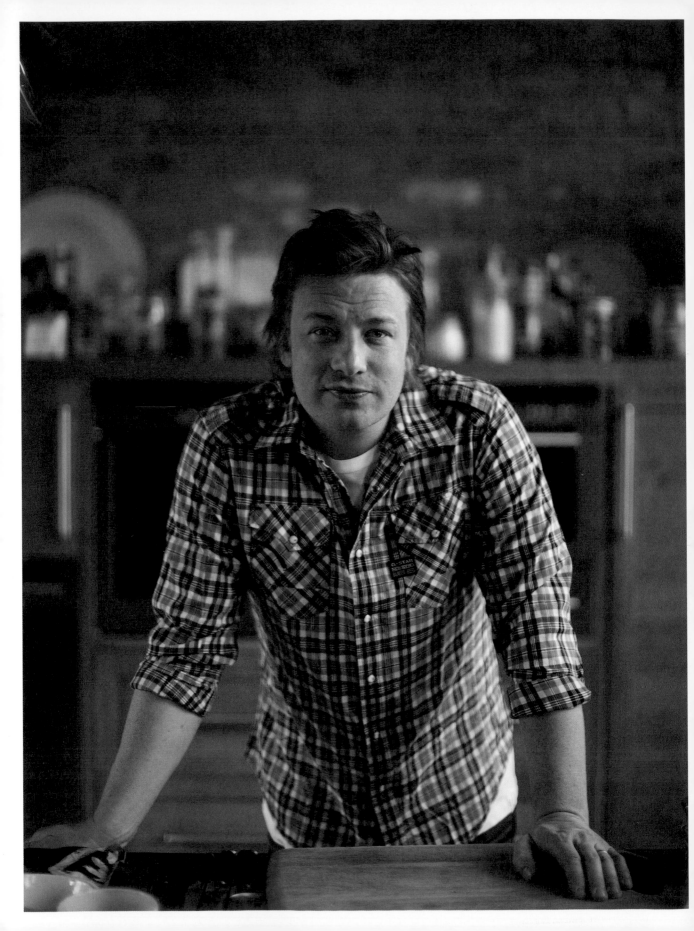

I'M TOO BUSY . . . IT'S TOO EXPENSIVE . . . I DON'T KNOW HOW . . .

These are the three excuses I always hear when I ask people why they don't cook at home more often. But I know that with the right kit, some organization and solid recipes, these excuses don't stand up. Regardless of whether you're a brilliant cook or a complete beginner, this book does what it says on the tin. I honestly believe that if you embrace my 30-minute meals, they will change the way you cook, for ever.

The most revolutionary thing about the meals in this book is not that they can be cooked quickly (they can), and it's not that they use loads of clever shortcuts and tricks (they do), it's that I've written them in a completely unique way. I'm going to walk you through every step needed to create a whole meal, so in 30 minutes you will be putting beautiful main dishes, exciting sides and salads, lovely drinks and puddings on the table at the same time – all from one recipe! I've come up with 50 incredible meals for you: meaty ones, vegetarian meals, quick pastas and puddings, lovely curries and things you might never have thought achievable in half an hour.

I want this book to help skyrocket you to another level, where you can nourish yourself and your family, and cook quickly, with a real sense of style. I'm going to ask you to use your kitchen in a completely new way, but it's different, it's fun, and the results will blow you away.

YOU DO HAVE THE TIME

You may be the busiest person in the world, but you still need to eat. In just 20 to 30 minutes – about the same amount of time it takes to warm up a ready meal in the oven, watch something on TV or order and pick up a takeaway – I want to show you that you can have an amazing home-cooked spread on the table.

I recently realized that the way I was cooking during the week wasn't very efficient. Because I can cook, I often freestyle my meals and make things up as I go, but this has meant that although the food tasted great, my approach was slightly chaotic and I ended up spending more time in the kitchen, and more time washing up, when I could have been putting the kids to bed and reading them a story. So I started making a plan and approaching Monday to Thursday's meals methodically. I haven't looked back.

Of course at the weekends I slow the pace down and really take my time in the kitchen, but with the week being such a busy time, it helps to be organized when it comes to shopping and cooking so you can have more fun with your free time. Family time seems to come way down the priority list these days, so I hope learning how to get beautiful, quick meals on the table will help to bring more people back together at mealtimes.

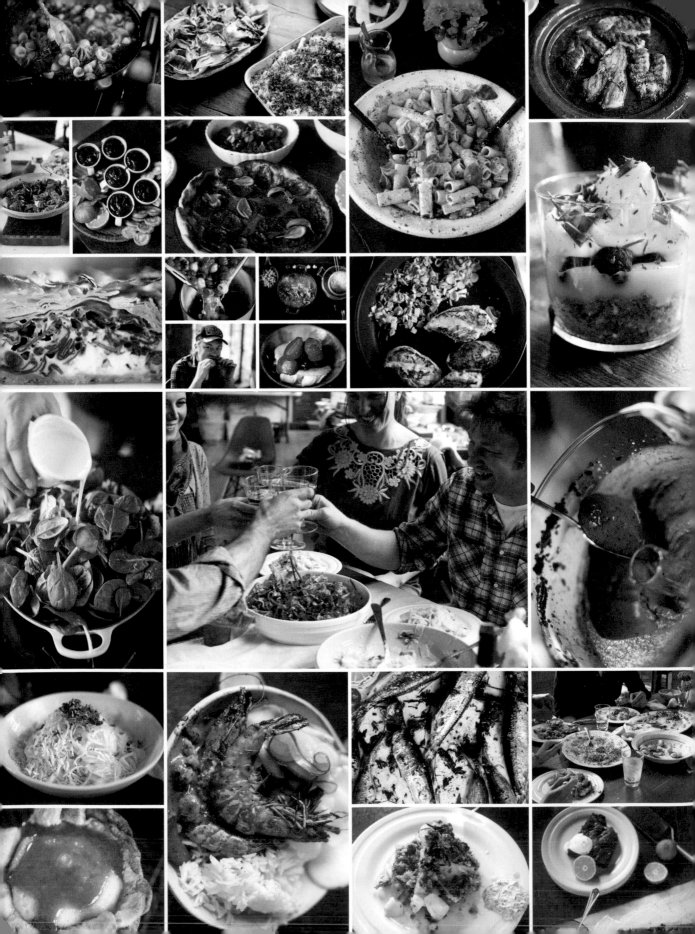

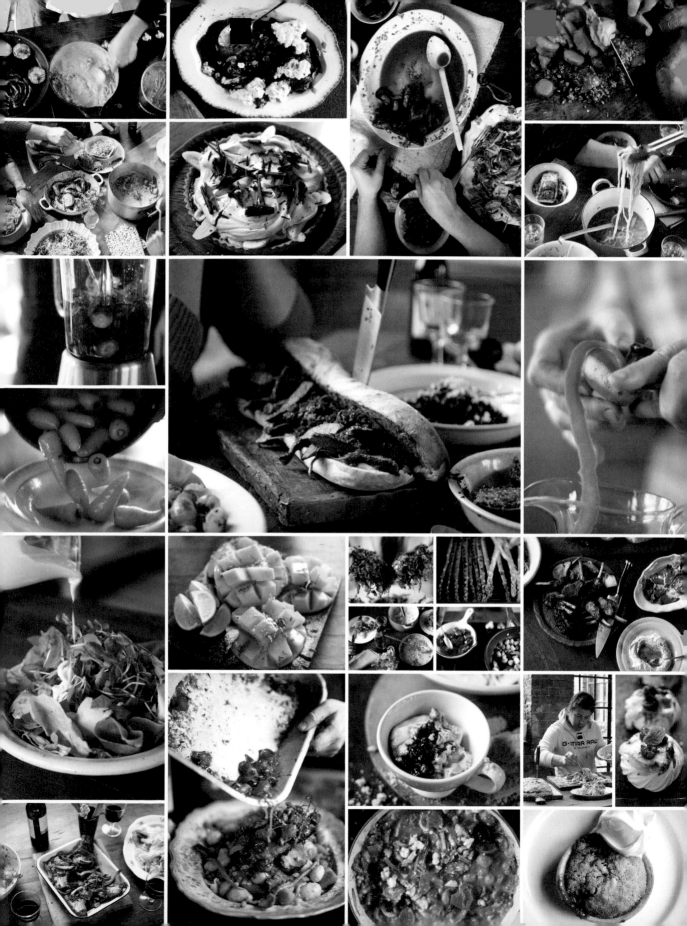

IT'S NOT TOO EXPENSIVE

I didn't set out to make this a budget cookbook; there are meals in here to satisfy the foodiest of foodies! But, because I was curious, I costed these meals against their equivalents on the high street, and it turns out that most of them are actually cheaper to make from scratch than they are to buy from your local takeaway, restaurant or ready-meal supermarket aisle. Just think: you can sit down with your favourite people in your own home and enjoy a fantastic spread for less than you'd spend anywhere else; you'll know exactly what went into it and it will be better for you. Just brilliant!

I've also discovered loads of cool tips and tricks by cooking this way which I've included in the recipes – I hope that they will help you to become a faster, more intelligent cook, no matter what you're making. In the long run, this will also help to save you money because you'll be able to cook anything from scratch in no time at all.

I'M GOING TO SHOW YOU HOW

These recipes are carefully choreographed so that no single minute is wasted. I've taken care of all the awkward, difficult stuff like menu planning and timing for you; all you have to do is follow my instructions, move quickly and enjoy the ride. If at first you run a little over time and your kitchen is a bit messy, please don't worry – it's all part of the process and you will radically improve the more you make these meals. Remember, this is about cooking in a whole new way. Like riding a bike, learning to drive or making 'beautiful love', you might not always get things right first time around, but the benefits when you finally crack it are incredible!

There's no denying that this is an energetic workhorse of a book. These 50 meals are going to keep you busy and make you multi-task, but you'll soon get used to it, and even find it slightly addictive. I don't want you to freestyle your way through the recipes, swap in different elements (at least not at the beginning) or use ingredients and measurements other than the ones I've used here, because they've been tested by my food team, my gang in the office and even complete strangers, so I know they work. Of course there will be nights when you just want to curl up on the sofa with your missus (or mister) and have a simple bowl of pasta or salad, and if that's the case you can pick and choose your favourite elements from these meals as they are clearly laid out and easy to extract. But this book is all about cooking meals, so on those weeknights or busy weekends when everyone is together, remember that with less than half an hour of organized energy you can create something truly special.

In order to knock these meals out quickly, I want you to get into the '30-minute meals frame of mind', which is all about organizing your kitchen and your equipment. On the next few pages I've outlined everything you need to do to make this happen. This is important stuff and it's there to help you, so please read it all before starting any of the recipes. See it as a call to action, and get excited about it!

You'll find that I'm being direct and to the point throughout the book, but there's good reason for that. I want you to end up with two things we all crave: beautiful, tasty food that shocks you because it's so good, and more time to spend with the people you love. So go on, and have fun with it!

Jamie O xx

PS When you see this symbol in the recipes go to www.jamieoliver.com/30MM, where you'll find a helpful video of that technique in the how-to section. There are also loads more great videos on my website (including one on knife skills), step-by-step pictures, hints, tips and all sorts of wonderful bonus material to help you become a lean, mean cooking machine.

RECLAIM YOUR KITCHEN FOR THE JOB IT WAS MEANT FOR!

Too many of us are trying to cook dinner with children's toys under our feet, magazines on the table, bills stacked up on our kitchen worktops and bags, keys, laundry, shoes and other bits of clutter around us. But that's all about to change, because my goal is to help you make your kitchen as pared-back, lean and relevant to its job as possible so that you can smash out incredible food any night of the week. Don't let the other rooms in your house invade your cooking space: if you see any of the clutter I'm talking about in your kitchen, find another home for it.

Sort out your equipment

Put aside an hour or two and pull out all your kitchen equipment. How much of it do you use? What bits of kit from the essential list on page 21 do you need? If you come across massive pots or fancy kitchen gadgets you only use once or twice a year, bung them into storage or well out of the way. Once this is done your cooking will flow so much better.

Arrange it sensibly

Before you cook one of these meals, read through the recipe to identify the other smaller bits of equipment you're going to need. Set everything out so it's on hand when you need it and think through the recipe. If you know you're going to need to put something into the freezer, make sure you've got the space before you start, so you don't get tripped up.

I find it really helpful to keep larger utensils, like tongs, fish slices and wooden spoons, in a big jar next to the stove so they're easy to reach when I'm cooking, but do whatever works best for you in the space you've got. Clear kilner jars are fantastic for storecupboard ingredients like flour, sugar, spices and herbs, because you can find the stuff you need right away.

Clear as you go

Cooking these meals is going to be busy and fast-paced, so having a bin or a large bowl for rubbish next to you as you prep is a great idea. Working into a clear sink or dishwasher as you go is also going to help keep your kitchen from looking like a bombsite after the meal is finished. These tips might sound basic, but they will make all the difference.

Make room for the meal

Clear your table before you start cooking. If it's cluttered, your lovely hot food is going to sit waiting while you sort it out. So clear it before you start and you'll be ready to cook some serious meals.

A QUICK WORD ABOUT INGREDIENTS

I hope that you lot know me well enough by now to realize that when I use eggs or chicken in a recipe, I want you to use eggs or meat from higher-welfare chickens. The same goes for pork. There are so many things to keep in mind when you're shopping for ingredients, and the food industry is constantly changing and evolving. To help make things a bit clearer, these are the standards I look for when I'm shopping:

Eggs: Always large, preferably higher welfare

Chicken: Preferably higher welfare

Pork: Preferably higher welfare

Gelatine: Beef or vegetable, not pork

Fish: Sustainably caught

Salmon: Preferably farmed higher welfare

Chicken, beef or vegetable stock: Preferably organic

Mayonnaise: Good-quality, preferably made with free-range eggs

Meringues: Preferably made with free-range eggs

Pre-made pastry cases: Preferably made with free-range eggs

Egg noodles: Preferably made with free-range eggs

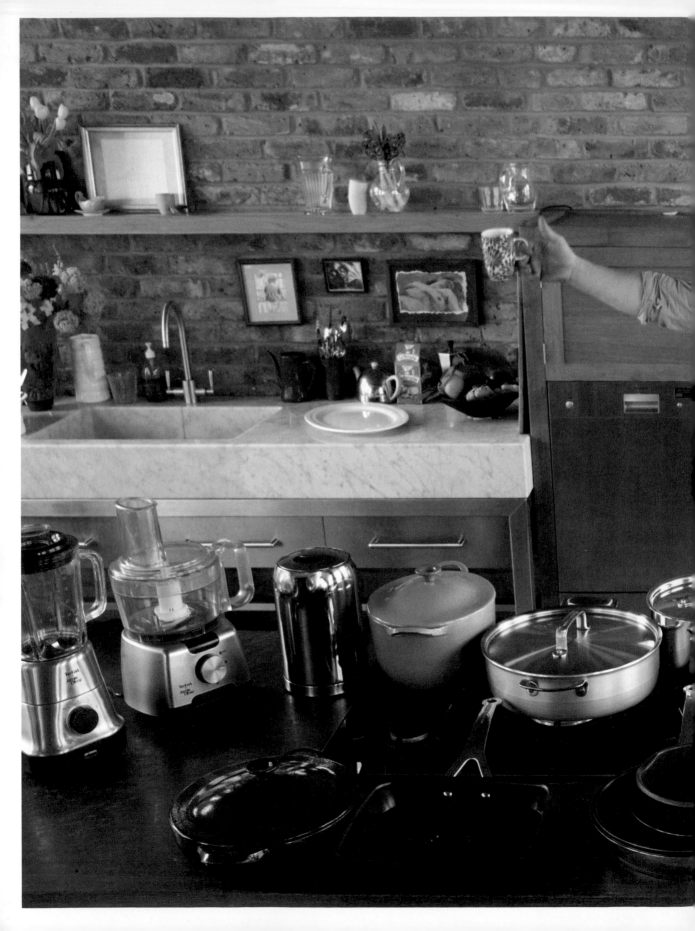

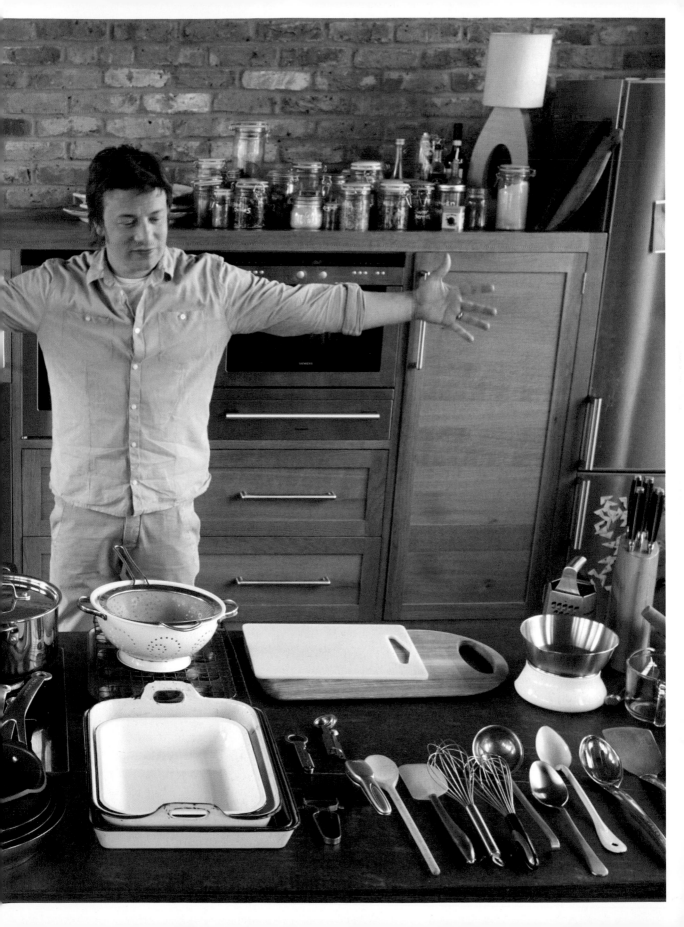

YOU NEED THIS KIT

Because it's my duty to help you achieve the meals in this book quickly and efficiently, I'm going to be straight with you: you've GOT to have the gear listed opposite in order to make the meals in this book in 30 minutes. Without certain bits of kit, like a food processor or a liquidizer, you simply won't be able to work fast enough.

I've priced the whole lot on the Argos, Debenhams and John Lewis websites and (as of the month this book went to print) if you're starting from scratch you can get absolutely everything on the list for around £300. That includes a food processor and a microwave, each for around £30, and a liquidizer for a tenner (about the same price as a small round of pints at the pub). Of course the products on those sites range from very cheap and basic to top-of-the-line gear, and everything in between. Whether you want to spend the bare minimum or invest a lot more, accumulating all this kit should not be seen as an unachievable goal. Start off with what you can and build the rest up over time, because the more you have, the more of these meals you'll be able to make and the faster and better your cooking will get.

Personally, when it comes to things like knives, pans and electrical equipment I think it's well worth spending a bit more and getting something decent that will last. So save up, or use birthdays, holidays or your wedding list to blag the bits you're missing. If you don't have a garlic crusher or a speed-peeler, skip your morning cappuccino and use that £2 to buy one.

Most of us eat three times a day, every day of our lives. Spending money on prepackaged food, takeaways or fast food because you don't want to invest the money in your own kitchen is a false economy. I know this kit will pay for itself 100 times over in the long run, so please – for the sake of yourself, your family and your future dinner guests – prioritize your kitchen. If you don't, you're only cheating yourself.

A QUICK WORD ABOUT MICROWAVES

Microwaves have sort of become synonymous with ready meals, so including one on my equipment list is definitely a first for me! But I've read that over 92 per cent of homes in the UK have a microwave, so it would be mad for me to think you don't have one. In this book, you're going to be using your microwave to free up space on the hob and help you cook fresh tasty food. The recipes in this book have all been tested using an 800W microwave, so you may need to adjust your timings or power levels depending on the wattage of yours.

THE LIST

Food processor with the following
    attachments: standard blade, thick
    and thin slicer discs, fine and coarse
    graters, whisk and beater

Liquidizer

Microwave

Electric whisk

Kettle

Large griddle pan (approx. 25 x 29cm)

Large non-stick ovenproof frying pan with
    lid (approx. 30cm)

Medium non-stick frying pan with lid
    (approx. 26cm)

Small non-stick frying pan with lid
    (approx. 20cm)

Large deep saucepan with lid
    (approx. 24cm)

Medium saucepan with lid (approx. 20cm)

Small saucepan with lid (approx. 16cm)

3-level steamer pan

Large deep sturdy roasting tray
    (approx. 28 x 35cm)

Medium roasting tray

Baking tin (approx. 26 x 32cm)

Non-stick baking tray

Wire rack

6-hole muffin tin

12-hole shallow bun tin (or jam tart tin)

3 good-quality knives: chef's knife, paring
    knife, bread knife

2 plastic chopping boards

2 large wooden chopping boards

Nest of mixing bowls

Colander

Fine sieve

Pestle and mortar

Garlic crusher

Tongs

Fish slice

Wooden spoons

Ladle

Slotted spoon

Spatula

Potato masher

Speed-peeler

Box grater

Fine hand-held grater

Measuring jug

Scales

Measuring spoons

Balloon whisk

Tin opener

Rolling pin

Pastry brush

Bottle opener

Ice cream scoop

Tin foil, greaseproof paper

Microwave-safe clingfilm

FAMILY-STYLE SHARING

This book is full of food you're going to share with your family and friends, and for that reason I see the table as the heart and soul of my *30-Minute Meals*. All the lovely dishes you create are going to come together here in one beautiful spread, and eating them together should be a fun, sociable experience. Because my job is to make you look good, I've given you a list below of some of the bits and pieces I use for serving all the time. These things aren't 'essential' in the same way as the kitchen kit, but to my mind they are incredibly important because they are going to help you create an exciting-looking table people want to sit around.

- Platters of all shapes and sizes – new or antique, whichever style you fancy

- Beautiful large serving bowls that work for salads, soups, vegetables and desserts

- Large wooden chopping boards that look good enough to double as serving boards

- Mats, boards or even cute ceramic tiles to put trays, pots and pans on so you can take them directly from the oven to the table

- Frying pans and saucepans that look good enough to go straight to the table (it's worth bearing this in mind when you shop for pans, so they can do two jobs for you)

- Teacups or cappuccino cups that can double as little dessert bowls (I think it's quite sweet when they're mismatched)

- Pint glasses or jars to put cutlery in (who says you have to set the table every night?)

- Little bowls for sauces and dips

- Gravy boats and little glass jugs for gravies and dressings

- A nice big 1-litre jug for drinks

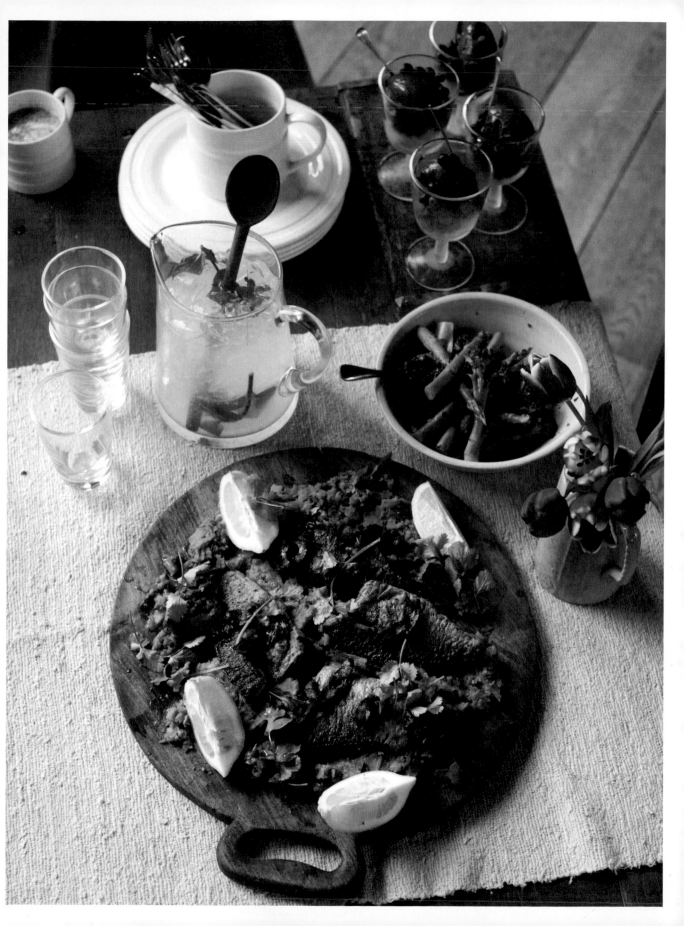

BROCCOLI ORECCHIETTE

COURGETTE &
BOCCONCINI SALAD

PROSCIUTTO &
MELON SALAD

SERVES 6

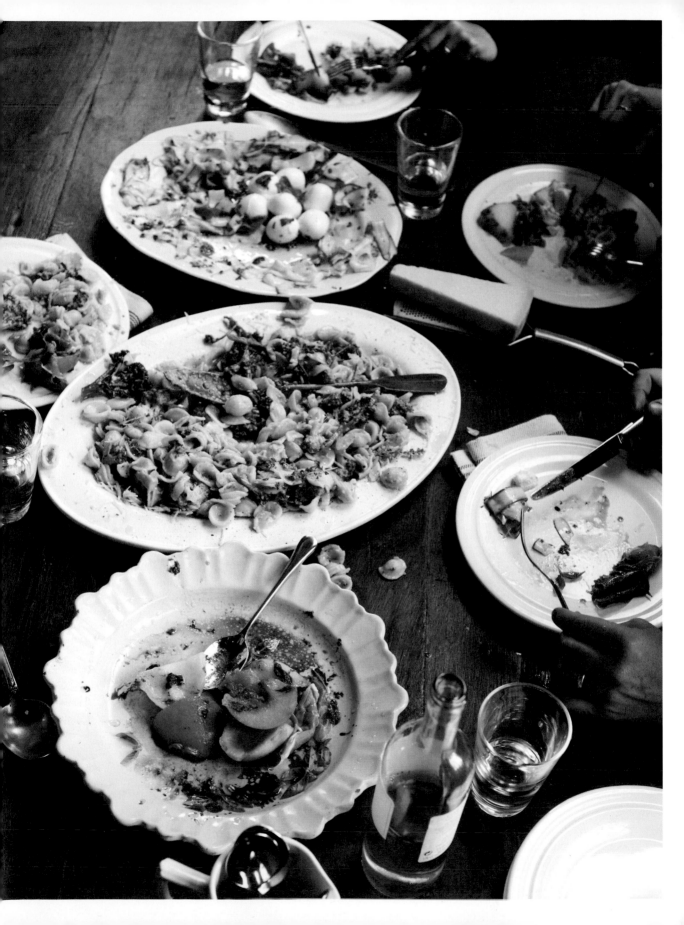

PASTA

125g Parmesan cheese
1 large head of broccoli
200g purple sprouting broccoli
1 x 30g tin of anchovies in oil
1 heaped tablespoon capers
1 small dried chilli
3 cloves of garlic
a few sprigs of fresh thyme
500g dried orecchiette

COURGETTE SALAD

3 large sprigs of fresh mint
½ a fresh red chilli
1 lemon
200g baby courgettes, mixed colours
1 x 125g tub of bocconcini di
  mozzarella (baby mozzarella balls)

SEASONINGS

olive oil
extra virgin olive oil
sea salt & black pepper

PROSCIUTTO & MELON SALAD

a small bunch of fresh basil
½ a lemon
2 x 115g packs of prosciutto
1 cantaloupe melon
balsamic vinegar

TO START Get all your ingredients and equipment ready. Put the fine grater attachment into the food processor. Fill and boil the kettle. Put a large frying pan on a low heat.

PASTA Trim the rind off your Parmesan and set aside. Grate the chunk of Parmesan in the food processor, then tip into a bowl. Slice all the florets off the stalk of the large head of broccoli. Trim off the florets from the purple sprouting broccoli and chop up just the tender stalks. Put all the broccoli to one side.

Fit the standard blade attachment to the processor. Halve the large broccoli stalk and put into the empty processor with the anchovies and their oil, and the drained capers. Crumble in the dried chilli. Peel and add the 3 cloves of garlic, then pulse it all to a paste. Pour the boiled water into a large deep saucepan and put on a high heat.

Put about 3 tablespoons of olive oil into the large frying pan and spoon in the broccoli paste. Stir, then pick and tear in some thyme leaves, discarding the woody stalks. Pour a wineglass of water into the pan and add the reserved Parmesan rind. Give it a good stir and turn the heat up to medium. Keep your eye on it, stirring every now and then. Half-fill the kettle and reboil.

Add the orecchiette to the saucepan of boiling water with a pinch of salt and cook according to packet instructions, with the lid askew. Now you've got about 12 minutes of pasta cooking time to make your 2 salads, so crack on!

COURGETTE SALAD Pick the mint leaves over a chopping board. Add ½ a red chilli. Zest over ½ the lemon, then chop the chilli and mint together until really fine. Spoon into the middle of a serving platter, drizzle over about 3 tablespoons of extra virgin olive oil and squeeze in the juice of ½ the lemon. Add a pinch of salt & pepper, then taste and adjust the flavours if necessary. Speed-peel the courgettes into ribbons over this dressing. Drain the tub of baby mozzarella, then tip over the courgettes and take to the table to toss and dress at the last minute.

PASTA Give the pasta a stir and top up with more water from the kettle, if needed. After 5 minutes add all the reserved broccoli florets and the chopped purple sprouting broccoli stalks to the pasta with a splash of water from the kettle.

PROSCIUTTO & MELON SALAD Pick the leaves from the basil, setting the smaller ones aside for later. Put the big leaves into a pestle & mortar with a pinch of salt and bash to a paste. Add 2 tablespoons of extra virgin olive oil, plus a good squeeze of lemon juice. Lay 12 slices of prosciutto on a platter, leaving a space in the middle. Halve the melon, spoon out the seeds, then use a spoon to quickly scoop chunks of flesh into the middle of the platter. Drizzle over a little balsamic, then scatter over the reserved small basil leaves. Squeeze the juices from the melon halves into the dressing and stir in, then take the platter to the table, with the mortar and a spoon for drizzling over the dressing.

PASTA Drain the pasta and broccoli in a colander, reserving some of the cooking water, and add to the frying pan of paste. Fish out the Parmesan rind and discard. Add a big handful or two of grated Parmesan and a ladle or two of the cooking water. Carefully and quickly stir around and keep it moving until you achieve shiny, loose, lovely pasta. Taste and correct the seasoning, then tip on to a serving platter and sprinkle over a handful of Parmesan. Drizzle with extra virgin olive oil and scatter over the rest of the small reserved basil leaves. Take to the table with the rest of the Parmesan for sprinkling over.

TO SERVE When everyone is ready to eat, use 2 forks to toss the courgette ribbons and baby mozzarella. Serve next to some of that lovely pasta and the prosciutto and melon salad.

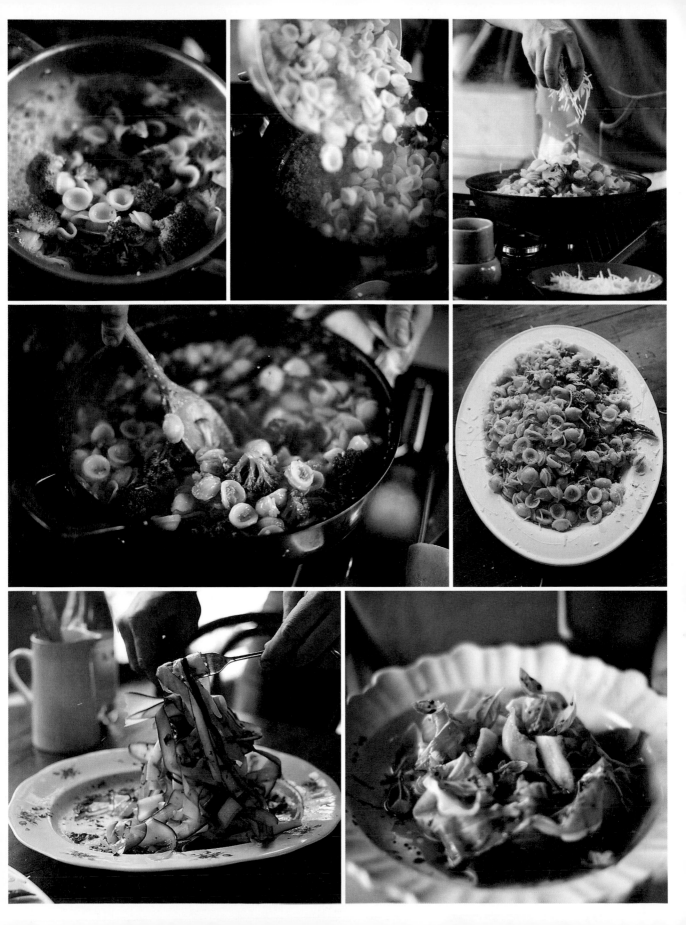

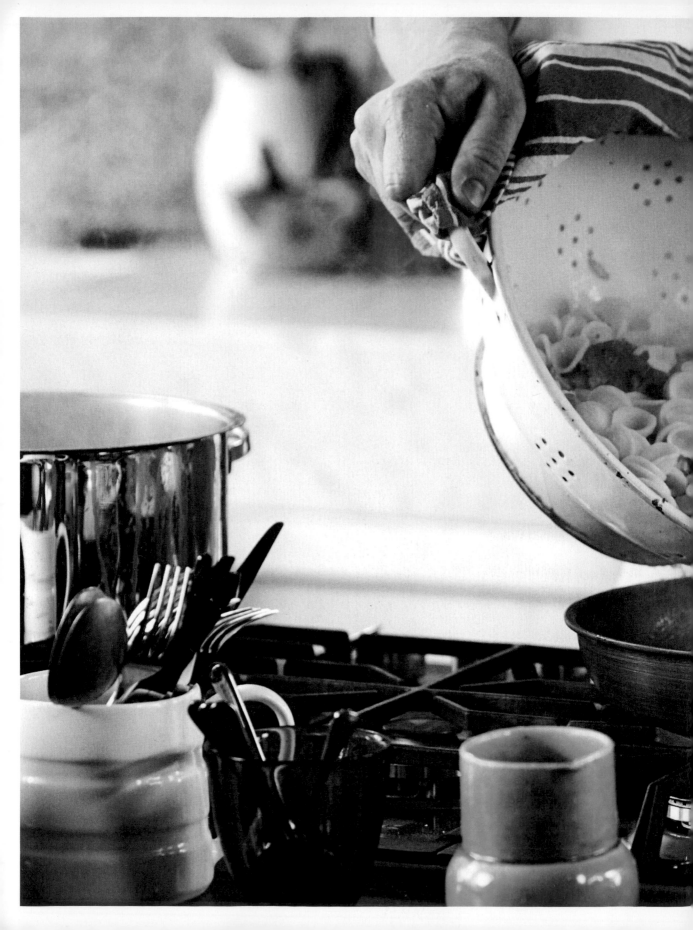

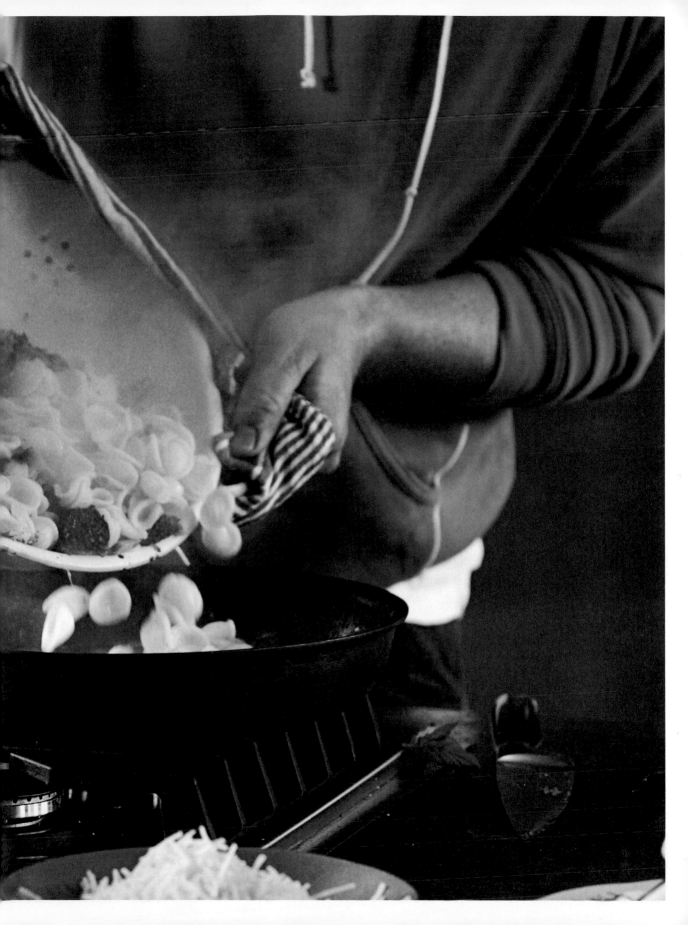

PREGNANT JOOLS'S PASTA

CRUNCHY CHICORY & WATERCRESS SALAD

LITTLE FRANGIPANE TARTS

SERVES 6

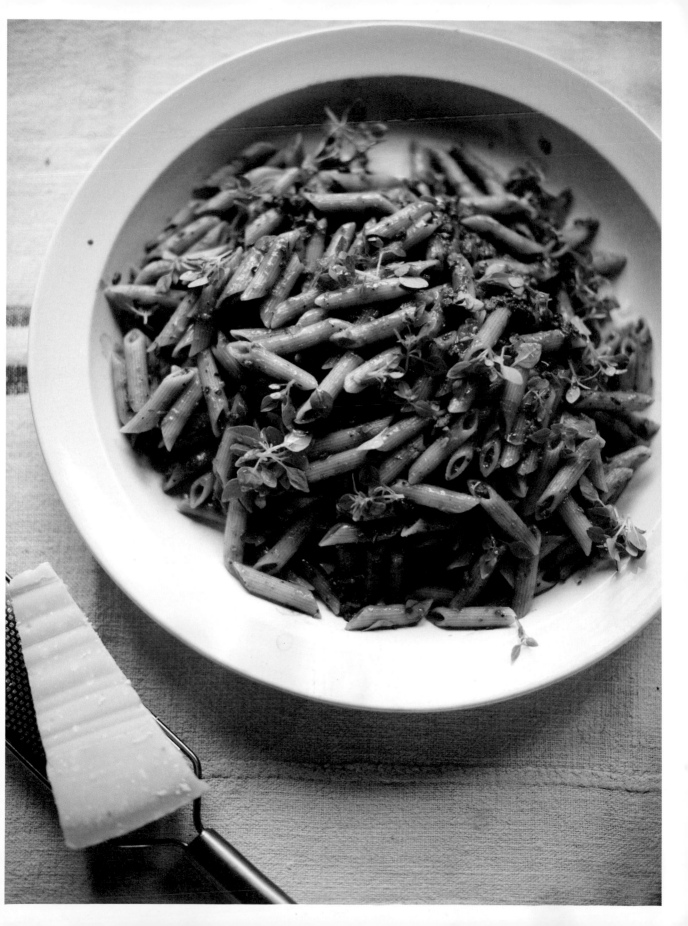

PASTA

4 spring onions
1 carrot
1 stick of celery
1–2 fresh red chillies
1 x 6-pack of good-quality sausages
  (approx. 400g)
1 heaped teaspoon fennel seeds
1 teaspoon dried oregano
500g dried penne
4 cloves of garlic
4 tablespoons balsamic vinegar
1 x 400g tin of chopped tomatoes
a few sprigs of Greek basil, or
  regular basil

SALAD

2 red chicory
1 x 100g mixed bag of prewashed
  rocket and watercress
Parmesan cheese, for shaving over
1 lemon

SEASONINGS

olive oil
extra virgin olive oil
sea salt & black pepper

TARTS

6 small deep shortcrust pastry cases
1 egg
100g ground almonds
100g butter
90g golden caster sugar
1 orange
1 tablespoon vanilla paste or extract
½ a 350g jar of good-quality
  raspberry jam
1 x 250g tub of crème fraîche, to serve

TO START Get all your ingredients and equipment ready. Turn your oven to 190°C/375°F/gas 5. Fill and boil the kettle. Put a large frying pan on a high heat. Put the standard blade attachment into the food processor.

PASTA Trim the spring onions, carrot and celery. Roughly chop all the vegetables, then blitz in the food processor with the chillies (stalks removed). Add the sausages, 1 heaped teaspoon of fennel seeds and 1 teaspoon of oregano. Keep pulsing until well mixed, then spoon this mixture into the hot frying pan with a lug of olive oil, breaking it up and stirring as you go. Keep checking on it and stirring while you get on with other jobs. Put a large deep saucepan on a low heat and fill with boiled water. Fill and reboil the kettle.

TARTS Put the 6 pastry cases on a baking tray. Make a frangipane mixture by cracking the egg into a mixing bowl and adding 100g of almonds, 100g of butter and 90g of golden caster sugar. Grate over the zest of ½ an orange and add 1 tablespoon of vanilla paste or extract. Use a spoon to mix everything together.

Spoon a small teaspoon of jam into each pastry base. Top with a heaped teaspoon of frangipane, add another small teaspoon of jam, then finally another heaped teaspoon of frangipane. Put the tray in the oven on the middle shelf and set the timer for 18 minutes exactly.

PASTA Top up the saucepan with more boiled water if needed. Season well then add the penne and cook according to packet instructions, with the lid askew.

SALAD Trim off the bases of the chicory, then click apart all the leaves and quarter the heart. Scatter over a platter, then sprinkle the rocket and watercress on top and toss quickly with your hands.

PASTA Crush 4 unpeeled cloves of garlic into the sausage mixture and stir in 4 tablespoons of balsamic vinegar and the tinned tomatoes. Add a little of the starchy cooking water from the pasta to loosen if needed.

SALAD Speed-peel or shave some of the Parmesan over the chicory salad and take it to the table with a bottle of extra virgin olive oil, salt, pepper and lemon wedges for dressing right before eating.

PASTA Drain the pasta, reserving about a wineglass worth of the cooking water. Tip the pasta into the pan of sauce and give it a gentle stir, adding enough of the cooking water to bring it to a silky consistency. Taste, correct the seasoning, then tip into a large serving bowl and take straight to the table with the rest of the Parmesan for grating over. Scatter over a few basil leaves.

TARTS When the little tarts are golden and cooked, turn the oven off and take them out. Serve them warm, with a dollop of crème fraîche on the side.

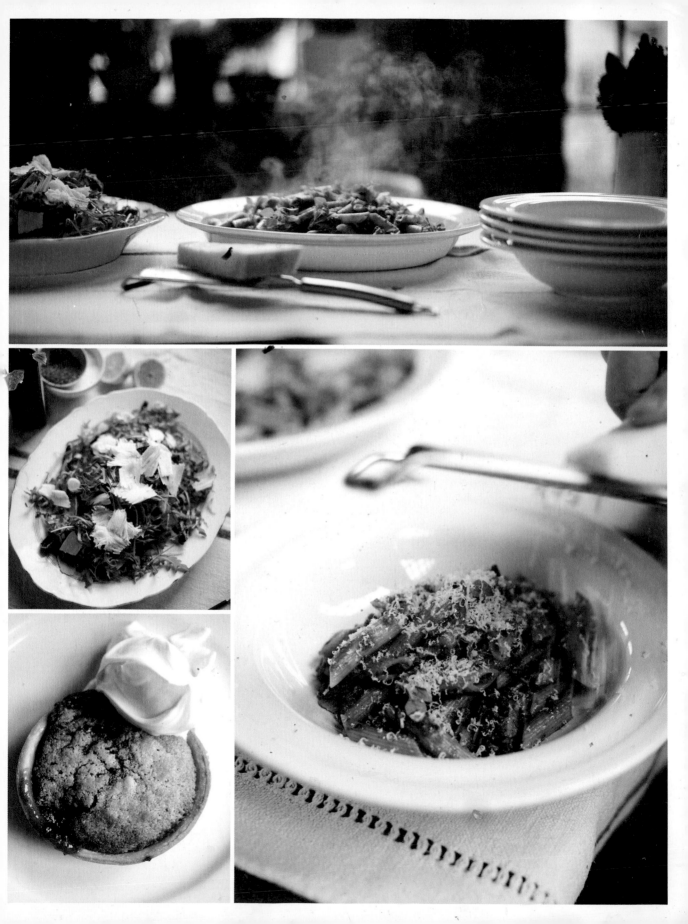

CAULIFLOWER MACARONI

SERVES 6

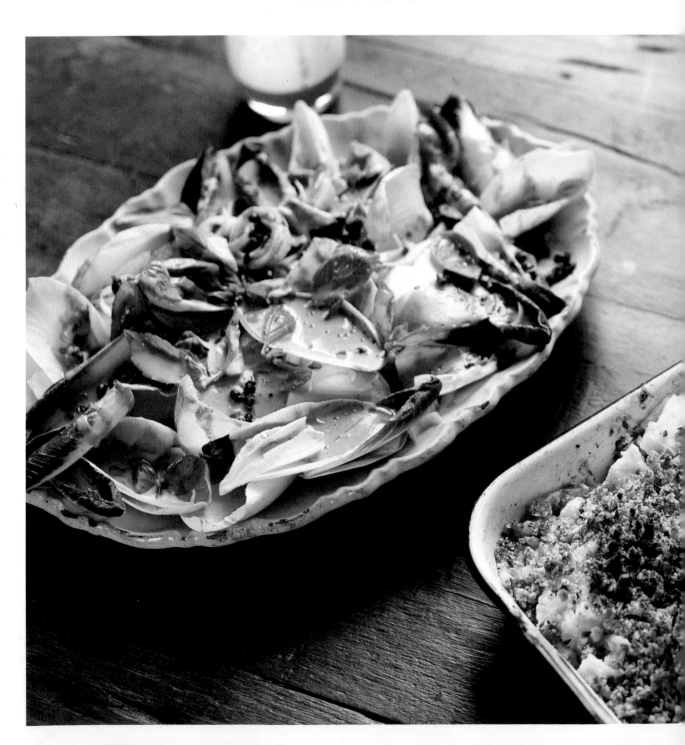

CHICORY SALAD WITH INSANE DRESSING
LOVELY STEWED FRUIT

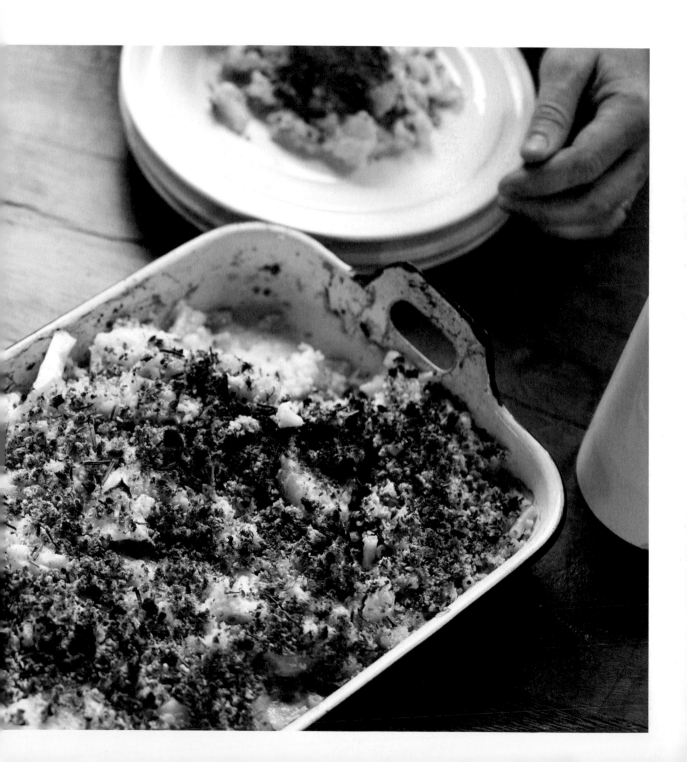

CAULIFLOWER MACARONI
8 rashers of pancetta
1 large head of cauliflower
500g dried macaroni
250g mature Cheddar cheese
4 thick slices of country bread
a few sprigs of fresh rosemary
2 cloves of garlic
1 x 250g tub of crème fraîche
Parmesan cheese, to serve

SALAD
2 large red chicory
2 large white chicory
a small bunch of fresh basil
1 clove of garlic
½ a 30g tin of anchovies in oil
1 teaspoon Dijon mustard
2 tablespoons natural yoghurt
3 tablespoons red wine vinegar
a small handful of capers, drained

SEASONINGS
olive oil
extra virgin olive oil
sea salt & black pepper

STEWED FRUIT
18 ripe plums or a mixture of
  any stone fruit you like, such as
  nectarines or apricots
1 teaspoon vanilla paste or extract
2 heaped tablespoons golden caster
  sugar
1 orange
1 cinnamon stick
optional: a good splash of brandy
1 x 500ml tub of good-quality vanilla
  ice cream

TO START Get all your ingredients and equipment ready. Fill and boil the kettle. Turn the oven on to 220°C/425°F/ gas 7. Put the coarse grater attachment into the food processor.

CAULIFLOWER MACARONI Lay the pancetta in a roasting tray (approx. 30 x 25cm, or large enough to bake the pasta in) and put on the top shelf of the oven. Get rid of any tatty outer leaves from the cauliflower, then trim off the tough base of the stalk and quarter the head. Put in a large saucepan, core down, with the pasta, on a high heat. Cover with boiling water, filling and reboiling the kettle if necessary. Season with a good pinch of salt, drizzle over a little olive oil, then stir and cook according to packet instructions, with the lid askew.

STEWED FRUIT Halve and stone the plums and put them into another large roasting tray with 1 teaspoon of vanilla paste or extract and 2 heaped tablespoons of caster sugar. Speed-peel in the zest from ½ the orange, then squeeze in all the juice. Add the cinnamon stick, snapped in half, and stir in a good swig of brandy, if using. Place on the bottom shelf of the oven. They will be perfect after about 15 minutes.

CAULIFLOWER MACARONI Grate the Cheddar in the food processor and tip into a bowl. Fit the standard blade attachment, then get your pancetta out of the oven and blitz in the processor with the bread, rosemary leaves and a good drizzle of olive oil until you have a coarse breadcrumb consistency.

Put a colander over a large bowl to catch the pasta water, then drain the pasta and cauliflower. Tip into the roasting tray you cooked your pancetta in, and put over a low heat. Add 400ml (or just under a pint) of the reserved pasta water from the bowl. Crush in the 2 unpeeled cloves of garlic and mix in the crème fraîche and grated Cheddar, gently breaking up the cauliflower with tongs or a potato masher. Have a taste and correct the seasoning. It should be nice and loose; if not, add another splash of the pasta water.

Spread out evenly and scatter over the breadcrumbs. Put on the top shelf of the oven for about 8 minutes, or until golden and bubbling.

STEWED FRUIT If the plums look soft and juicy, take them out of the oven and set aside. If not, leave them in a little longer.

SALAD Trim the bases of the chicory and click the leaves over a serving platter. Quickly pick the basil leaves and scatter the small ones all over the salad. Put a small frying pan on a medium to low heat.

Put the bigger basil leaves into a liquidizer. Crush in the unpeeled garlic clove, then add a good pinch of salt & pepper, ½ the tin of anchovies plus a little of their oil, 1 teaspoon of mustard, 2 tablespoons of yoghurt, 3 tablespoons of red wine vinegar and about the same amount of extra virgin olive oil. Add a small splash of water and whiz until smooth.

Add a splash of olive oil and the capers to the hot frying pan. Fry for a few minutes until crispy. Taste the dressing to check for acidity, then pour into a jug. Sprinkle the crispy capers all over the chicory leaves and take to the table with the jug of dressing. You won't need all the dressing – keep any extra in the fridge for another day.

TO SERVE When the cauliflower macaroni is golden and bubbling, take it to the table and shave over some Parmesan. If the fruit is still in the oven, take it out and put it to one side. Take the ice cream out of the freezer to soften. When ready, serve the fruit in small glasses, layered up with vanilla ice cream.

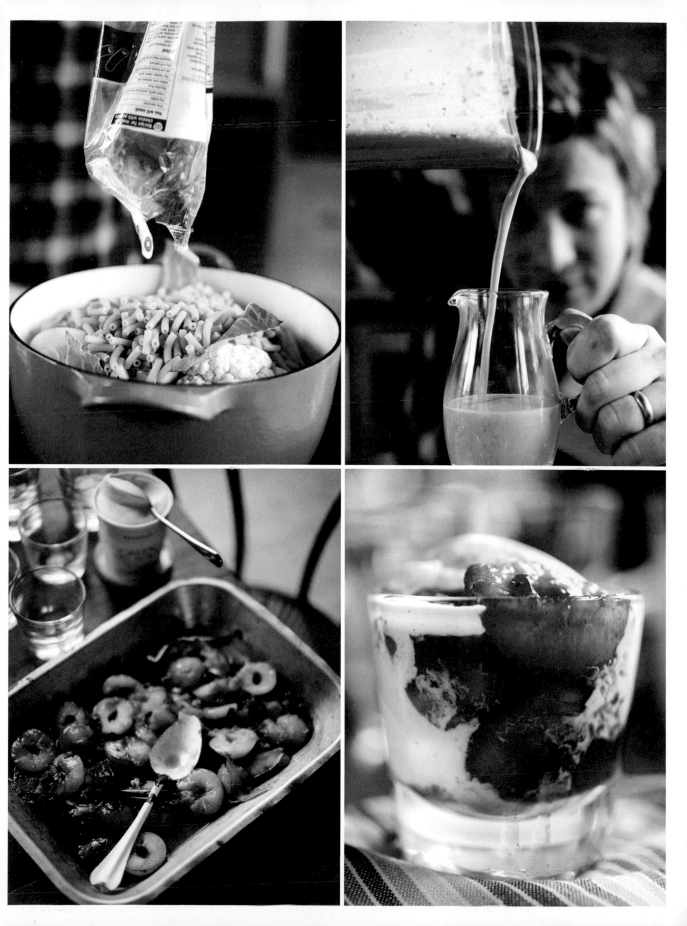

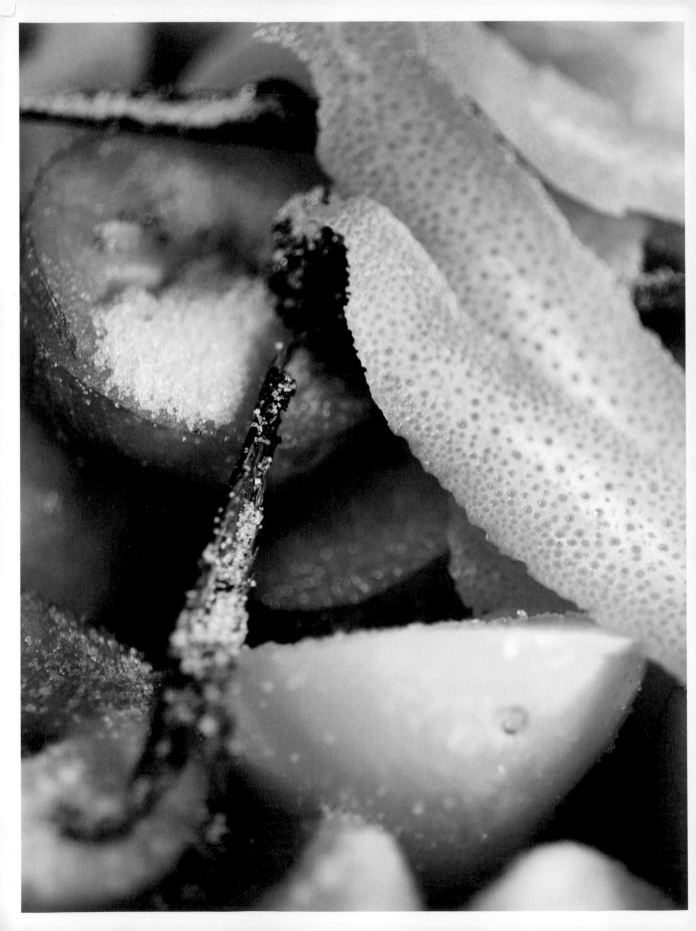

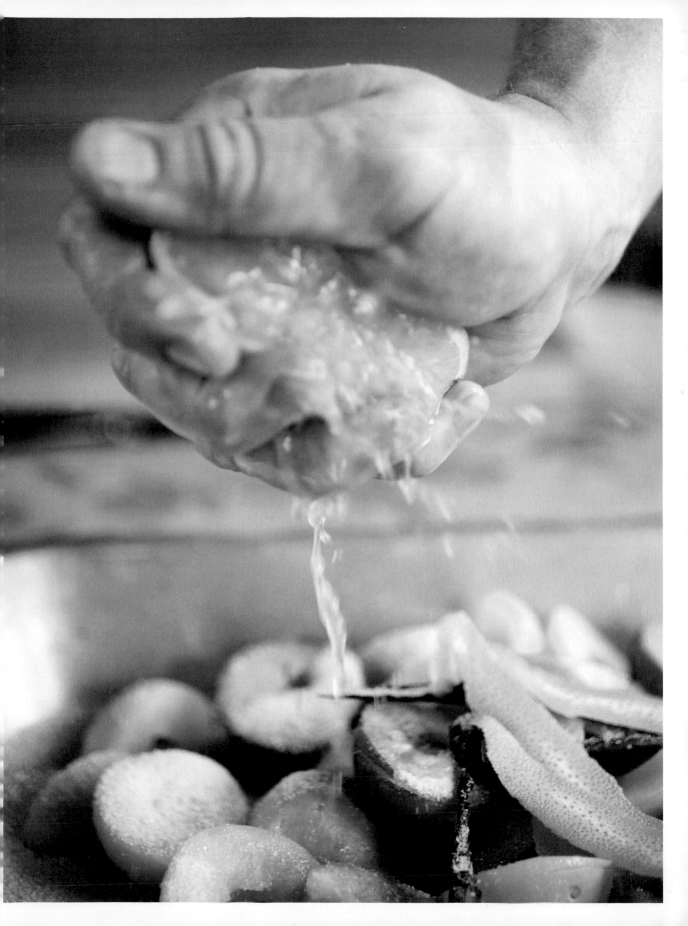

TRAPANI-STYLE RIGATONI

GRIDDLED CHICORY SALAD

ROCKET & PARMESAN SALAD

LIMONCELLO KINDA TRIFLE

SERVES 6

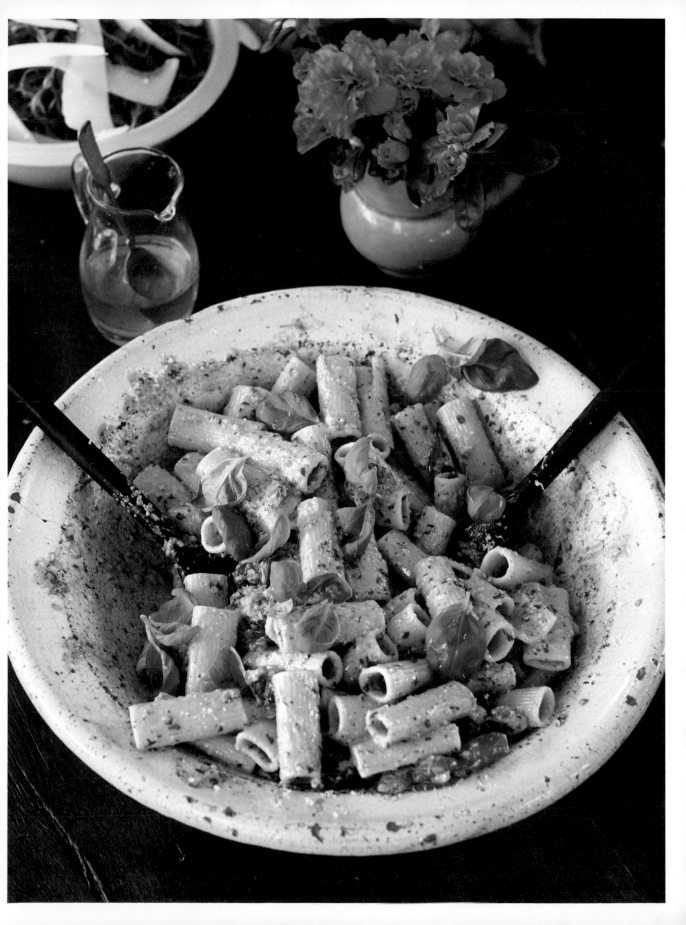

CIABATTA
1 ciabatta loaf
1 heaped teaspoon dried thyme

PASTA
500g dried rigatoni
40g Parmesan cheese
100g whole blanched almonds
2 cloves of garlic
1–2 fresh red chillies
2 large bunches of fresh basil
4 anchovy fillets in oil
450g cherry tomatoes, red and
  yellow if possible

CHICORY SALAD
2 red chicory
2 white chicory
balsamic vinegar
a few sprigs of fresh rosemary
½ a clove of garlic

ROCKET SALAD
1 x 100g bag of prewashed wild rocket
40g Parmesan cheese
½ a lemon

SEASONINGS
olive oil
extra virgin olive oil
sea salt & black pepper

TRIFLE
3 oranges
75ml limoncello
100g sponge fingers
250g mascarpone
2 heaped tablespoons icing sugar,
  plus extra for dusting
100ml semi-skimmed milk
1 lemon
1 teaspoon vanilla paste or extract
1 punnet of raspberries, or other
  seasonal fruit
1 x 100g bar of good-quality dark
  chocolate (approx. 70% cocoa
  solids), for shaving over

TO START Get all your ingredients and equipment ready. Fill and boil the kettle. Turn the oven on to 180°C/350°F/gas 4. Put a couple of inches of hot water into a large saucepan on a medium heat. Put a griddle pan on a high heat. Put the standard blade attachment into the food processor.

CIABATTA Drizzle the ciabatta with olive oil and sprinkle over the dried thyme and a good pinch of salt. Place in the oven.

TRIFLE Squeeze the juice from 3 oranges into an appropriately sized serving dish. Stir in the limoncello and taste to check the balance of sweetness and booze, adjusting if necessary. Cover the base of the dish with a layer of sponge fingers. Put the mascarpone and icing sugar into a separate bowl with the milk. Finely grate over the zest of the lemon, then squeeze in the juice from one half. Add the vanilla paste or extract to the bowl and whisk well. Spread this mixture all over the sponge fingers, then scatter over the raspberries and finely scrape over a little dark chocolate. Put into the fridge.

CHICORY SALAD Trim the chicory and halve each one lengthways. Lay them flat side down on the griddle pan. Turn every few minutes and take the pan off the heat once nicely charred on both sides.

PASTA Add the pasta and boiling water to the large saucepan, turn up to a high heat, and cook according to the packet instructions, with the lid askew. Fill and reboil the kettle for topping up, if needed.

ROCKET SALAD Put the rocket into a bowl. Use a speed-peeler to shave the Parmesan over. In a small jug, mix 3 tablespoons of extra virgin olive oil with the juice of ½ a lemon, then season to taste. Take the salad and dressing to the table.

PASTA Put the Parmesan, 100g of almonds, 2 peeled cloves of garlic and 1 or 2 chillies (stalks removed) into a food processor and whiz until fine. While the processor is still running, add 1½ bunches of basil, 4 anchovies and two-thirds of the cherry tomatoes. Whiz to a paste, then add a lug or 2 of extra virgin olive oil. Taste and season if needed, then put aside. Halve or quarter the remaining tomatoes, then put aside. By now the pasta should be perfectly cooked, so drain, reserving some of the cooking water, and return it to the hot pan. Add the paste, mixing well to coat the pasta. Add a splash of water to make it silky and loose.

CHICORY SALAD Move the chicory to the board. Roughly chop it, then dress it with a couple of splashes of balsamic vinegar and a couple of lugs of extra virgin olive oil. Season with salt & pepper. Pick and finely chop the rosemary leaves and crush over ½ a peeled clove of garlic. Toss together and take to the table.

CIABATTA Remove the bread from the oven, put it on a board and take to the table.

PASTA Tip the pasta into a large serving bowl, toss quickly then scatter the reserved cherry tomatoes and basil on top and take to the table.

TRIFLE After dinner take the dessert out of the fridge. Sieve over a little icing sugar, then serve. If you're feeling a bit indulgent you can melt the rest of the chocolate in the microwave and drizzle it over the top.

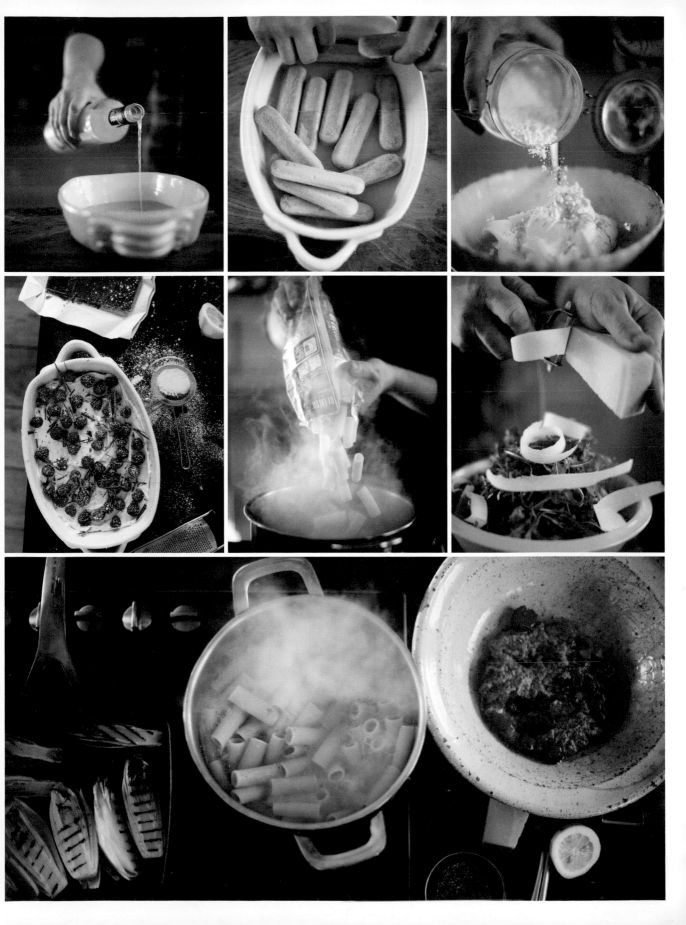

WONKY SUMMER PASTA

SERVES 4

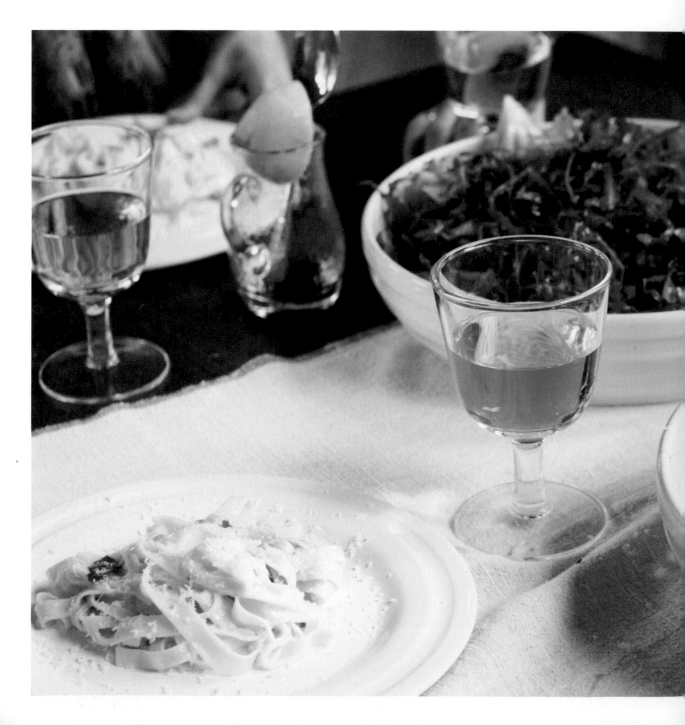

HERBY SALAD
PEAR DROP TARTLETS

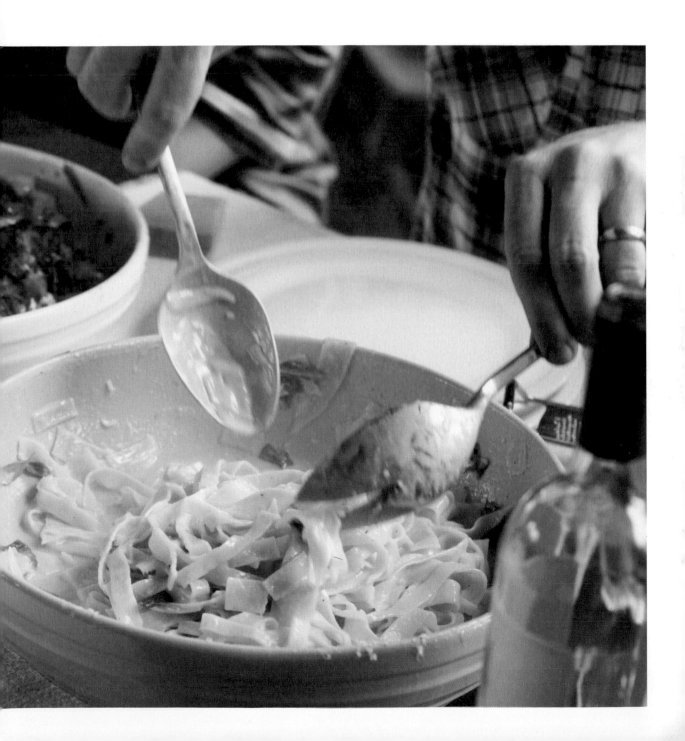

PASTA
2 egg yolks
125g Parmesan cheese, plus extra
  for serving
zest and juice of 2 lemons
a small bunch of fresh basil
500g fresh lasagne sheets

SALAD
8 rashers of pancetta
1 clove of garlic
1 tablespoon fennel seeds
1 x 100g bag of prewashed rocket
  and/or watercress

a small bunch of fresh mint
a small bunch of fresh tarragon
a large handful of red, green or
  mixed grapes
2 tablespoons balsamic vinegar
½ a lemon

SEASONINGS
olive oil
extra virgin olive oil
sea salt & black pepper

TARTLETS
4 small, deep shortcrust pastry cases
4 dessertspoons raspberry jam
1 x 400g tin of pear halves in natural
  juice
optional: 2 sprigs of fresh lemon
  thyme
2 egg whites
100g white caster sugar
1 teaspoon vanilla paste or extract
1 small tub of good-quality vanilla ice
  cream, to serve

TO START Get all your ingredients and equipment ready. Turn the oven on to 190°C/375°F/gas 5. Fill a large saucepan with hot water, put it on a high heat and cover with a lid. Put the fine grater attachment into the food processor.

TARTLETS Put the pastry cases into a roasting tray and spoon 1 dessertspoon of raspberry jam into each one. Slice 4 pear halves and divide between the pastry cases. Scatter a few lemon thyme leaves over each, if using.

PASTA Carefully separate 2 eggs and put the yolks into a big serving bowl. Put the whites into a whisking bowl.

TARTLETS Add the caster sugar and a pinch of salt to the whisking bowl with the egg whites, turn on the electric whisk and leave running at full whack until the mixture is glossy and stiff.

PASTA Add 3 tablespoons of extra virgin olive oil and a good pinch of salt & pepper to the bowl of egg yolks. Grate the Parmesan in the processor and tip it into the bowl of egg yolks with the lemon zest and juice. Reserve some of the small basil leaves, then split the rest of the bunch into 2 halves. Pound one half in a pestle & mortar until you have a green paste, and roughly chop the other half. Add both to the bowl. Stir until everything is mixed together, then season with salt & pepper.

TARTLETS The egg whites should be glossy, smooth and thick by now, so mix in the vanilla paste or extract, then spoon and smooth the meringue over the tartlets so you get lovely peaks. Put into the oven on the middle shelf and set the timer for 6 minutes, or until golden and lovely.

SALAD Put the pancetta into an empty frying pan on a medium heat and add a squashed, unpeeled clove of garlic. Once the rashers are golden, turn them over and add the tablespoon of fennel seeds. Meanwhile, empty the bag of

salad leaves on to a serving platter or into a large bowl. Quickly tear in some mint and tarragon leaves, and add a large handful of whole or halved grapes. When the pancetta is nice and crispy, take the pan off the heat. Toss the salad together and put on a platter, with the crispy pancetta and fennel seeds on top.

Make the dressing. Pour 4 tablespoons of extra virgin olive oil and 2 tablespoons of balsamic vinegar into a small jug or jam jar. Add a pinch of salt & pepper and squeeze in the juice of ½ a lemon, then take to the table with the salad so you can dress it right before tucking in.

PASTA Stack the lasagne sheets on a chopping board and carefully slice them into fairly thin strips – do this in batches. Add to the pan of boiling water with a good pinch of salt. Stir, then put the lid on slightly askew and keep it at a hard boil for just 1½ minutes.

TARTLETS Check on your tartlets and take them out to cool if cooked. Take the ice cream out of the freezer so you can serve it with your tartlets when ready.

PASTA This pasta must be eaten ASAP to be enjoyed properly, so call everyone around the table now. I like to use tongs to move the pasta to the egg mixture, because the cooking water that comes with it is what really makes the sauce incredible. If you find that tricky, just drain the pasta in a colander, but save the water. Toss the pasta and sauce together quickly, then add 2 or 3 more spoonfuls of cooking water to make it silkier if needed. Fresh pasta is constantly sucking up water so make it slightly looser than it needs to be and it will be perfect at the table. Have a taste. Does it need more salt or Parmesan to balance the lemon juice? If so, adjust then sprinkle over the reserved basil leaves and grate over some extra Parmesan. Take to the table, quickly dress the salad and eat straight away.

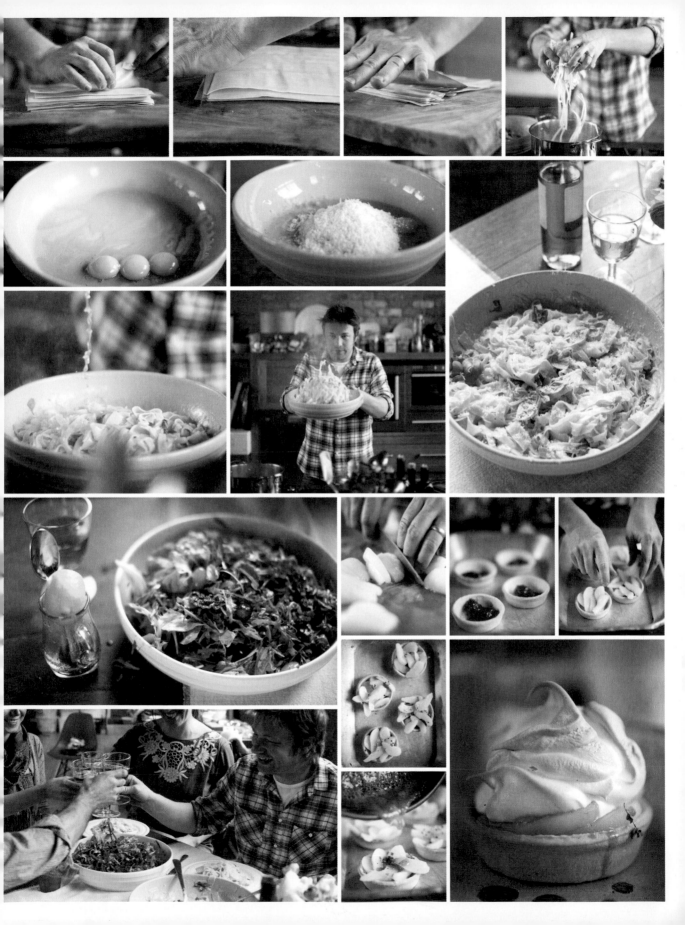

SUMMER VEG LASAGNE

SERVES 6–8

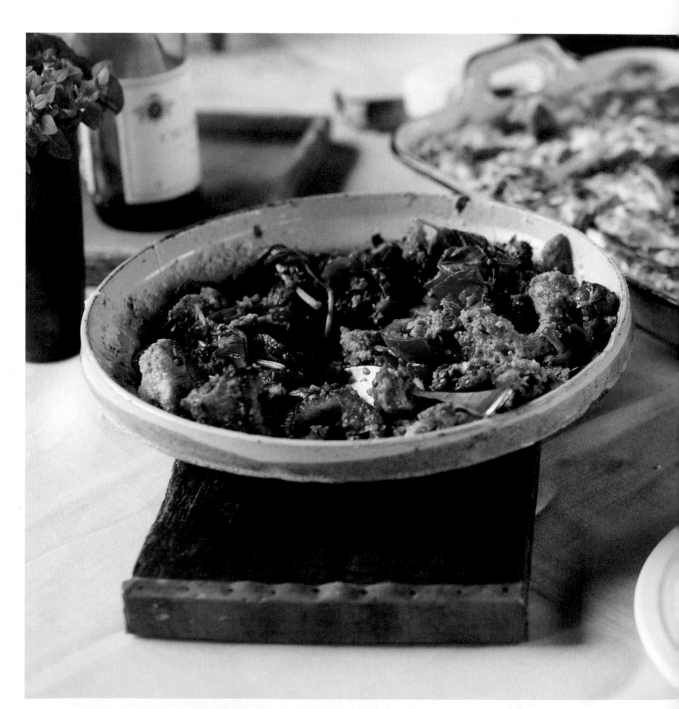

TUSCAN TOMATO SALAD
QUICK MANGO FROZEN YOGHURT IN BABY CORNETS

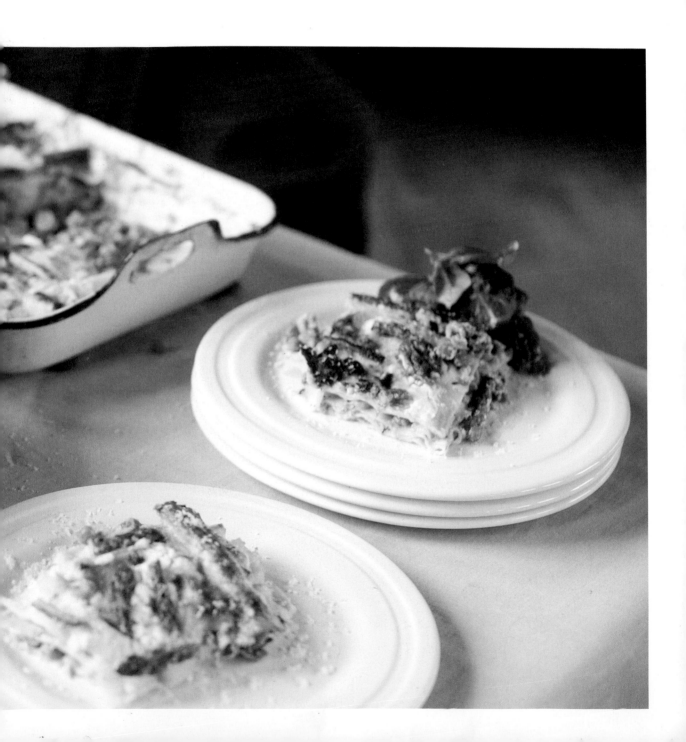

LASAGNE

a bunch of spring onions
½ a 30g tin of anchovies in oil
6 cloves of garlic
700g asparagus
500g frozen peas
300g frozen broad beans
a large bunch of fresh mint
300ml single cream
1 lemon
300ml organic vegetable stock
2 x 250g tubs of cottage cheese
2 x 250g packs of fresh lasagne
 sheets
Parmesan cheese
a couple of sprigs of fresh thyme

TUSCAN SALAD

½ a ciabatta loaf
1 teaspoon fennel seeds
a few sprigs of oregano or rosemary
1 tablespoon small capers
½ a 30g tin of anchovies in oil
a small bunch of fresh basil
6 jarred red peppers
1 clove of garlic
4 vines of cherry tomatoes, red and
 yellow if you can get them
3 large tomatoes
red wine vinegar
Parmesan cheese, to serve

SEASONINGS

olive oil
extra virgin olive oil
sea salt & black pepper

MANGO DESSERT

1 x 500g bag of frozen mango chunks
2 tablespoons runny honey
1 lime
a few sprigs of fresh mint
250g natural yoghurt
6–8 small ice cream cornets
good-quality dark chocolate (70%
 cocoa solids), for grating over

TO SERVE

a bottle of chilled white wine

TO START Get all your ingredients and equipment ready. Half-fill and boil the kettle. Put a large frying pan on a high heat. Turn the grill on to full whack. Put the standard blade attachment into the food processor.

LASAGNE Trim and finely slice the spring onions. Pour the oil from the tin of anchovies into the frying pan with half the tin of anchovies, add the spring onions, crush in 6 unpeeled cloves of garlic and toss well. Trim the ends off the asparagus and finely slice the stems, leaving the tips whole. Set the tips aside and add the stems to the pan with a pinch of salt & pepper. Add a splash of boiled water. Keep stirring so nothing catches.

TUSCAN SALAD Quickly tear the ciabatta into 2cm pieces. Put into a roasting tray, drizzle with olive oil, and toss with the fennel seeds, a few sprigs of oregano or rosemary and a pinch of salt. Mix so the bread is coated, then put under the grill on the middle shelf for around 10 minutes, or until golden.

LASAGNE Add the peas and broad beans to the pan of asparagus and stir occasionally. Pick and roughly chop the mint leaves and add to the pan with the cream. Finely grate in the zest of ½ a lemon.

TUSCAN SALAD Don't forget to check the croutons. Once golden and crisp, tip into a large bowl and set aside.

LASAGNE Roughly mash and squash everything in the pan, tasting and tweaking if necessary. Cover with stock and bring back to the boil. Add 1 tub of cottage cheese to the vegetable mixture. The consistency should be quite creamy and loose. Put a large deep sturdy roasting tray (approx. 30 x 35cm) on a medium heat. Spoon in about a quarter of the veggie mixture, to cover the bottom of the tray. Top with a layer of fresh lasagne sheets and a really good grating of Parmesan. Quickly repeat the layers till the vegetables run out, finishing with lasagne.

Mix a splash of water into the second tub of cottage cheese and spread it all over the top layer of lasagne. Toss the asparagus tips in the empty frying pan with a drizzle of olive oil. Tip on to the lasagne. Push everything down with the back of a spoon to help compact it, and finish with the thyme leaves, a drizzle of olive oil and a generous grating of Parmesan. Turn the heat up under the tray until bubbling, then place under the grill on the middle shelf for 8 minutes, or until golden and gorgeous.

TUSCAN SALAD Get a large chopping board and roughly chop and mix 1 tablespoon of capers with ½ the tin of anchovies, most of the leaves from the bunch of basil and 4 of the jarred peppers. Crush over an unpeeled clove of garlic and add all of the tomatoes and hack everything up. Sweep it all into a large serving bowl, add a splash of red wine vinegar, a good drizzle of extra virgin olive oil and a good pinch of salt & pepper.

Add the croutons, then tear in the remaining 2 peppers and scrunch and squeeze everything with your hands. Taste and tweak as necessary, adding more red wine vinegar if needed. Top with the rest of the basil leaves, then finely grate over a little Parmesan and take to the table.

MANGO DESSERT Whiz the frozen mango chunks in the food processor with 2 tablespoons of honey, the juice of 1 lime, a good pinch of mint leaves and 250g of yoghurt. Once smooth, pop into the freezer until ready to serve.

TO SERVE Once the lasagne is bubbling and golden on top, take to the table with the Parmesan for grating over. Serve with a bottle of chilled white wine. When you're ready for dessert get the frozen yoghurt out of the freezer, divide between cornets and grate over a little chocolate before tucking in.

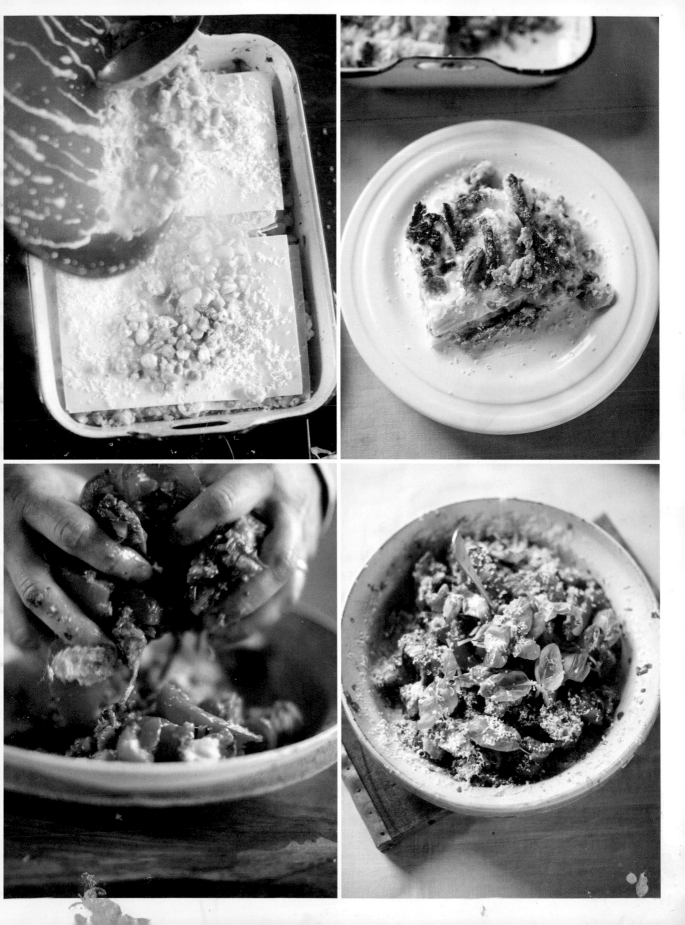

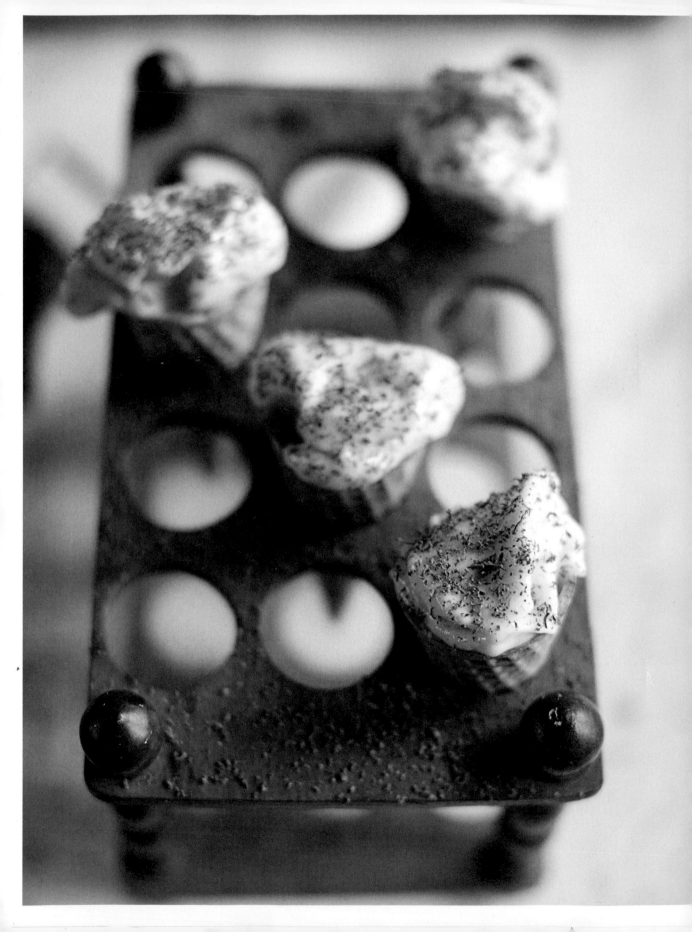

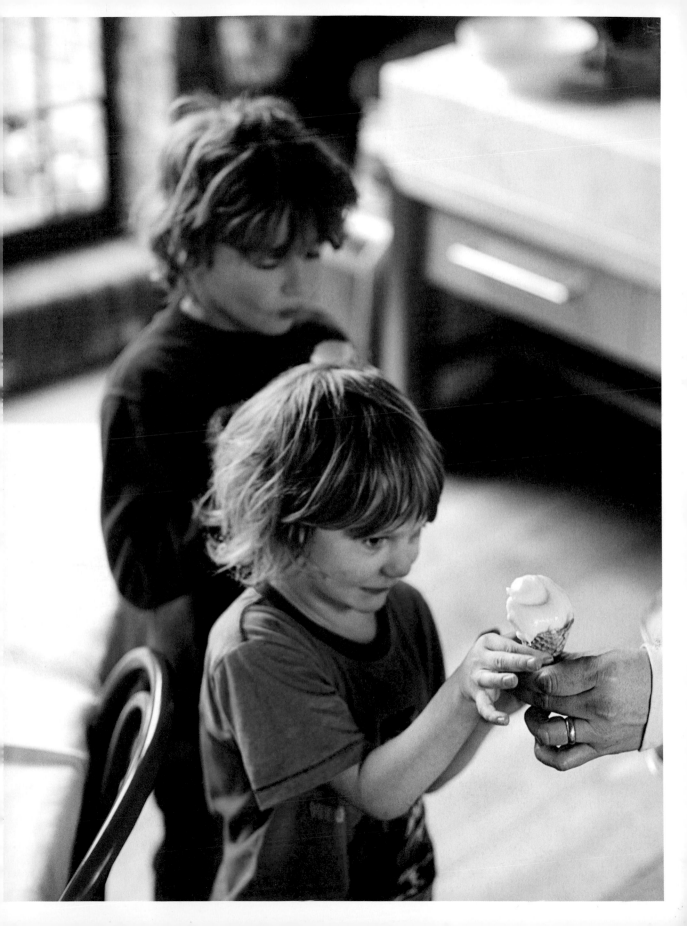

SPAGHETTI ALLA PUTTANESCA

CRUNCHY SALAD

GARLIC BREAD

SILKY CHOCOLATE GANACHE

SERVES 4–6

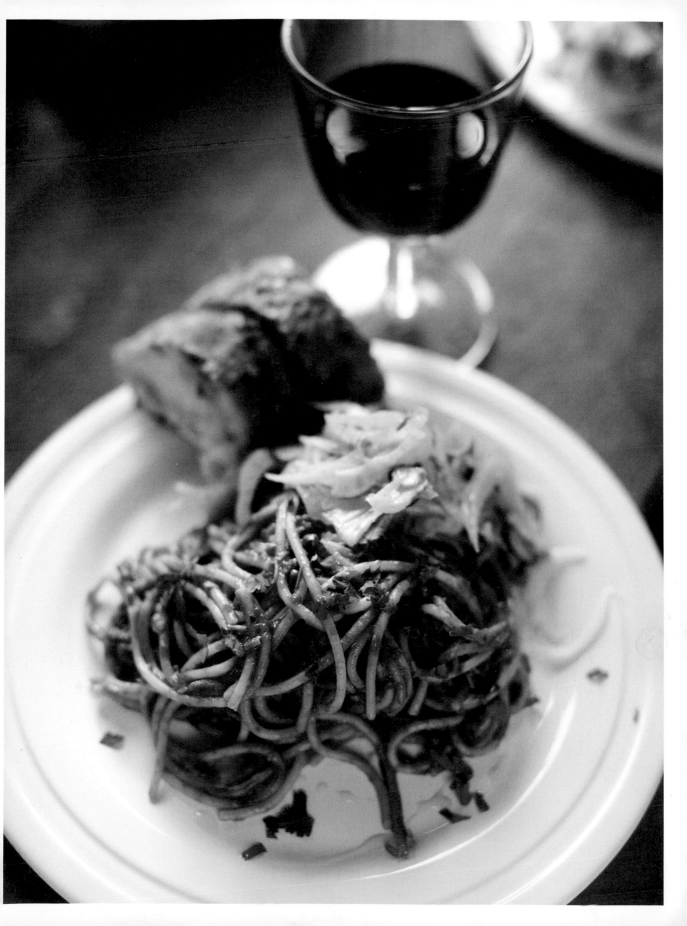

GARLIC BREAD
1 ciabatta loaf
a small bunch of fresh flat-leaf parsley
3–4 cloves of garlic

SALAD
2 bulbs of fennel
a bunch of radishes
1 lemon

SEASONINGS
olive oil
extra virgin olive oil
sea salt & black pepper

SPAGHETTI
500g dried spaghetti
1 x 225g jar of tuna in oil
2 cloves of garlic
1 tablespoon capers, drained
1 x 30g tin of anchovy fillets in oil
1–2 fresh red chillies
a small bunch of fresh flat-leaf parsley
8 jarred black olives, stoned
ground cinnamon
1 x 700g jar of passata or 2 x 400g tins
  of chopped tomatoes
1 lemon

GANACHE
2 x 100g bars of good-quality dark
  chocolate (approx. 70% cocoa solids)
a large knob of butter
300ml single cream
3 clementines
12 palmiers or other nice biscuits,
  for dipping

TO SERVE
a bottle of chilled Valpolicella

TO START Get all your ingredients and equipment ready. Fill and boil the kettle. Turn the oven on to 180°C/350°F/gas 4. Put a large frying pan and a large deep saucepan on a low heat. Put the thick slicer disc attachment into the food processor.

GARLIC BREAD Slice the ciabatta at 2cm intervals, three-quarters of the way through. Finely chop the bunch of parsley. Scrunch up a large sheet of greaseproof paper under the tap, then lay it flat. Scatter it with the parsley and a pinch of salt & pepper. Drizzle generously with olive oil, crush 3 or 4 unpeeled cloves of garlic on top, and smear this mixture all over the bread with your hands, pushing it down into the cuts. Wrap it up well, put it into the oven and check on it every so often.

GANACHE Pour the boiled water into the saucepan for the pasta and place a large heatproof bowl on top (don't let the bowl touch the water). Smash up the chocolate bars in their wrappers, then unwrap and empty into the bowl. Add the butter, cream and a pinch of salt. Finely grate in the zest of 1 clementine, gently stir and leave to melt.

SPAGHETTI Lift up the chocolate bowl and add the spaghetti to the water with a pinch of salt and cook according to the packet instructions. Put the bowl back on top. Keep an eye on it – if it looks like bubbling over, reduce the heat a little. Pour the tuna oil into the frying pan, keeping the tuna in the jar. Crush in 2 unpeeled cloves of garlic and add the capers, anchovies and their oil. Finely chop the chillies and parsley stalks and add them to the pan. Quickly check your spaghetti and give it a stir. Roughly chop the parsley leaves and put aside. Cook for 2 minutes, stirring well, then add the tuna, breaking it up as you go and the black olives. Stir in a large pinch of ground cinnamon and the passata or tinned tomatoes.

GANACHE Once melted, give the chocolate a good stir and divide between 6 espresso cups. Halve the remaining 2 clementines and arrange them on a board next to the palmiers. Take to the table.

SALAD Trim and quarter the fennel. Trim any leaves off the radishes. Put the fennel and radishes into the food processor and shred. Tip into a large bowl. Squeeze in the juice of a lemon, add 2 lugs of extra virgin olive oil and a pinch of salt & pepper, then toss and scrunch with your hands. Taste and tweak as necessary, then take to the table.

SPAGHETTI Once the pasta is cooked, drain it and reserve some of the cooking water. Carefully tip the pasta into the pan of sauce. Add most of the reserved parsley, squeeze in the juice of a lemon, drizzle over the extra virgin olive oil and toss really well. Add some of the cooking water to loosen it if needed. Tip on to a platter, scatter over the remaining parsley and take to the table.

TO SERVE Take the garlic bread straight to the table from the oven and unwrap. Pour the red wine into glasses and let everyone help themselves.

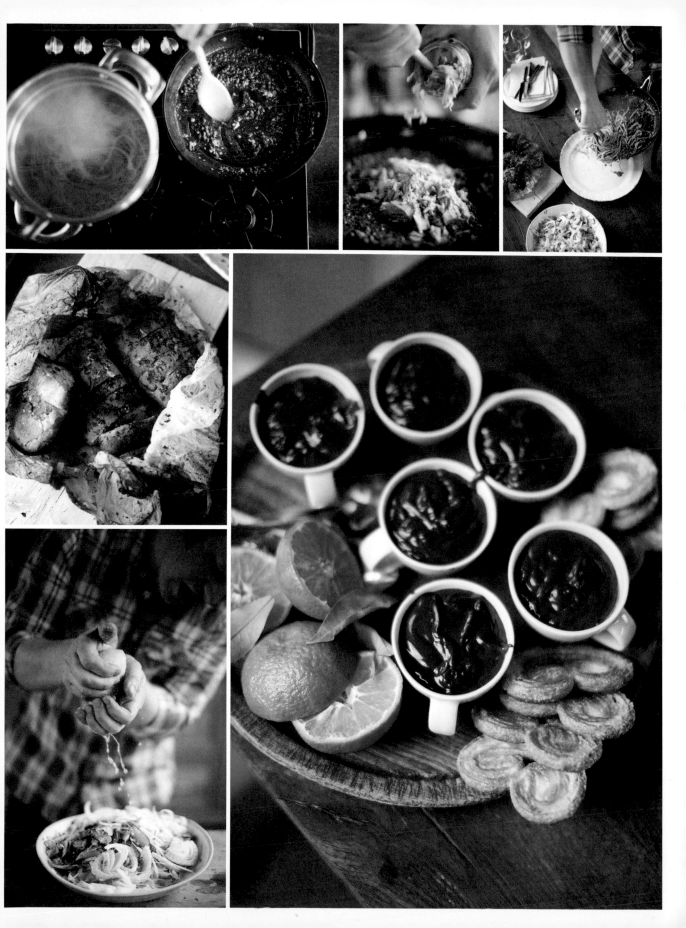

CHEAT'S PIZZA

3 DELISH SALADS

SQUASHED CHERRIES &

VANILLA MASCARPONE CREAM

SERVES 4

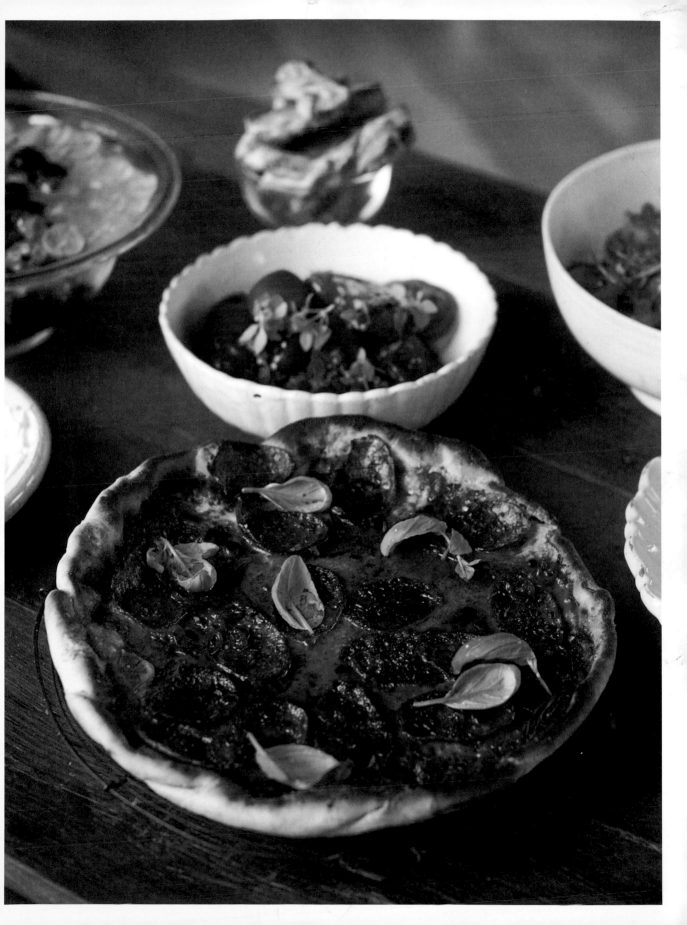

PIZZA
1 mug of self-raising flour, plus extra
  for dusting
½ a mug of tepid water

TOPPING
1 x 400g tin of chopped tomatoes
a few sprigs of fresh basil
½ a clove of garlic
red wine vinegar
½ a 125g ball of buffalo mozzarella
Parmesan cheese, for grating over
8 slices of salami
1 teaspoon fennel seeds
½ a fresh red chilli

ROCKET SALAD
1 x 100g bag of prewashed wild rocket
½ a lemon

TOMATO SALAD
500g mixture of interesting
  tomatoes such as cherry, plum
  and salad, mixture of colours if
  you can get them
½ a fresh red chilli
a few sprigs of fresh basil
1 tablespoon balsamic vinegar
½ a clove of garlic

MOZZARELLA SALAD
1½ x 125g balls of buffalo mozzarella
¼ of a jar of green pesto
a few sprigs of fresh basil
1 lemon

SEASONINGS
olive oil
extra virgin olive oil
sea salt & black pepper

CHERRY DESSERT
2 good handfuls of ice
300g cherries or other seasonal fruit
125g mascarpone
50ml milk
1 heaped tablespoon icing sugar
1 clementine
1 teaspoon vanilla paste or extract
a few palmiers or other nice biscuits,
  to serve

TO START Get all your ingredients and equipment ready. Turn the grill on to full whack. Put a large (30–32cm diameter) ovenproof frying pan on a low heat. Put the standard blade attachment into the food processor.

TOMATO SALAD Scrunch the cherry tomatoes into a bowl with your hands. Roughly slice the larger tomatoes and add to the bowl. Finely slice the chilli and add, then tear in the larger leaves from a few sprigs of basil. Add 3 tablespoons of extra virgin olive oil, 1 or 2 tablespoons of balsamic vinegar, then season to perfection. Finely grate in ½ a peeled clove of garlic. Mix and take to the table with the smaller basil leaves sprinkled on top.

PIZZA Turn the heat under the frying pan up to high and dust a clean surface with flour. Put 1 mug's worth of flour into a food processor, then half-fill the same mug with tepid water and add to the flour with a pinch of salt and a lug of olive oil. Whiz until smooth, then tip on to the floured board. Sprinkle the top of the dough and the rolling pin with flour (the dough will be quite wet, so be generous with the flour). Roll the dough to a 1cm thickness. Drizzle olive oil into the pan, then dust the dough with flour again and very lightly fold it over into a half-moon shape. Lightly fold the half-moon in half, then move the dough to the pan and unfold it, pushing it down into the sides of the pan. If you don't have a pan this big, don't cook all of the dough at once, halve it and make two pizzas.

TOPPING Put a third of the tinned tomatoes into a liquidizer with a few sprigs of basil, ½ a peeled clove of garlic, a splash of red wine vinegar, a drizzle of extra virgin

olive oil and a pinch of salt. Whiz until smooth. Pour over the middle of the pizza base and spread out evenly. Tear ½ a mozzarella ball into small pieces and dot around the base. Finely grate a layer of Parmesan over, then top with the salami slices. I like to bash the fennel seeds in a pestle & mortar and finely chop the chilli, then scatter them over the pizza. Put the pan under the hot grill for 4 or 5 minutes, until golden and cooked through.

MOZZARELLA SALAD Tear 1½ balls of mozzarella into chunks and arrange on a large platter. Spoon a little pesto over each chunk. Sprinkle with pepper and pick over the basil leaves. Finely grate over the lemon zest and drizzle with extra virgin olive oil. Take to the table.

ROCKET SALAD Open the bag of rocket and drizzle in extra virgin olive oil, squeeze in the juice of ½ a lemon and season with salt & pepper. Toss the rocket in the bag with your hands, then tip into a bowl and take to the table.

PIZZA Remove it from the grill, transfer it to a wooden board and scatter over the reserved baby basil leaves. Drizzle over a little extra virgin olive oil and take straight to the table.

CHERRY DESSERT Put a little cold water into a large bowl. Add the ice and cherries. Spoon the mascarpone into a separate bowl, add the milk and mix with the icing sugar. Finely grate in the zest of the clementine. Add vanilla paste or extract to the bowl. Mix well. Divide the cream between some serving bowls, squash over the cold cherries, then put on the table with some biscuits for dipping.

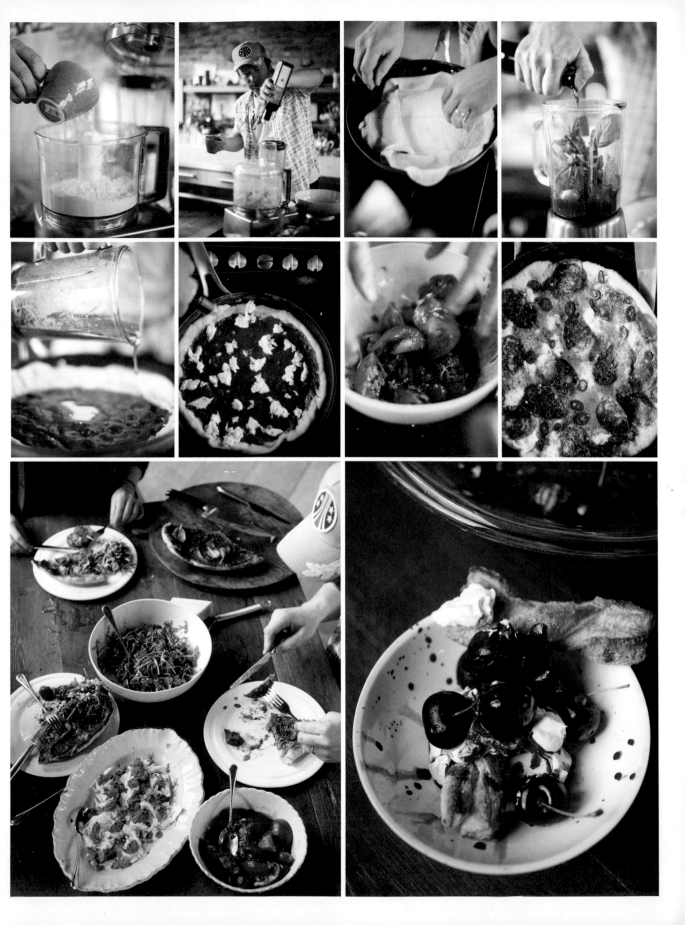

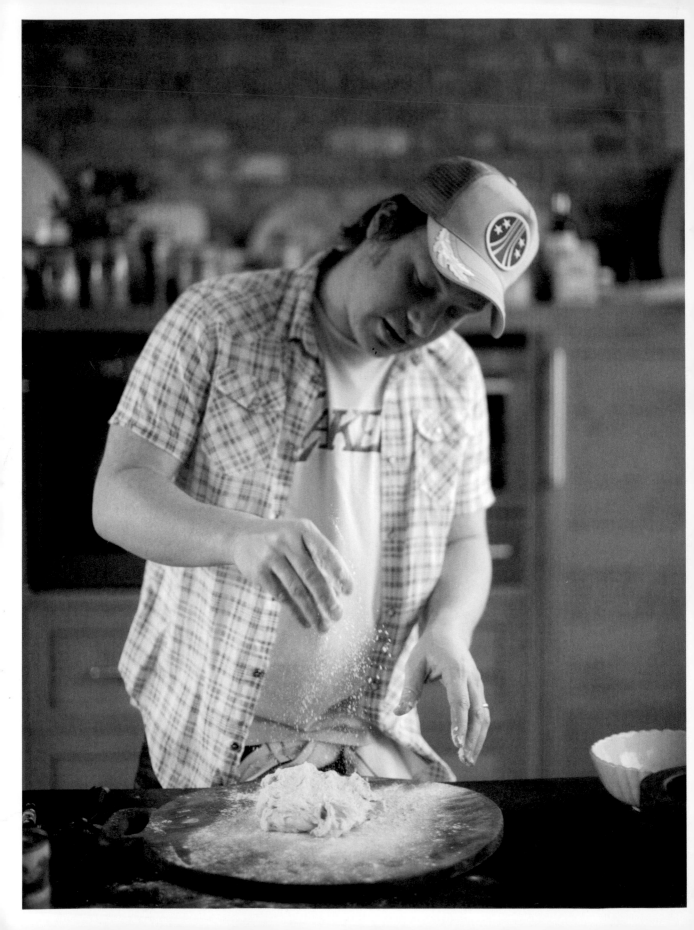

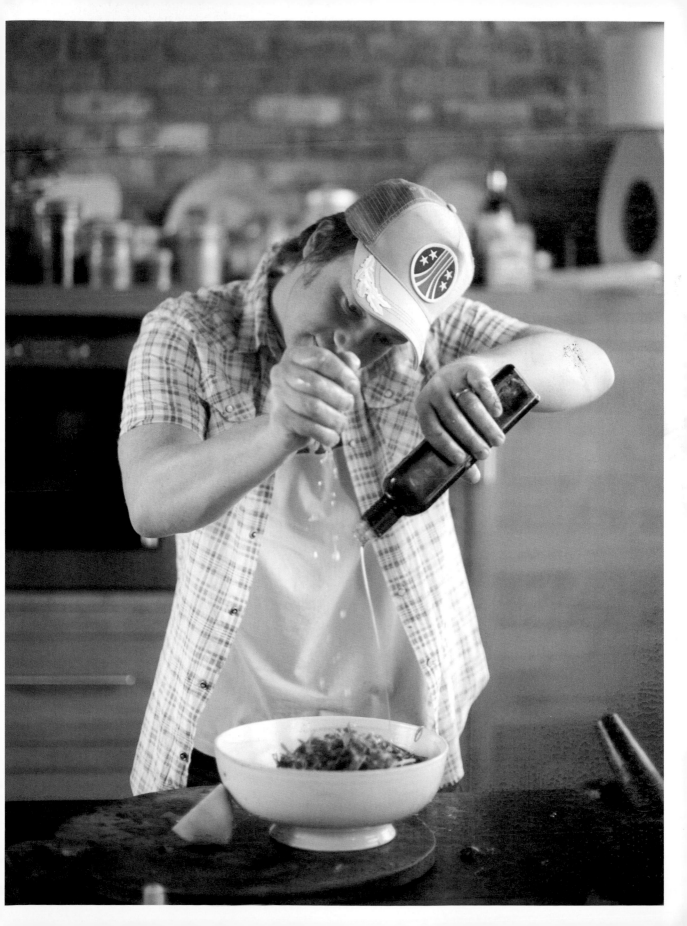

OOZY MUSHROOM RISOTTO
SPINACH SALAD
QUICK LEMON & RASPBERRY CHEESECAKE

SERVES 4

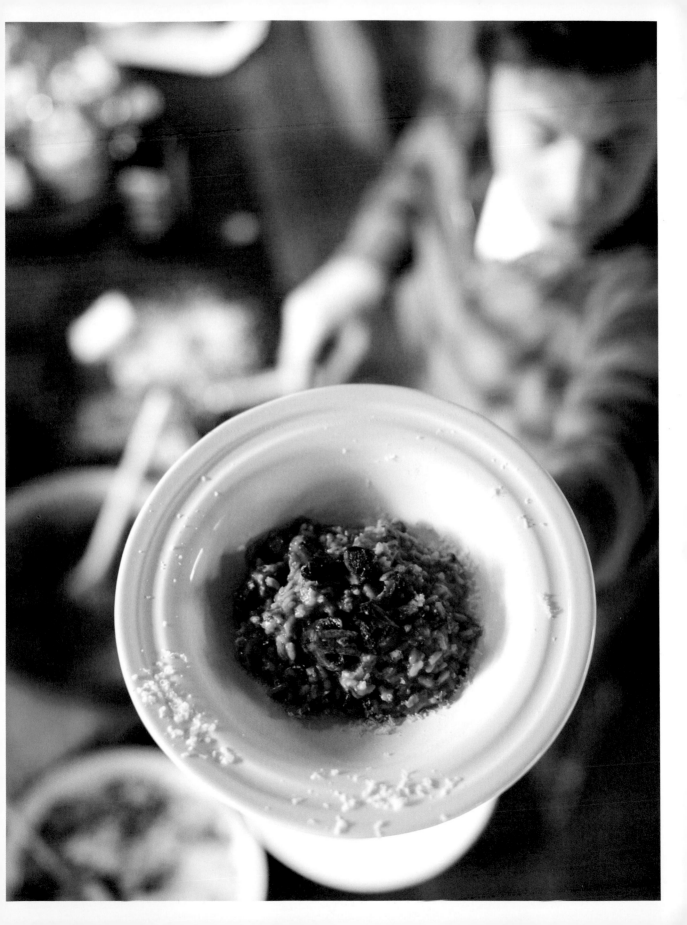

RISOTTO

1 large white onion
1 stick of celery
2 sprigs of fresh rosemary
15g dried porcini mushrooms
300g risotto rice
½ a glass of white wine
1 organic veg or chicken stock cube
500g mixed mushrooms, such as
  chestnut, oyster, shiitake
1 clove of garlic
a small bunch of fresh thyme
a large knob of butter
a 40g chunk of Parmesan cheese
½ a lemon
½ a small bunch of fresh
  flat-leaf parsley

SALAD

100g pinenuts
1 tablespoon balsamic vinegar
½ a lemon
200g prewashed baby spinach
3 large sprigs of fresh mint
5 jarred sun-dried tomatoes
1 medium cucumber

SEASONINGS

olive oil
extra virgin olive oil
sea salt & black pepper

CHEESECAKE

50g butter
50g blanched hazelnuts
8 gingernut biscuits
1 lemon
4 heaped teaspoons good-quality
  lemon curd
1 punnet of raspberries (approx. 150g)
250g light or low-fat cream cheese,
  mascarpone cheese or crème fraîche
1 teaspoon vanilla paste or extract
a splash of milk
1 tablespoon icing sugar
good-quality dark chocolate
  (approx.70% cocoa solids), for grating

TO START Get all your ingredients and equipment ready. Fill and boil the kettle. Put a large high-sided saucepan on a medium heat. Turn the grill to full whack. Put 4 tumblers for the puddings into the freezer. Put the standard blade attachment into the food processor.

RISOTTO Halve and peel the onion, then put into the food processor with the celery and dried porcini and pulse until finely chopped. Drizzle a couple of lugs of oil into the saucepan, then scrape in the veg and stir regularly.

SALAD Put the pinenuts into a large ovenproof frying pan on a medium heat and toast, tossing occasionally, until lightly golden, then tip into a small bowl and set aside.

RISOTTO Pick and finely chop the rosemary leaves and add to the saucepan with the rice. Stir well for 1 minute, then pour in the white wine and crumble in the stock cube, stirring until the wine is absorbed. Season, then add a mug of boiling water and stir in well. Your job now is to get into the habit of coming back to the risotto and adding good swigs of boiling water, or stock if you've got it (you'll probably use about 1 litre in total), every minute or so for around 16 to 18 minutes as you're getting on with other jobs. To make it oozy and lovely, you're going to massage starch out of the rice and stop it from sticking.

Put the large ovenproof frying pan you used for the pinenuts back on a high heat. Rinse the mushrooms in their pack if they look dirty. Tear half of them into the risotto pan and the other half into the hot frying pan with a couple of good lugs of extra virgin olive oil and a good pinch of salt & pepper. Crush over 1 unpeeled clove of garlic. Pick the leaves from a few sprigs of thyme into the pan, stir them in, then take off the heat. Pick the remaining thyme leaves into the risotto.

CHEESECAKE Put the butter into a medium frying pan on a high heat. Wrap the hazelnuts and biscuits in a clean tea towel and quickly bash with a rolling pin. Turn the heat off under the melted butter, tip in the bashed nuts and

biscuits and stir. Finely grate in the lemon zest and mix well. Take the tumblers out of the freezer and divide the mixture between them, gently patting it down until firm.

RISOTTO Put the frying pan of mushrooms under the grill on the top shelf to crisp up. Keep stirring the risotto.

SALAD Put 3 tablespoons of balsamic vinegar, the juice of ½ a lemon, 3 tablespoons of extra virgin olive oil and a good pinch of salt & pepper into a nice large salad bowl with the toasted pine nuts. Season to taste. Grab handfuls of spinach, roughly slice them 1cm thick, along with some picked mint leaves, and add to the bowl. Roughly chop the sun-dried tomatoes and add. Use a fork to score the cucumber lengthways, then halve and slice 1cm thick at an angle. Add to the bowl, then take to the table but don't toss until the last minute.

CHEESECAKE Put 1 heaped teaspoon of lemon curd into each tumbler and top with a few raspberries. Spoon the cream cheese, mascarpone or crème fraîche into a bowl and add the vanilla paste or extract and a splash of milk. Stir, then add the icing sugar and another splash of milk and mix really well until it looks soft and silky smooth. Divide between the tumblers, scrape over a few gratings of dark chocolate and set aside until you're ready to serve.

RISOTTO Check the mushrooms and remove from the grill if golden and crispy. Turn off the grill. The risotto should be porridge-like. Stir in the butter, finely grate over most of the Parmesan and add a good squeeze of lemon juice. Season with salt & pepper and add a splash more water or stock if needed to make it oozy and delicious. Chop the parsley and sprinkle ½ over the risotto and ½ over the crispy mushrooms. Put the lid on the risotto and take to the table with the crispy mushrooms.

TO SERVE Divide the risotto between your bowls, then top with a big pinch of crispy mushrooms. Toss and quickly dress the salad. Finish off with a good grating of Parmesan, and serve.

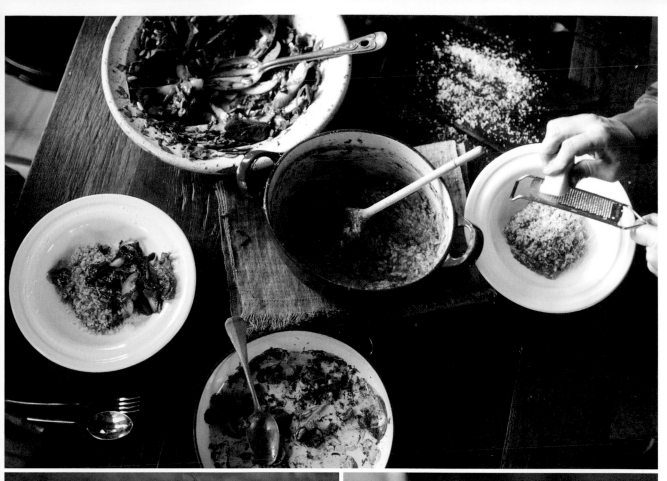

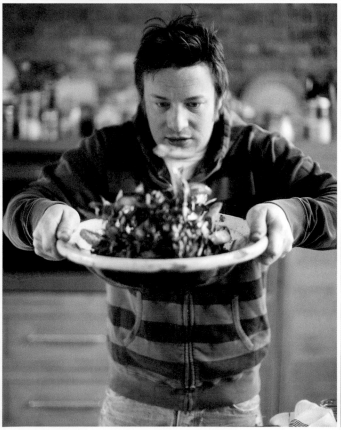

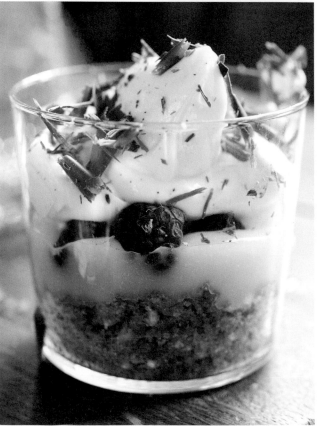

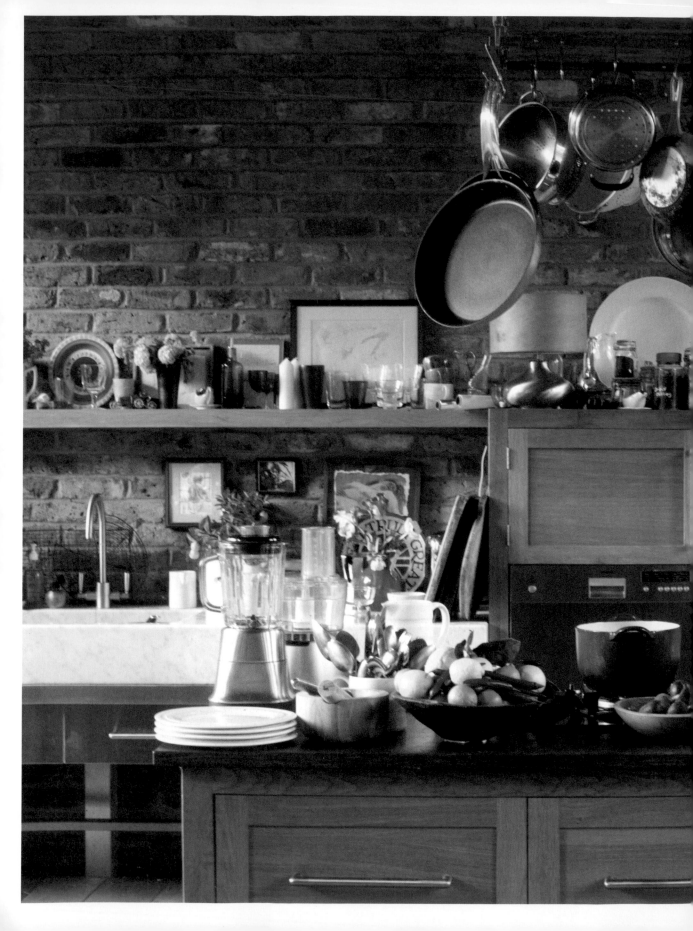

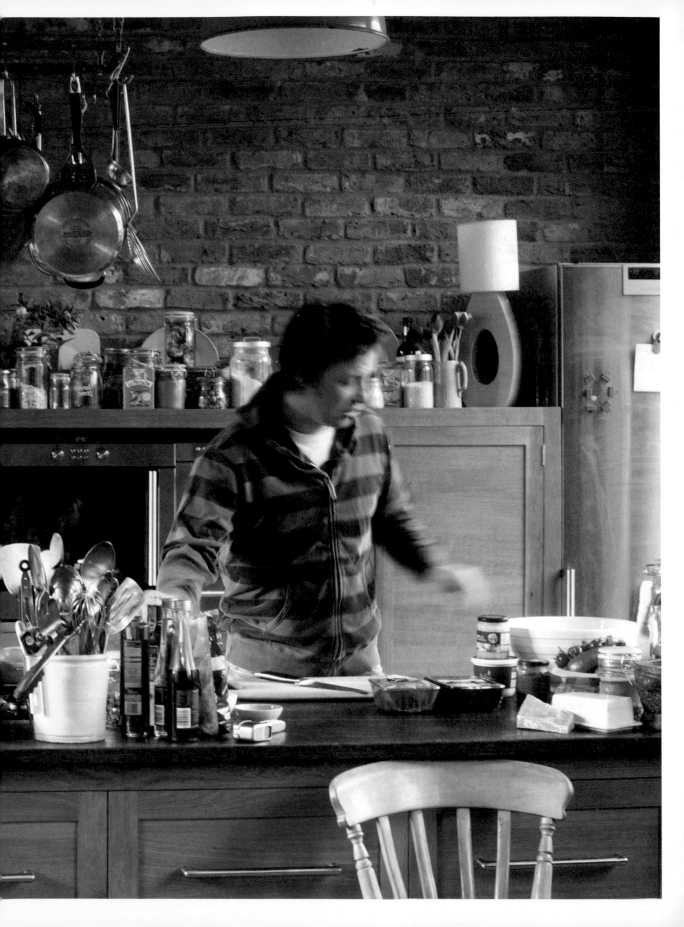

SPINACH & FETA FILO PIE

CUCUMBER SALAD

TOMATO SALAD

COATED ICE CREAM

SERVES 4–6

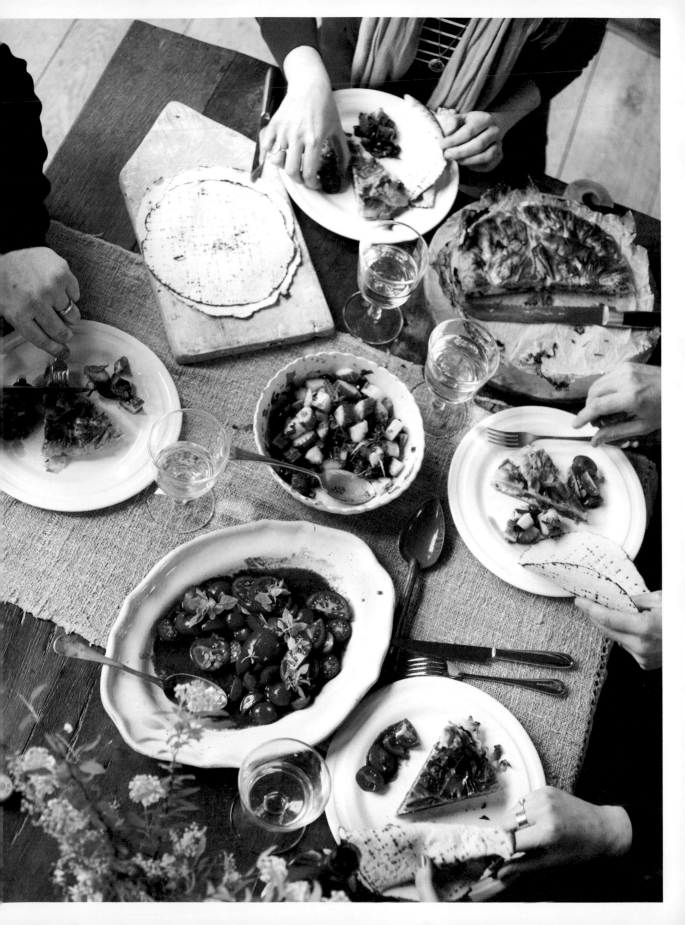

SPINACH & FETA PIE

100g pinenuts
5 eggs
300g feta cheese
50g Cheddar cheese
dried oregano
1 lemon
a knob of butter
400g prewashed baby spinach
1 x 270g pack of filo pastry
cayenne pepper
1 whole nutmeg, for grating

CUCUMBER SALAD

1 cucumber
10 black olives
2 tablespoons balsamic vinegar
3 spring onions
½ a lemon
½ a fresh red chilli
5 or 6 sprigs of fresh mint

TOMATO SALAD

a small bunch of fresh basil
1 clove of garlic
white wine vinegar
300g mixed cherry tomatoes

optional: a small bunch of fresh Greek basil

SEASONINGS

olive oil
extra virgin olive oil
sea salt & black pepper

COATED ICE CREAM

4 tablespoons coffee beans
100g hazelnuts
1 x 100g bar of good-quality dark chocolate (70% cocoa solids)
good-quality vanilla ice cream

TO START Get all your ingredients and equipment ready. Turn the oven on to 200°C/400°F/gas 6. Put a medium (approx. 26cm diameter) ovenproof frying pan on a medium heat. Put the standard blade attachment in the food processor.

SPINACH & FETA PIE Put the pinenuts into the dry ovenproof frying pan to toast, tossing occasionally. Keep an eye on them. Crack 5 eggs into a mixing bowl and crumble in 300g of feta. Grate in 50g of Cheddar. Add a pinch of pepper, a couple of pinches of dried oregano, zest of 1 lemon and a lug of olive oil. Once the nuts are light golden, add them to the egg mixture and mix well.

Put the empty frying pan back on the heat, add a little olive oil and a knob of butter and pile in half of the spinach. Gently push and move it around and add more as it wilts down. Make sure it doesn't catch on the bottom and when there's room, start adding the rest, stirring frequently.

Meanwhile, take the pastry out of the fridge. Lay a large sheet of greaseproof paper, approximately 50cm long, on the worktop, rub a little olive oil all over it, then scrunch it up and lay it out flat again. Arrange 4 filo pastry sheets in a large rectangle, overlapping at the edges, so they almost cover the paper. Rub some olive oil over them. Sprinkle over a good pinch of salt & pepper and a pinch of cayenne. Repeat until you have 3 layers. Don't worry about any cracked bits. Remember to keep stirring the spinach.

Once the spinach is really nice and dense, take the pan off the heat. Add the wilted spinach to the egg mixture and grate in ½ a nutmeg. Mix well. Carefully move the greaseproof paper and filo into the empty frying pan so the edges spill over. Push it down into the sides of the pan, then pour in the egg mixture and spread it out. Fold the filo sheets over the top and let them fall where they will (🍳II). Put the pan back on a medium heat for a couple of minutes to get the bottom cooking, then put the pan into the oven on the top shelf to cook for 18 to 20 minutes, or until golden and crisp.

CUCUMBER SALAD Run a fork down the length of the cucumber all around it, then halve and quarter it lengthways and cut the quarters across into 1cm chunks. Put them into a mixing bowl and set aside. Drain 10 black olives, squeeze out their stones, and tear them into another bowl. Pour over 2 tablespoons of balsamic vinegar and push down on the olives so the vinegar starts pulling out their saltiness. Trim and finely slice the spring onions, then add to the olives.

Drizzle 4 tablespoons of extra virgin olive oil and the juice of ½ a lemon into the olive mixture and stir really well. Deseed and finely slice ½ a red chilli and add to the bowl of cucumber. Pick the leaves from the sprigs of mint, finely slice them and add to the cucumber. Pour over the dressing, toss quickly, drizzle over a little more extra virgin olive oil and take to the table.

SPINACH & FETA PIE Check on the pie.

COATED ICE CREAM Pour the coffee beans into a liquidizer and blitz. Add the hazelnuts and blitz to a powder. While that's going on, really bash the chocolate, still in its wrapper, against the work surface (this works best if it's straight from the fridge). Unwrap and add to the food processor. Whiz again, then tip into a bowl and put to one side.

TOMATO SALAD Quickly rinse out the liquidizer. Rip the top off the bunch of basil, reserving a few of the smaller leaves, and put into the liquidizer with a pinch of salt & pepper, a peeled clove of garlic, a couple of good lugs of extra virgin olive oil and a splash of white wine vinegar. Whiz until you have a dark green oil. Taste and adjust the seasoning if needed. Halve or quarter the tomatoes. Pour this dressing over a platter and sit the tomatoes on top. Scatter over some Greek basil leaves or smaller basil leaves and a pinch or two of salt, then take to the table and toss right before serving.

TO SERVE Take the ice cream out of the freezer to soften. Take the pie to the table with your beautiful salads and divide up between your guests. After dinner, take the ice cream to the table with the bowl of powdered topping. Roll a scoop of ice cream in the powder to coat, and eat at once. Store any leftover powder in an airtight container and use another time.

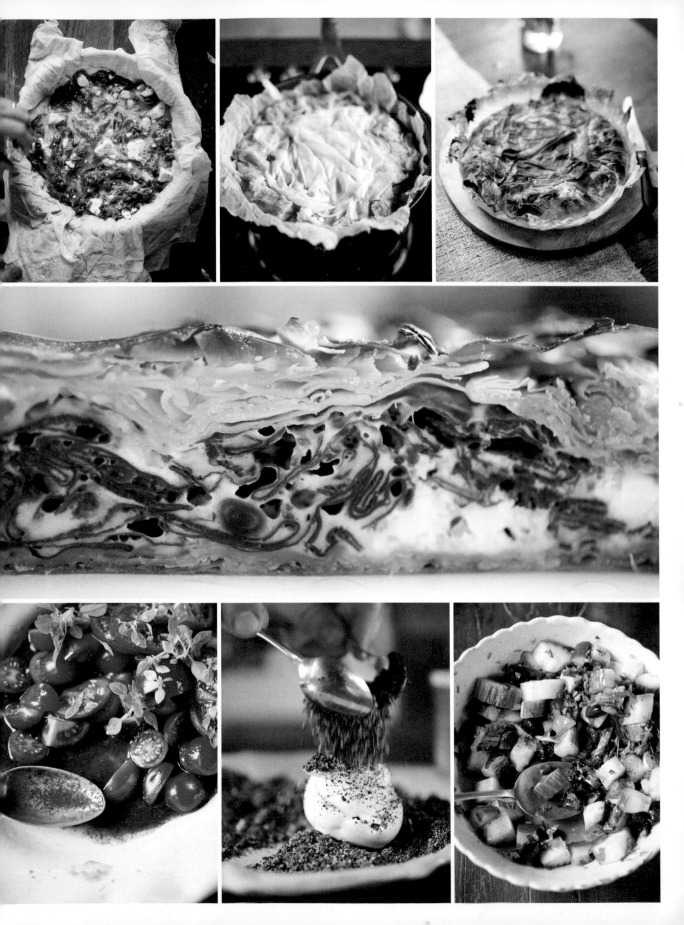

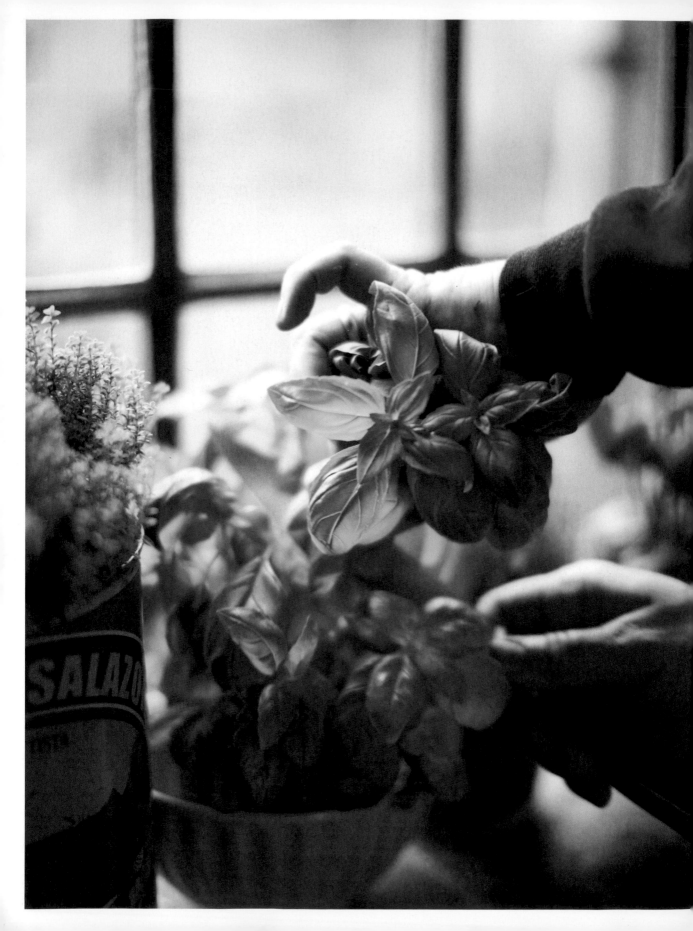

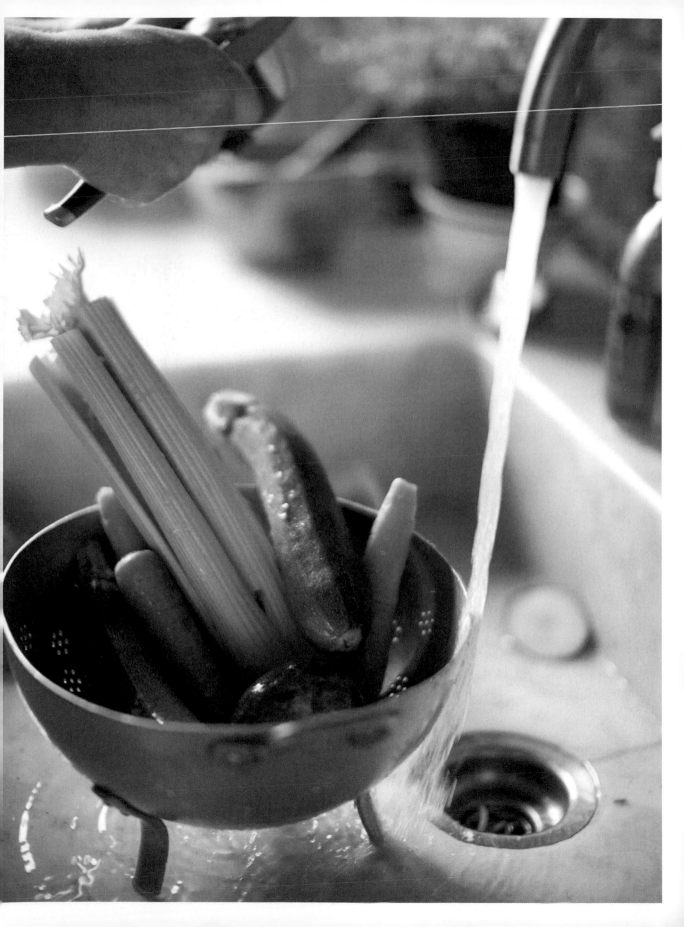

TOMATO SOUP

CHUNKY CROUTONS

CRUNCHY VEG & GUACAMOLE

STICKY PRUNE SPONGE PUDDINGS

SERVES 4

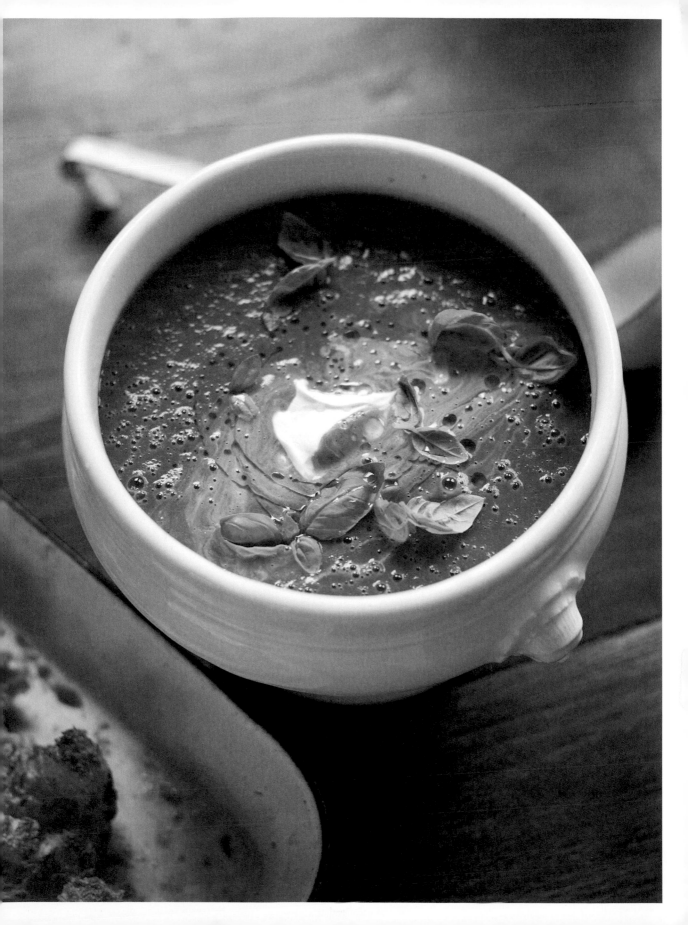

TOMATO SOUP & CROUTONS

1kg ripe cherry tomatoes on the vine, red and yellow if you can get them
4 large tomatoes
1 fresh red chilli
4 cloves of garlic
1 ciabatta loaf
2 small red onions
4 tablespoons balsamic vinegar
a small bunch of fresh basil
a few dollops of crème fraîche, to serve

SEASONINGS

olive oil
extra virgin olive oil
sea salt & black pepper

GUACAMOLE PLATTER

a handful of mixed-colour cherry tomatoes
1–2 fresh red chillies
a handful of fresh coriander
2 ripe avocados
2 limes
½ a bulb of fennel
1 carrot
½ a cucumber
½ a 125g pack of grissini or other breadsticks

PRUNE PUDDINGS

1 x 290g tin of pitted prunes
100g plain flour
50g soft dark brown sugar
50g unsalted butter, room temperature
1 heaped teaspoon ground ginger
½ a level teaspoon bicarbonate of soda
1 egg
75ml milk
golden syrup, to serve
a few dollops of crème fraîche, to serve

TO START Get all your ingredients and equipment ready. Turn the oven on to 220°C/425°F/gas 7 and put a large saucepan on a low heat. Put the standard blade attachment into the food processor.

TOMATO SOUP Pull the tomatoes off the vines, but leave some of their green tops on. Quarter the larger tomatoes, then put all the tomatoes into a roasting tray. Drizzle over a good lug of olive oil and season. Halve and deseed the red chilli and add to the tray. Crush in 4 peeled cloves of garlic. Quickly toss everything, then put on the top shelf of the oven for 12 to 15 minutes.

CROUTONS Get another roasting tray and rip the ciabatta loaf into 8 equal chunks. Add a good lug of olive oil, a pinch of salt and whack on to the bottom shelf of the oven.

TOMATO SOUP Peel and roughly chop the onions and put them into the hot saucepan with a lug of olive oil and a good pinch of salt. Turn the heat up to medium and leave to soften, stirring occasionally.

PRUNE PUDDINGS Get 4 cups that will all fit into your microwave at the same time. Tip the prunes into a bowl, then spoon 1 tablespoon of their syrupy juice into each of the cups. Divide all the prunes between the 4 cups.

TOMATO SOUP Stir 4 tablespoons of balsamic vinegar into the onions and let it cook away and reduce down.

PRUNE PUDDINGS Put the flour, sugar, butter, ground ginger and bicarbonate of soda into a food processor and whiz. Crack in the egg, then add the milk. Let it whiz until smooth (you may need to scrape round the edge and whiz again), then divide between the cups (they should be two-thirds full) and put to one side.

GUACAMOLE Squeeze a handful of cherry tomatoes on to the biggest board you have, then finely chop up the flesh with 1 to 2 red chillies and a handful of coriander leaves, including the top part of the stalks.

TOMATO SOUP Take the tray of tomatoes out of the oven and add everything to the pan of onions.

CROUTONS Check them – if they are crisp and golden turn off the oven, but leave them in there to keep warm.

GUACAMOLE Halve and stone the avocados, then squeeze them over a board so the flesh comes out of the skins. Discard the skins, add a pinch of salt, squeeze over the juice of 2 limes and chop everything together until fine. Taste and adjust the flavours if needed, then use your knife to sweep everything to one side of the board. Cut the ½ bulb of fennel into wedges. Peel the carrot, quarter lengthways and cut into batons, then do the same with the cucumber. Sprinkle over a pinch of salt, then arrange the vegetables next to the guacamole. Put a handful of grissini into a glass and take them to the table with the board of guacamole.

TOMATO SOUP In 2 batches, carefully pour the vegetables from the saucepan into a liquidizer. Add most of the basil, put the lid on, cover with a tea towel and whiz to a fairly rustic consistency, pouring the mixture into a large pan or serving bowl as you go. Once finished, mix well, season to taste and top with a dollop of crème fraîche, a few basil leaves and a drizzle of extra virgin olive oil. Take to the table with a stack of soup bowls and the tray of croutons from the oven.

PRUNE PUDDINGS Just before serving, pop the puddings into the microwave to cook on full power for 6 minutes.

TO SERVE Put a crouton or two in the bottom of each soup bowl. Ladle the soup on top, then dig in and let everyone help themselves to the guacamole. When the desserts are ready, bring to the table, drizzle over a little golden syrup, top with crème fraîche and go for it (use a spoon to turn them upside down in the cups and you'll be in for a treat).

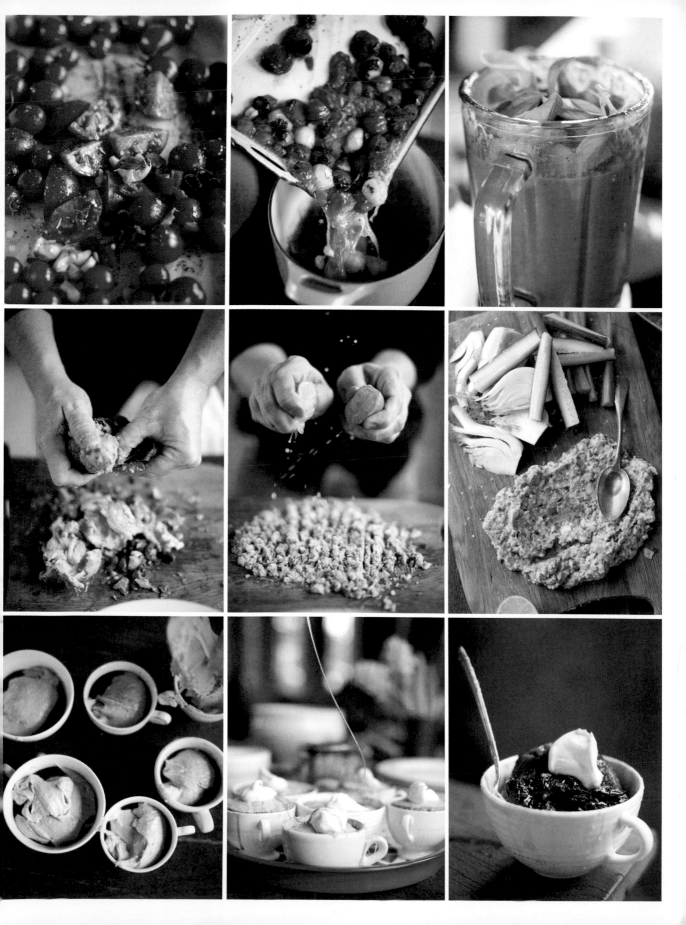

CURRY

ROGAN JOSH

FLUFFY RICE

CARROT SALAD

POPPADOMS

FLATBREAD

BEER

SERVES 4–6

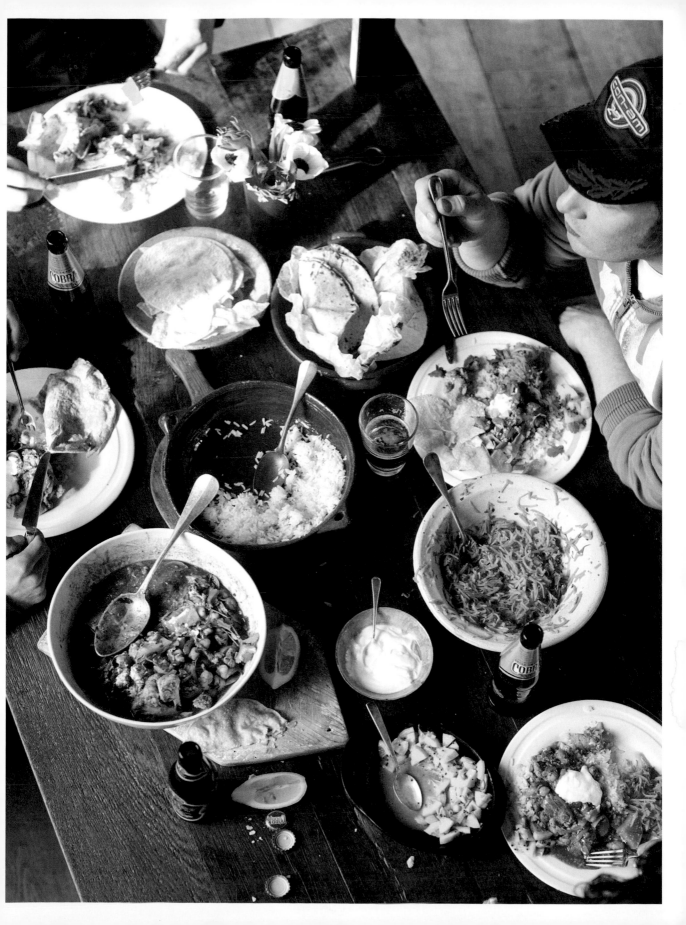

CURRY

2 onions
1 medium butternut squash
1 small cauliflower
optional: 1 fresh red chilli
4 cloves of garlic
a bunch of fresh coriander
½ a 283g jar of Patak's rogan josh
   paste
1 x 400g tin of chickpeas
100g prewashed baby spinach
1 x 500g tub of natural yoghurt

RICE

1 mug of basmati rice
a few whole cloves

CARROT SALAD

a handful of flaked almonds
5 or 6 carrots
1 fresh red chilli
a bunch of fresh coriander
a 2cm piece of fresh ginger
1 lemon

CHAPATTIS

1 pack of chapattis
turmeric, for dusting

LEMON PICKLE

1 lemon
2 teaspoons mustard seeds
1 level teaspoon turmeric
¼ of a fresh red chilli
1 small dried chilli

SEASONINGS

olive oil
extra virgin olive oil
sea salt & black pepper

TO SERVE

1 packet of poppadoms
cold beer

TO START Get all your ingredients and equipment ready. Fill and boil the kettle. Put a large saucepan on a high heat. Turn the oven on to 180°C/350°F/gas 4. Put the coarse grater attachment into the food processor.

CURRY Peel and slice the onions and add to the large pan with a splash of water and a few good lugs of olive oil. Carefully cut the butternut squash in half across the middle (for speed I'm only using the seedless neck), wrap up the base and put in the fridge for another day. Quarter the neck lengthways, then slice it into 1cm chunks – no need to peel them (🐷). Add to the pan. Trim the cauliflower and remove the outer leaves. Cut it into bite-sized chunks, and throw them into the pan. If you want some extra heat, slice up the chilli and add it now. Crush in the unpeeled garlic. Finely chop the coriander (stalks and all). Reserve a few leaves for garnish and add the rest to the pan with a couple of generous splashes of boiled water. Add the rogan josh paste and the tin of chickpeas, with their juices. Season and stir well, then put a lid on. Cook hard and fast, stirring occasionally.

RICE Put the mug of rice into a medium saucepan with a lug of olive oil and a few cloves, then cover with 2 mugs of boiled water (use the same mug you used for the rice). Add a pinch of salt, then put the lid on and boil on a medium heat for 7 minutes. Fill and reboil the kettle.

CHAPATTIS Scrunch up a large sheet of greaseproof paper under the tap. Flatten it out, then layer the chapattis on top, drizzling each lightly with a little olive oil and a sprinkling of turmeric. Wrap them in the paper and put them on the middle shelf of the oven.

CARROT SALAD Toast the almonds in a small pan on a medium heat, tossing occasionally until golden. Tip into a small bowl. Wash and trim the carrots. Grate them in a food processor, using the coarse grater attachment, with the chilli (stalks and seeds removed), the top third of a bunch of coriander and a peeled 2cm piece of ginger. Tip into a serving bowl.

CURRY Check and add a splash of water if it looks a bit dry. Stir, then replace the lid.

RICE By now the 7 minutes should be up, so take the rice off the heat and leave it to sit with the lid on for 7 minutes. This will let it steam and will give you beautiful fluffy nutty rice.

CARROT SALAD Drizzle a lug of extra virgin olive oil over the salad and add a pinch of salt. Finely grate in a little lemon zest, then add a good squeeze of lemon juice. Toss well. Sprinkle over the toasted almonds and half of the reserved coriander leaves, and take to the table.

CURRY Take the lid off. Do you need to adjust the consistency at this point? If so, you can add a generous splash of boiled water, depending on whether you want it drier or wetter. Or mash up some of the veg for different textures. Taste and add a pinch of salt, if needed, then add the spinach and stir through.

LEMON PICKLE Cut the lemon into eighths, then deseed and finely slice. Finely slice the red chilli quarter. Put the small pan you toasted the almonds in back on to a medium to high heat. Add a drizzle of olive oil to the pan and the mustard seeds, turmeric and the sliced chilli. Crumble in the dried chilli. When everything starts to sizzle, add the sliced lemon and a pinch of salt, count to ten, then take off the heat and put in a bowl to cool.

TO SERVE Tip half the tub of yoghurt into a small bowl. Drizzle over a little extra virgin olive oil and take to the table with the poppadoms and the bowl of lemon pickle. Remove the chapattis from the oven and take them straight to the table. Transfer the rice and curry into large serving bowls. Spoon the remaining yoghurt over the curry, sprinkle with the rest of the coriander leaves and take both bowls to the table. Crack open your beers and go for it!

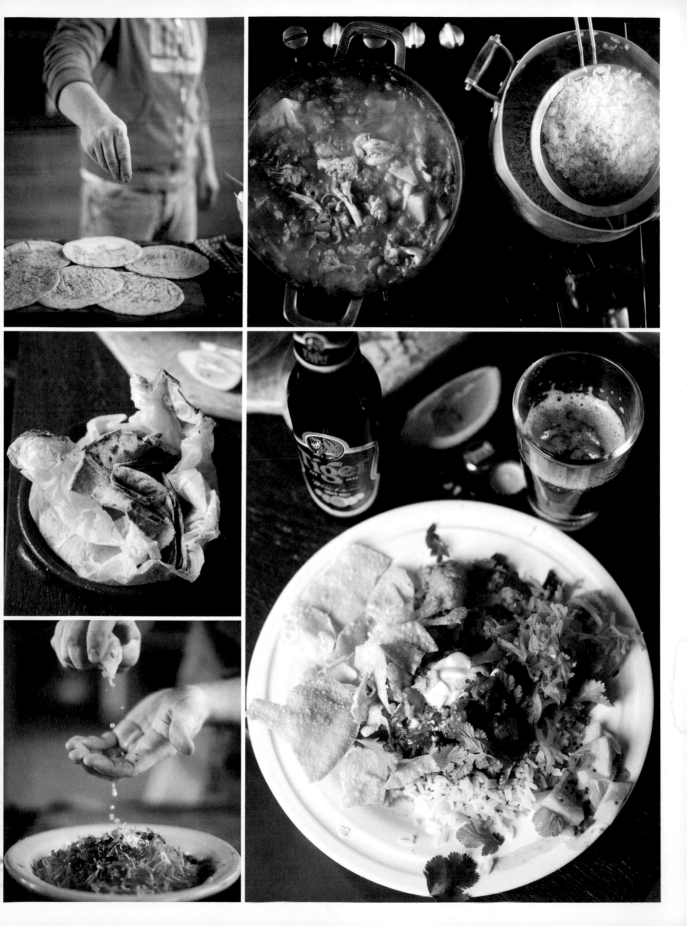

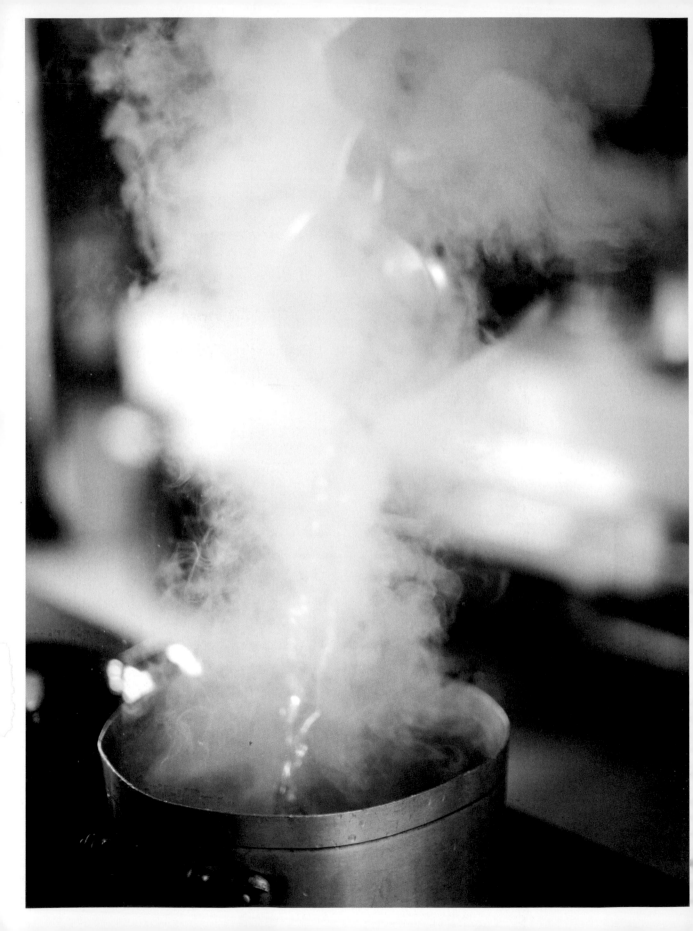

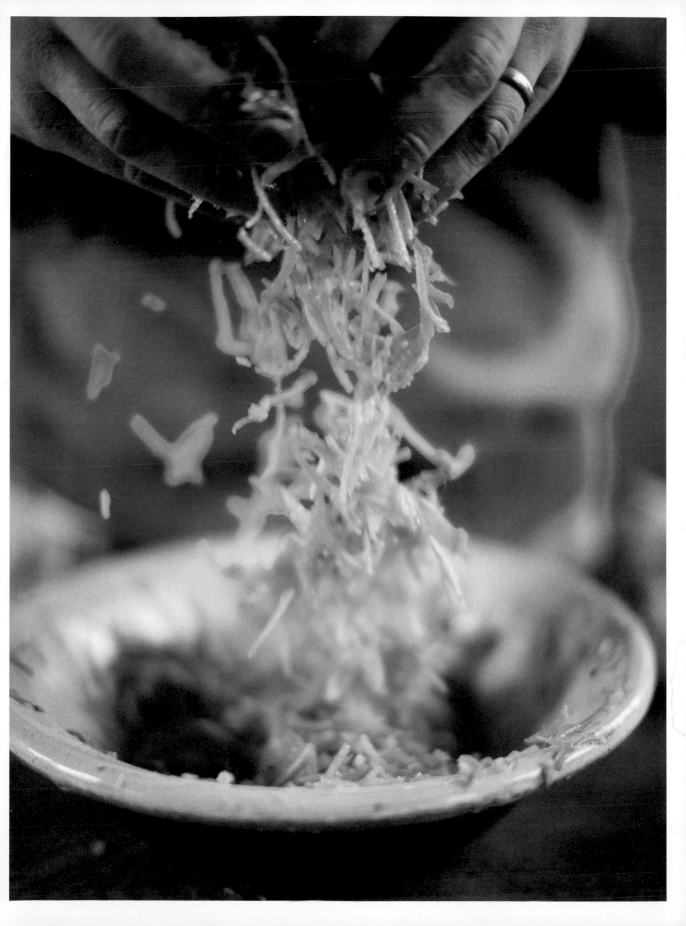

GREEN CURRY

CRISPY CHICKEN

KIMCHEE SLAW

RICE NOODLES

SERVES 4

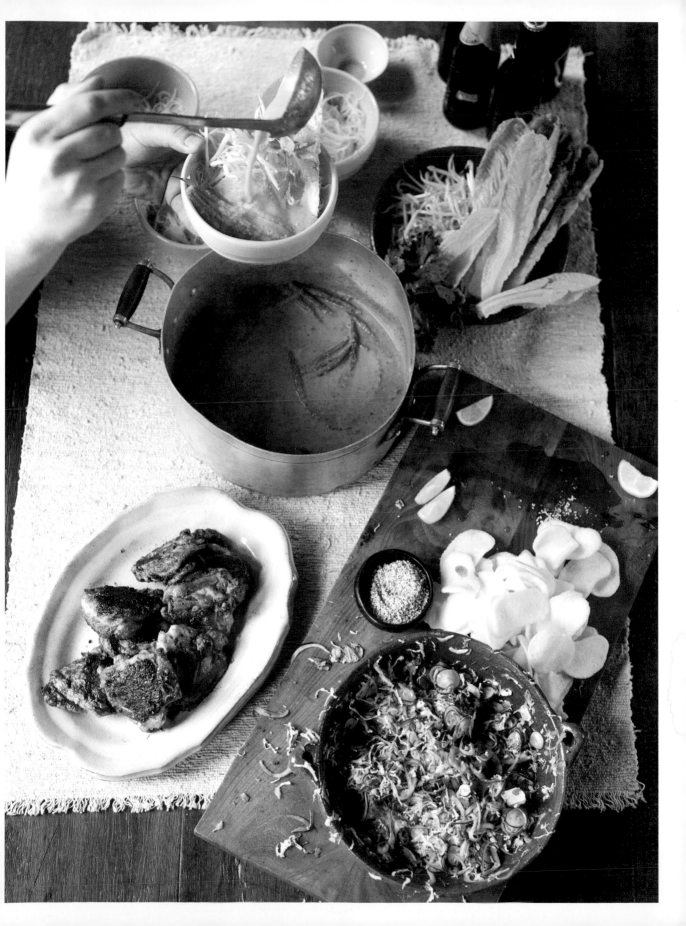

CHICKEN
8 chicken thighs, skin on and bone in
2 tablespoons sesame seeds
2 large tablespoons runny honey

KIMCHEE SLAW
a small bunch of radishes
1 red onion
½ a Chinese cabbage
a small bunch of fresh coriander
1 fresh red chilli
1 fresh green chilli
a 2cm piece of fresh ginger
2 limes
sesame oil

CURRY SAUCE
a 2cm piece of fresh ginger
2 fresh red chillies
optional: a few fresh kaffir lime leaves
a bunch of fresh coriander
4 cloves of garlic
1 stick of lemongrass
a small bunch of spring onions
sesame oil
300ml organic chicken stock
200g fine green beans
1 x 400ml tin of coconut milk
lime juice
soy sauce

NOODLES
250g rice noodles
1 lime

SEASONINGS
olive oil
sea salt & black pepper

GARNISHES
prawn crackers
chilli sauce
1 lime
½ a cos or romaine lettuce
½ a bag of beansprouts
a few sprigs of fresh coriander

TO START Get all your ingredients and equipment ready. Put 1 large and 1 smaller frying pan on a high heat. Put the thin slicer disc attachment into the food processor.

CHICKEN Tip the chicken thighs into the largest frying pan, skin side down. Drizzle with olive oil, add a pinch of salt & pepper and leave to cook, turning every minute or so for 18 to 20 minutes, or until cooked through. Wash your hands.

KIMCHEE SLAW Wash the radishes well. Peel and halve the red onion. Shred the radishes, red onion and Chinese cabbage in the food processor. Tip into a serving bowl. Add the bunch of coriander and the chillies (stalks removed) to the processor and whiz. Peel and crush in the ginger, then tip into the bowl.

CHICKEN Put some greaseproof paper on top of the chicken then place the smaller frying pan on top of that, with something heavy like a pestle & mortar in it to weight it down. The heat from the smaller pan will get the chicken cooking on both sides and make it dead crispy.

CURRY SAUCE Put the slicer attachment into the food processor. Peel the ginger and put it into the food processor with the chillies (stalks removed), lime leaves and most of the coriander. Crush in 4 unpeeled cloves of garlic. Halve the lemongrass and discard the outer leaves, trim the spring onions, and add both to the processor. Blitz to a paste, adding a good drizzle of sesame oil and a good few lugs of olive oil as you go.

CHICKEN Move the top pan to a medium heat and get rid of the greaseproof paper. Carefully drain away the fat and turn the chicken pieces skin side up. Add 2 tablespoons of sesame seeds to the empty frying pan and leave to toast until golden, tossing occasionally, then put into a small bowl and take the pan off the heat.

KIMCHEE SLAW Squeeze in the juice from both limes, and add a pinch of salt and a splash of sesame oil. Really scrunch together with your hands. Taste to check the balance, then put a large saucepan on a medium heat.

CHICKEN Carefully drain the fat again, then wipe the pan with kitchen paper and reduce the heat. Add 2 tablespoons of curry paste from the food processor, toss to coat and glaze the chicken, then turn the chicken over and carry on cooking to make it sticky and delicious. Fill and boil the kettle.

CURRY SAUCE Tip the rest of the curry paste into the hot saucepan and stir in the chicken stock. Trim the green beans and add. Turn up the heat under the saucepan. Shake the tin of coconut milk then add and stir in. Bring to the boil, then turn down and leave to tick away.

NOODLES Put the noodles into the empty frying pan with a pinch of salt and cover with boiled water. Leave for a few minutes and as soon as the noodles are soft enough to eat, quickly drain, then rinse under cold water and return to the frying pan. Drizzle over some sesame oil and a good squeeze of lime juice. Add a pinch of salt and toss.

CHICKEN Check the chicken is cooked through then add 2 tablespoons of honey and toss, flipping the chicken skin side down again.

GARNISHES Pile some prawn crackers on a serving board with a good pool of chilli sauce. Cut the lime into wedges, put some on the side and squeeze one of them over. Click off the lettuce leaves, wash and spin dry. Put into a bowl and add the beansprouts and coriander. Take to the table.

CURRY SAUCE Taste and correct the seasoning with lime juice and soy sauce, cook for another minute or so if you want a thicker sauce then take straight to the table.

TO SERVE Divide the noodles between 4 bowls. Put the chicken on a platter and let everyone layer up noodles, chicken, beansprouts, kimchee slaw, and sauce. Finish with a pinch of toasted sesame seeds.

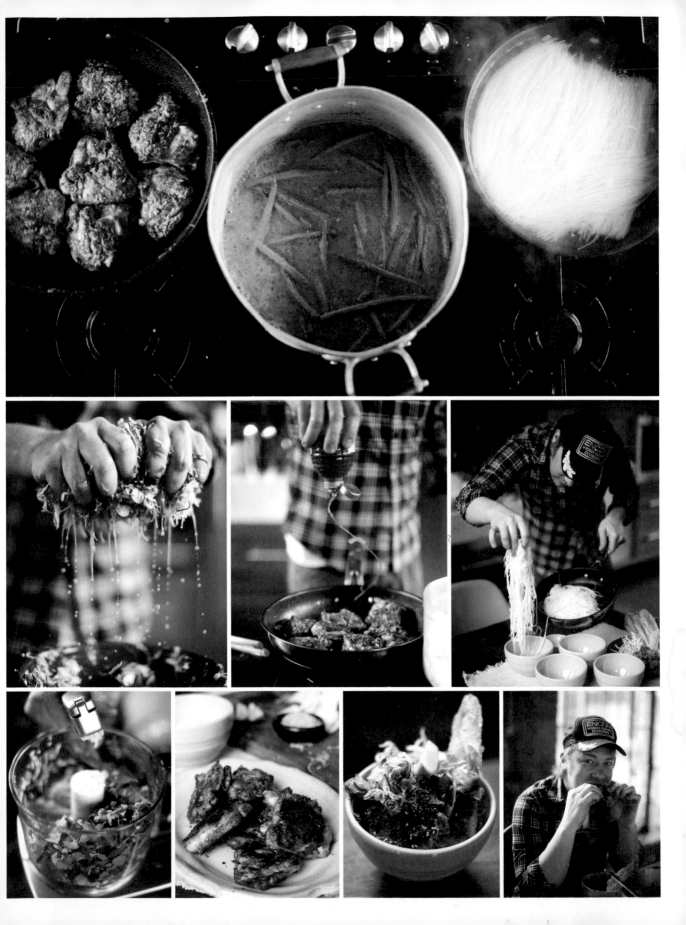

CHICKEN PIE

FRENCH-STYLE PEAS

SWEET CARROT SMASH

BERRIES, SHORTBREAD & CHANTILLY CREAM

SERVES 6

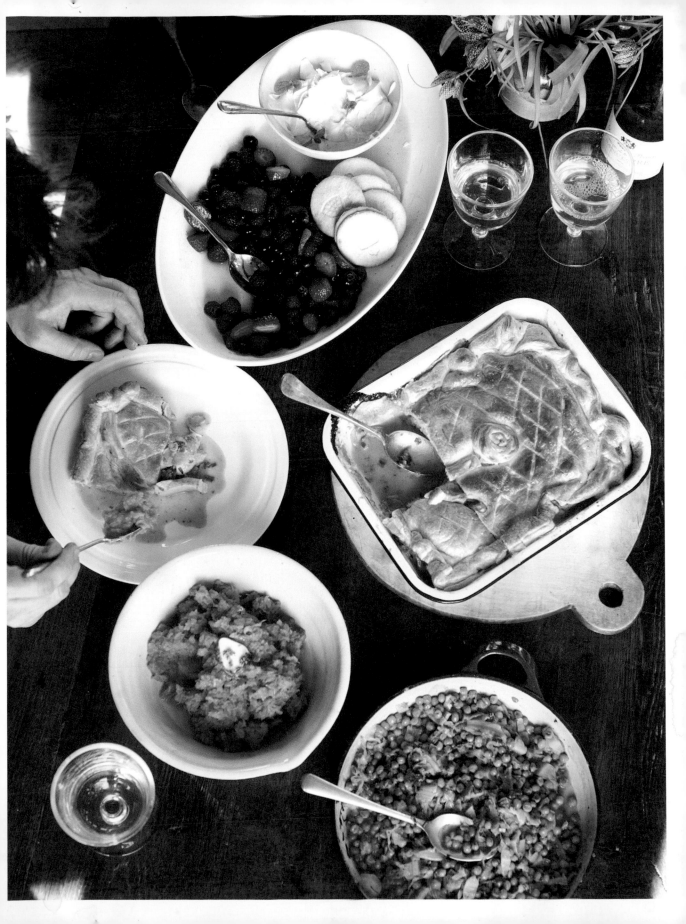

CHICKEN PIE

4 x 180g skinless chicken breasts
a knob of butter
a bunch of spring onions
150g button mushrooms
1 heaped tablespoon plain flour, plus
  extra for dusting
2 teaspoons English mustard
1 heaped tablespoon crème fraîche
300ml organic chicken stock
a few sprigs of fresh thyme
⅓ of a nutmeg, for grating
1 sheet of pre-rolled puff pastry
1 egg

SMASH

600g carrots
a few sprigs of fresh thyme

PEAS

2 little gem lettuces
a knob of butter
1 tablespoon flour
300ml organic chicken stock
a few sprigs of fresh mint
480g frozen peas
½ a lemon

SEASONINGS

olive oil
extra virgin olive oil
sea salt & black pepper

BERRIES & CREAM

400g mixed berries, such as
  blueberries, raspberries or
  strawberries
elderflower cordial
½ a lemon
2 sprigs of fresh mint
a few shortbread biscuits, to serve
150ml double cream
1 heaped tablespoon icing sugar
1 tablespoon vanilla paste or extract

TO START Get all your ingredients and equipment ready. Turn the oven on to 200°C/400°F/gas 6. Fill and boil the kettle. Put a large wide pan on a medium heat and a large saucepan with a lid on a low heat. Put the thick slicer disc attachment into the food processor.

CHICKEN PIE Put the chicken breasts on a plastic board and slice into 1cm strips. Put a lug of olive oil and a knob of butter into the hot, large, wide pan. Add the chicken and cook for 3 minutes or so. Meanwhile, quickly trim the spring onions and wash the mushrooms, then slice together in the food processor. Add to the pan with 1 heaped tablespoon of flour and stir. Add 2 teaspoons of mustard, 1 heaped tablespoon of crème fraîche and 300ml of chicken stock and stir well. Pick the thyme leaves and stir into the pan with a few fine gratings of nutmeg and a good pinch of salt & pepper. Leave to simmer.

SMASH Trim the carrots, then quickly slice in the food processor. Add to the saucepan with a lug of extra virgin olive oil, a good pinch of salt & pepper and a few thyme tips. Just cover with boiled water, then cover with a lid and turn the heat to high. Cook for 15 minutes, or until tender.

CHICKEN PIE Lightly dust a clean surface with flour and unroll the sheet of puff pastry. Use a small knife to lightly crisscross and score it. Take the pan of chicken off the heat. Tip the filling into an ovenproof baking dish slightly smaller than the sheet of pastry (approx. 30 x 25cm). Cover the filling with the pastry sheet, tucking it in at the edges (like in the picture). Quickly beat the egg, then brush it over the top of the pie. Put into the oven and cook on the top shelf for around 15 minutes, or until golden and gorgeous. Fill and reboil the kettle.

PEAS Return the empty chicken pan to a high heat. Quickly wash the lettuces then slice them in the food processor. Add a knob of butter and 1 tablespoon of flour to the pan, then pour in 300ml of chicken stock, tear in the mint leaves and use a balloon whisk to mix to a smooth and bubbling sauce. Add the peas and sliced lettuce. Squeeze over the juice of ½ a lemon, pour in a splash of boiled water, season with salt & pepper, stir, then put the lid on.

BERRIES & CREAM Slice any larger strawberries, if using, then put all the fruit into a large serving dish. Add a little swig of elderflower cordial and squeeze over the juice of ½ a lemon. Mix to coat all the fruit, then pick the mint leaves and tear over. Take to the table with the biscuits. Using an electric whisk, mix the double cream with the icing sugar and vanilla paste or extract until thick. Put next to the berries on the table.

SMASH Check the carrots are cooked through, then drain and return to the pan. Taste, correct the seasoning and leave as they are or smash up. Take to the table.

TO SERVE Take the peas to the table, then get the pie out of the oven and tuck in!

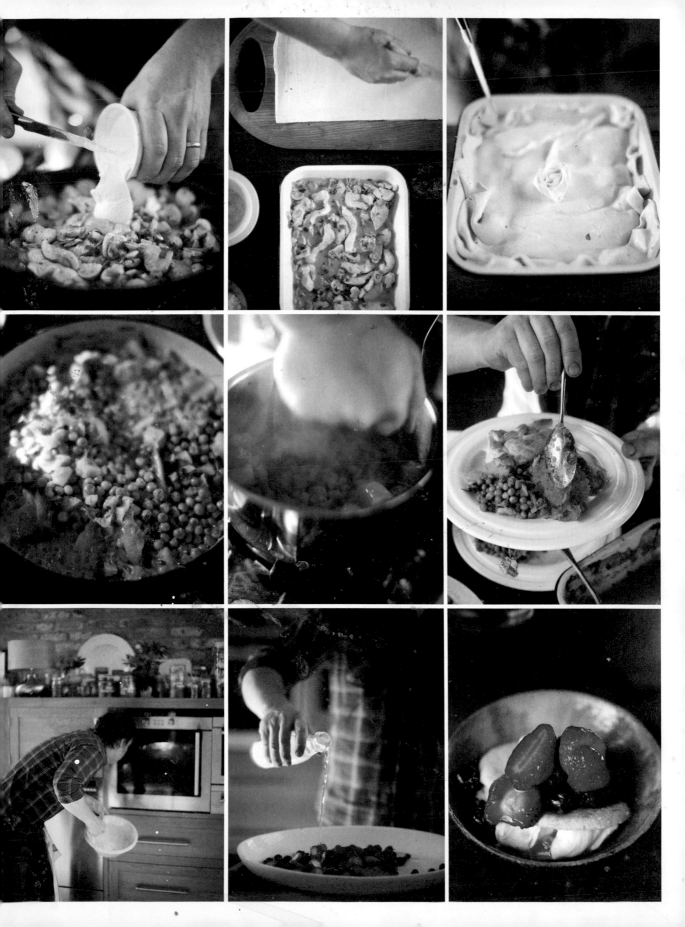

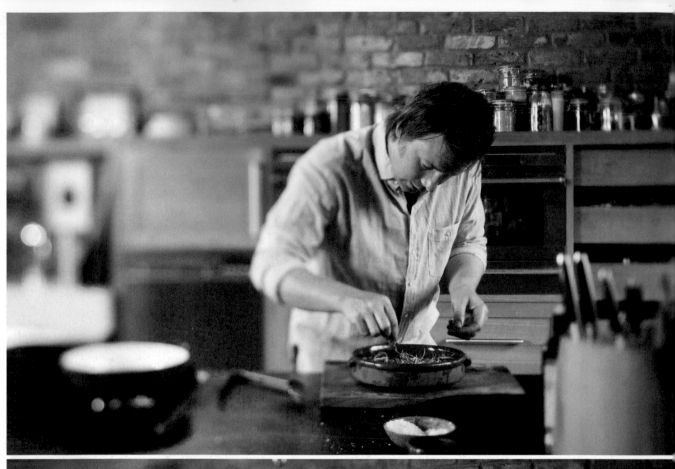

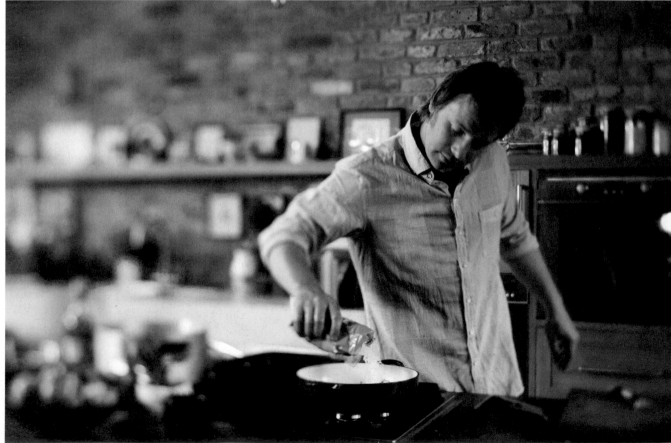

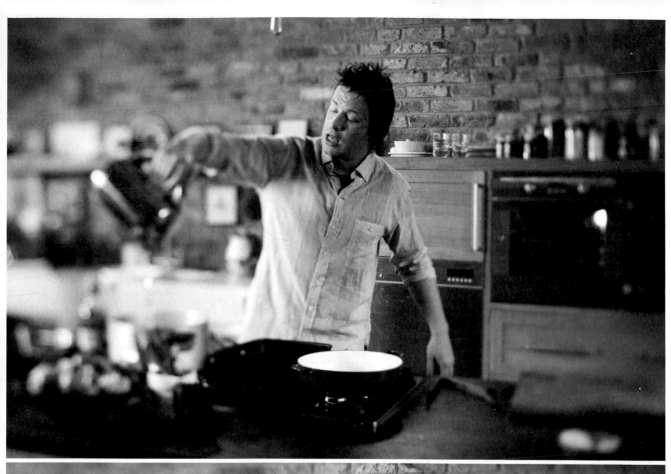
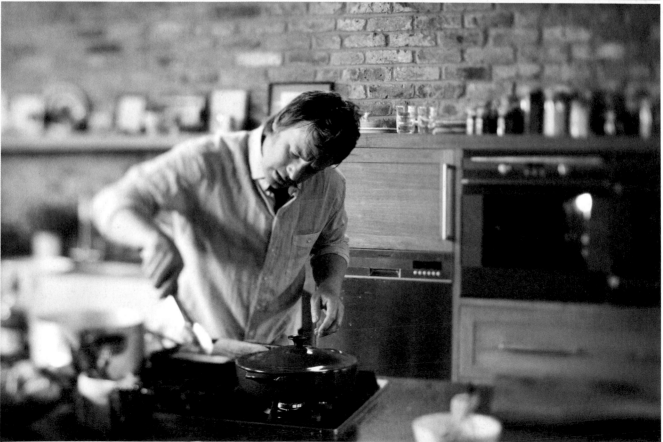

MUSTARD CHICKEN

SERVES 4–6

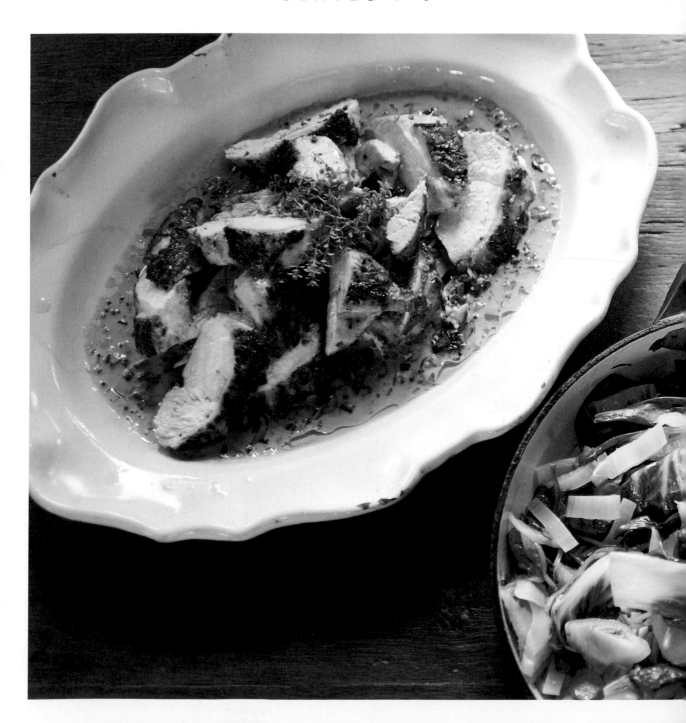

QUICK DAUPHINOISE
GREENS
BLACK FOREST AFFOGATO

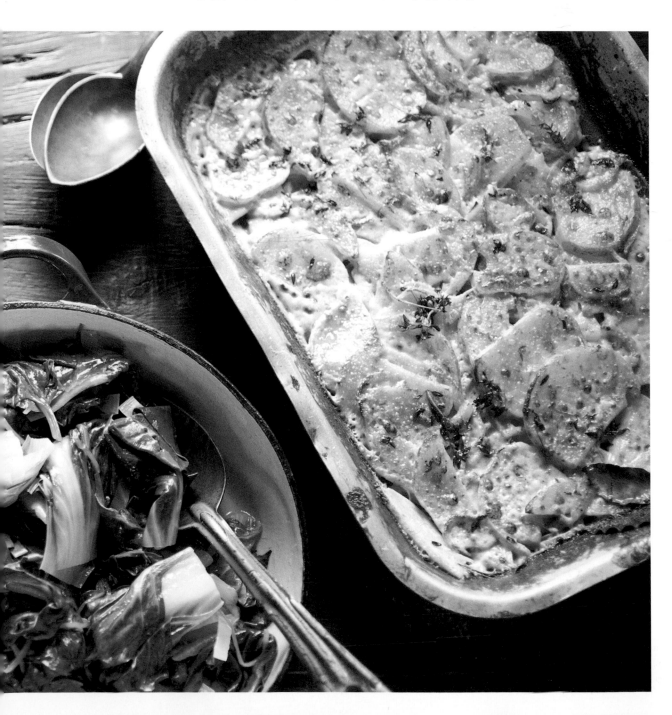

DAUPHINOISE
1 red onion
1kg Maris Piper potatoes
1 nutmeg
2 cloves of garlic
1 x 300ml tub of single cream
4 anchovies in oil
Parmesan cheese
2 bay leaves
a very small bunch of fresh thyme

SEASONINGS
olive oil
extra virgin olive oil
sea salt & black pepper

CHICKEN
a few sprigs of fresh rosemary
4 x 180g chicken breasts, skin on
4 teaspoons Colman's mustard powder
3 baby leeks or 1 large leek
4 cloves of garlic
white wine
75ml single cream (taken from cream
 for dauphinoise)
1 heaped teaspoon wholegrain mustard

GREENS
200g Swiss chard or other greens
1 x 200g bag of prewashed baby
 spinach
1 lemon

AFFOGATO
1 tablespoon instant coffee (or you
 could use 4–6 shots of espresso)
3 teaspoons golden caster sugar
4–6 round shortbread biscuits
1 x 425g tin of pitted black cherries
 in juice
1 x 100g bar of good-quality dark
 chocolate (70% cocoa solids)
1 x 500g tub of good-quality vanilla
 ice cream

TO START Get all your ingredients and equipment ready. Put a medium saucepan and a large ovenproof frying pan on a low heat. Fit the thick slicer disc attachment into the food processor and turn the oven on to 220°C/425°F/gas 7. Fill and boil the kettle.

DAUPHINOISE Peel and halve the red onion. Wash the potatoes, leave their skins on and slice in the food processor with the onion. Tip into a large sturdy roasting tray (approx. 35 x 25cm) and season. Grate over $\frac{1}{4}$ of the nutmeg, crush in 2 unpeeled cloves of garlic and pour in 225ml of single cream. Tear in the anchovies and finely grate over a large handful of Parmesan. Add the bay leaves, pick the leaves from a few thyme sprigs and add a good drizzle of olive oil. Use your clean hands to quickly mix and toss everything together, then put the tray over a medium heat. Pour in 200ml of boiled water, cover tightly with tin foil and leave on the heat.

CHICKEN Turn the heat under the frying pan up to medium. Pick and finely chop the leaves from the rosemary sprigs and sprinkle them into the pack of chicken. Sprinkle 1 teaspoon of mustard powder over each breast, then season and drizzle some olive oil over the chicken and into the frying pan. Massage and rub these flavours all over the meat. Put the chicken breasts in the pan, skin side down. Wash your hands well. Use a fish slice to press down on the chicken to help it cook. It should take around 18 minutes in total.

DAUPHINOISE Give the tray a shake so nothing catches.

GREENS Finely slice the stalks so they cook quickly. Wash the leaves. Put the stalks into the saucepan, cover with boiling water, add a good pinch of salt and put the lid on.

DAUPHINOISE Remove the tin foil. Finely grate over a layer of Parmesan. Drizzle the remaining thyme sprigs with oil, scatter on top and put into the oven on the top shelf to cook for 15 minutes, or until golden brown and bubbling.

CHICKEN Quickly trim the leeks and halve lengthways. Wash them under the cold tap, then finely slice them and add to one side of the chicken pan.

GREENS Add the chard leaves to the saucepan. Add another splash of boiled water if needed.

CHICKEN Crush 4 unpeeled cloves of garlic into the pan of chicken. Flip the chicken breasts skin side up, then press down on them again. Stir the leeks and add a good swig of white wine.

GREENS Empty the bag of spinach into a colander and pour the greens and the boiling water over the spinach. Add a lug of olive oil to the empty saucepan, squeeze in the juice of 1 lemon, then return all the drained greens to the pan and use tongs to toss and dress in the flavours. Season to taste, then take straight to the table.

CHICKEN Check the chicken is cooked through, then pour 75ml of cream into the frying pan. Cover the pan with tin foil. Quickly check on the dauphinoise.

AFFOGATO Put 1 tablespoon of instant coffee into a small jug with 3 teaspoons of sugar. Half-fill the kettle and boil. Crumble the shortbread biscuits into the bottom of 4 espresso cups. Drain the cherries and divide them between the cups. Bash the bar of chocolate up and add a few chunks to each cup. Take the cups to the table.

CHICKEN Turn the heat off. Transfer the chicken breasts to a board and slice into uneven pieces. Stir 1 heaped teaspoon of wholegrain mustard into the sauce, then taste and adjust the seasoning if necessary. Spoon the sauce on to a platter and put the sliced chicken on top. Drizzle over some extra virgin olive oil and take straight to the table.

DAUPHINOISE Take to the table. Get your ice cream out of the freezer to soften for later.

TO SERVE After dinner, stir some boiling water into the jug of coffee and sugar. Take to the table with the ice cream and spoon a scoop into each espresso cup. Grate over some chocolate, then pour over just enough hot coffee (or espresso) to start melting the chocolate. So delicious!

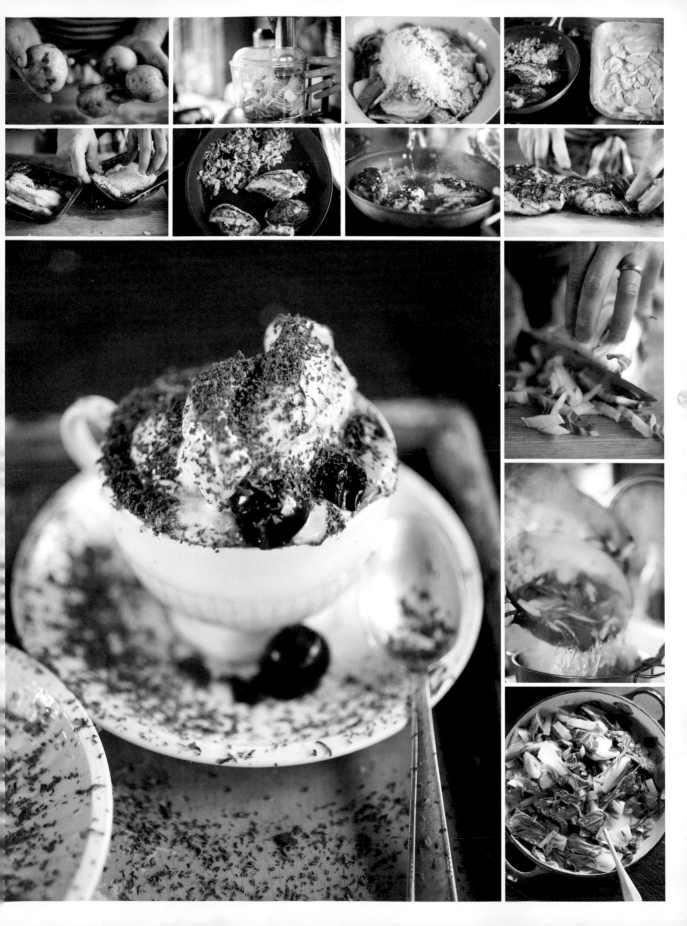

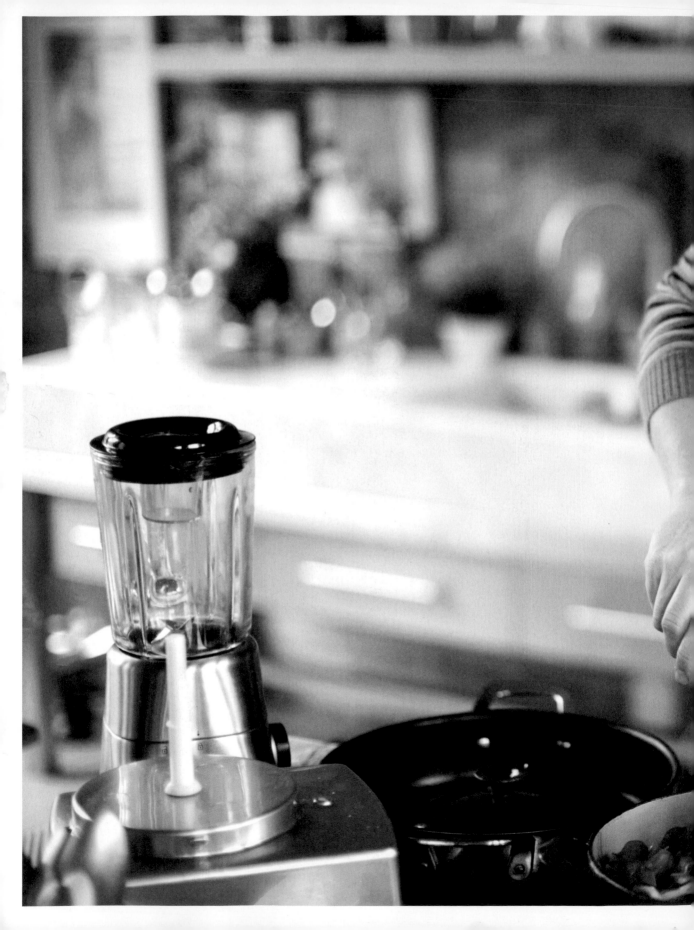

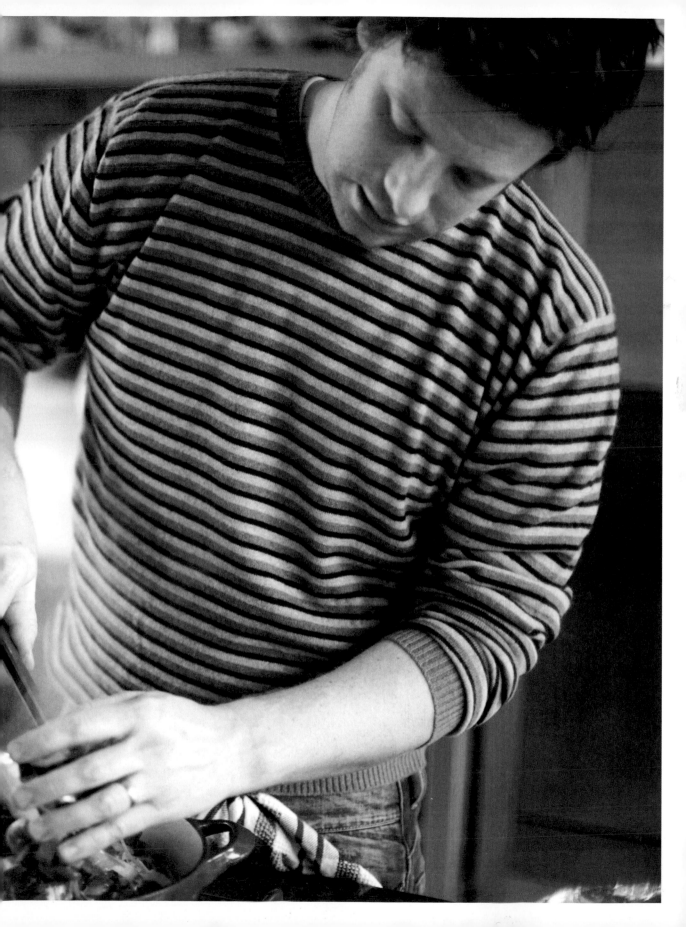

TRAY-BAKED CHICKEN

SQUASHED POTATOES

CREAMED SPINACH

STRAWBERRY SLUSHIE

SERVES 4

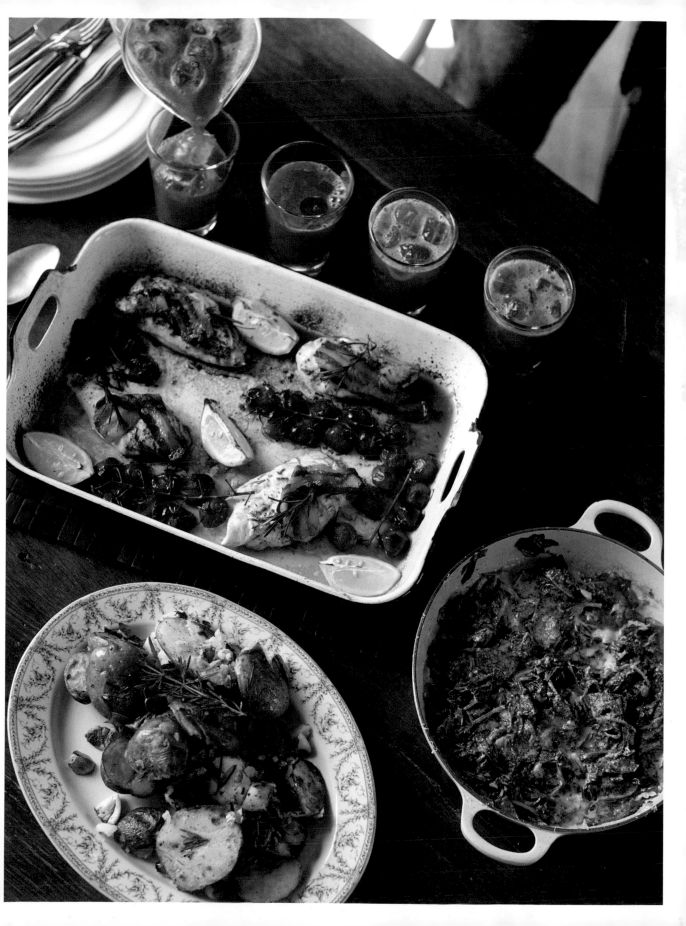

POTATOES
700g small red-skinned potatoes or
   new potatoes
a few sprigs of fresh rosemary
a couple of fresh bay leaves
6 cloves of garlic

SPINACH
a bunch of spring onions
3 cloves of garlic
a few fresh thyme tips
1 whole nutmeg, for grating
a large knob of butter
400g prewashed baby spinach

100ml single cream
25g Parmesan cheese

CHICKEN
dried oregano
sweet paprika
a knob of butter
4 x 180g skinless chicken breasts
1 lemon
300g cherry tomatoes on the vine
4 rashers of smoked streaky bacon
a couple of sprigs of fresh rosemary

SEASONINGS
olive oil
extra virgin olive oil
sea salt & black pepper

DRINK
400g strawberries, fresh or frozen
a few sprigs of fresh mint
½ a lemon
ice cubes
caster sugar, to taste

TO START Get all your ingredients and equipment ready. Fill and boil the kettle. Put a medium saucepan on a medium heat, a large frying pan on a low heat and a large shallow pan on a medium heat. Turn the grill to full whack.

POTATOES Wash the potatoes, then halve lengthways (or leave whole if using new potatoes) and add to the saucepan with a pinch of salt. Cover with boiled water, put the lid on and boil hard for around 12 to 14 minutes, or until cooked through.

SPINACH Trim and finely slice the spring onions. Add to the large shallow pan with a splash of olive oil. Crush in 3 cloves of unpeeled garlic and add a swig of boiled water. Pick in the leaves from a few sprigs of thyme, finely grate in ¼ of a nutmeg and add the knob of butter. Leave to tick away for around 3 minutes, stirring occasionally.

CHICKEN Turn the heat under the empty frying pan to high. Get out a large sheet of greaseproof paper. Sprinkle over a good pinch of dried oregano, salt & pepper and paprika, then drizzle over some olive oil and add a lug to the hot frying pan now too, along with the knob of butter. Lay the chicken breasts on top of the greaseproof paper and roll them in the flavours. Add to the hot pan and fry for 4 to 5 minutes, or until golden on both sides. While this is happening, clear away the greaseproof paper and wash your hands.

SPINACH Pile the spinach into the pan with the spring onions and leave to wilt. You may need to do this in batches but it will wilt quickly. Keep stirring so nothing catches.

CHICKEN Get out a nice roasting tray, then quarter the lemon and chuck it in the tray along with the vine tomatoes. Tip in the chicken breasts and any juices from the pan. Use tongs to arrange everything nicely, then lay the bacon on top of the breasts. Put the frying pan back on a medium heat, add the sprigs of rosemary to the pan and move them around so that they get coated in the juices. Pop them into the tray, then whack the tray under the grill for at least 14 minutes.

POTATOES Check the potatoes are cooked, then drain and let them steam dry for a minute or two. Add a couple of lugs of olive oil, leaves from a few sprigs of rosemary and the bay leaves to the empty frying pan. Put the potatoes on top of the herbs in a flat layer, drizzle over some olive oil and sprinkle over some salt. Crush in 6 unpeeled cloves of garlic, then turn the heat up to high. Get a flat lid from a smaller pan and really press down so you burst and squash the potatoes. Leave to colour, then toss after about 3 minutes and squash down again.

SPINACH Stir to help it along. Pour in the cream. Turn down the heat to low. Finely grate in the Parmesan and stir well.

POTATOES Keep checking, squashing and turning so the potatoes get golden all over.

DRINK Hull the strawberries and add them to the liquidizer with a handful of ice cubes, a few mint leaves and the juice of ½ a lemon. Add enough water to cover and whiz. Meanwhile, half fill a large jug with ice. Taste the mixture in the liquidizer and sweeten if necessary. Pour into the jug and stir with a wooden spoon. Take to the table.

POTATOES Check and squash down again.

TO SERVE Take the tray of chicken out from under the grill. Check the breasts are cooked through, then take straight to the table with the pan of spinach. Tip the potatoes on to a platter, take to the table and tuck in!

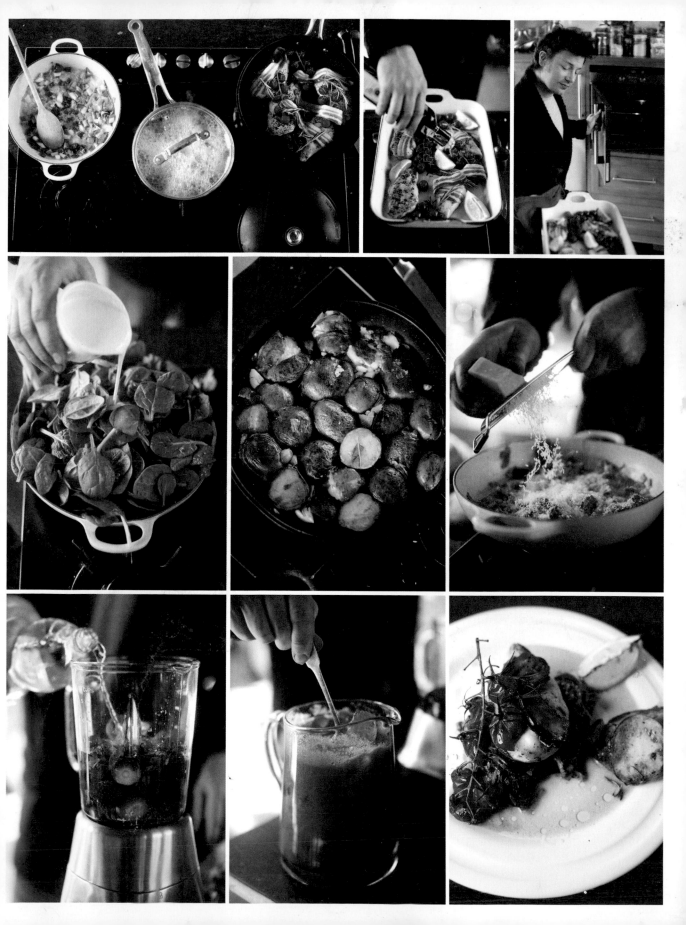

KILLER JERK CHICKEN

RICE & BEANS

REFRESHING CHOPPED SALAD

CHARGRILLED CORN

SERVES 4

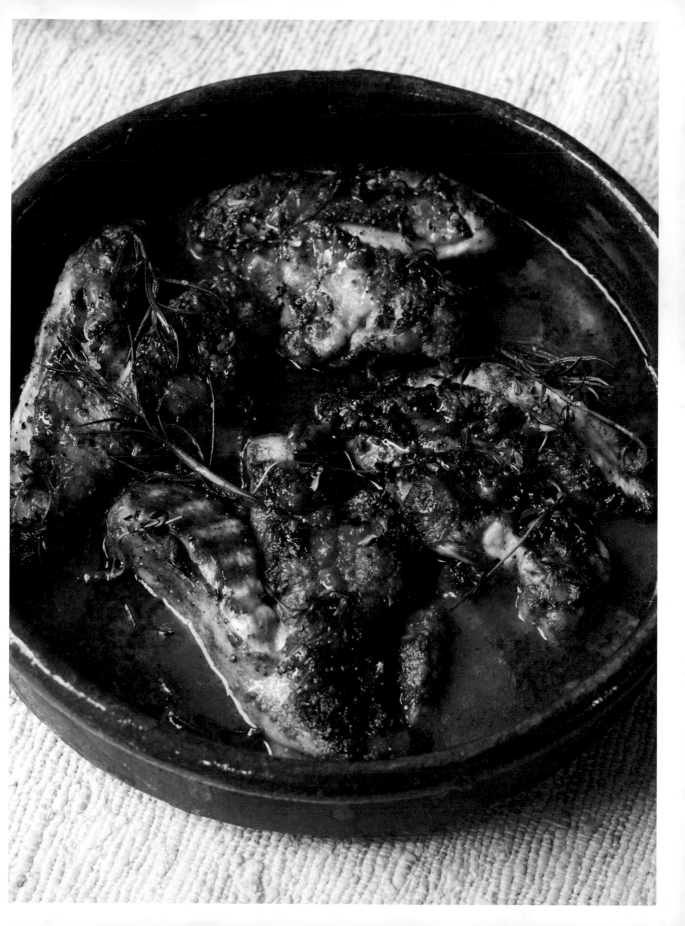

CHICKEN
4 x 180g chicken breasts, skin on
1 tablespoon runny honey
a few sprigs of fresh rosemary
a few sprigs of fresh coriander

CORN
4 large corn on the cob, husks
  removed

RICE & BEANS
2 spring onions
1 cinnamon stick
250g long-grain rice
600ml organic chicken stock
1 x 400g carton of black beans

JERK SAUCE
4 spring onions
a small bunch of fresh thyme
3 fresh bay leaves
ground cloves
ground nutmeg
ground allspice
6 tablespoons golden rum
6 tablespoons white wine vinegar
1 tablespoon runny honey
1 Scotch bonnet chilli
4 cloves of garlic

SEASONINGS
olive oil
extra virgin olive oil
sea salt & black pepper

SALAD
1 red pepper
1 red chicory
1 cos or romaine lettuce
2 limes
¼ of a red onion
a small bunch of fresh coriander
1 punnet of cress

YOGHURT
1 x 250g pot of natural yoghurt
a few sprigs of fresh coriander
1 lime

TO SERVE
cold beer

TO START Get all your ingredients and equipment ready. Fill and boil the kettle. Put a large griddle pan and a large saucepan on a high heat. Turn the oven on to 220°C/425°F/ gas 7.

CHICKEN Put the chicken breasts on a plastic board and halve each one, leaving them joined at the top of the breast. Drizzle with olive oil, sprinkle with salt & pepper, then rub all over both sides of the chicken. Put into the hot griddle pan, skin side down, and leave to cook. Clear away the board and wash the knife and your hands.

CORN Put the corn into the saucepan with a good pinch of salt and cover with boiling water. Put the lid on.

JERK SAUCE Trim and roughly chop the onions and put into the liquidizer with the leaves from most of the bunch of thyme, 3 bay leaves (stalks removed), a large pinch each of ground cloves, nutmeg and allspice, 6 tablespoons each of rum and vinegar, 1 tablespoon of honey and 2 teaspoons of salt. Remove the stalks and seeds from the Scotch bonnet chilli and add the chilli to the liquidizer, then quickly crush in 4 unpeeled cloves of garlic and blitz with the lid on until you have a really smooth paste. Add a drizzle of extra virgin olive oil to loosen, if needed.

CHICKEN The undersides should be golden now, so turn the chicken over. Pour the jerk sauce into a snug-fitting baking dish and use tongs to lay the chicken on top, skin side up. Drizzle over 1 tablespoon of runny honey and scatter over a few sprigs of rosemary and the remaining thyme sprigs. Put on the top shelf of the oven and cook for 15 minutes, or until cooked through. Carefully pour away the oil from the griddle pan and wipe clean with kitchen paper, then put back on a high heat.

RICE & BEANS Put a large wide saucepan with a lid on a medium heat. Trim and finely slice the spring onions and put in the saucepan with the cinnamon stick, a good lug of olive oil and a big pinch of salt & pepper. Stir and let soften for a minute or so, then add the rice and chicken stock. Drain and rinse the beans, then add to the pan. Stir gently. Bring to the boil, then reduce to a medium heat. Pop the lid on and leave for 12 minutes.

YOGHURT Tip the yoghurt into a small serving bowl. Finely chop a few sprigs of coriander and add to the bowl with a pinch of salt and a good lug of extra virgin olive oil. Finely grate over the zest of ½ the lime and squeeze in the juice. Stir in, then take to the table with the other lime half for squeezing over.

CORN Use tongs to move the corn to the hot griddle pan and drizzle over a little olive oil. Cook and turn frequently until charred. Once ready, put on a platter and take to the table.

SALAD Get a very large board that you're happy to serve on. Deseed and roughly chop the red pepper. Put the red chicory and cos lettuce on top and keep chopping until everything is fairly fine. Make a well in the centre. Pour in a few lugs of extra virgin olive oil and squeeze in the juice of 2 limes. Finely grate over the red onion quarter, season to taste, then toss everything together. Tear over the coriander, snip over the cress and take to the table.

RICE & BEANS Take the lid off the rice after 12 minutes and give it a stir. All the liquid should have been absorbed. Taste and correct the seasoning if need be, then take to the table.

TO SERVE Take the chicken out of the oven, sprinkle over some coriander leaves and take straight to the table. When serving, spoon over the jerk sauce from the bottom of the baking dish. Crack open a few cold bottles of beer and enjoy.

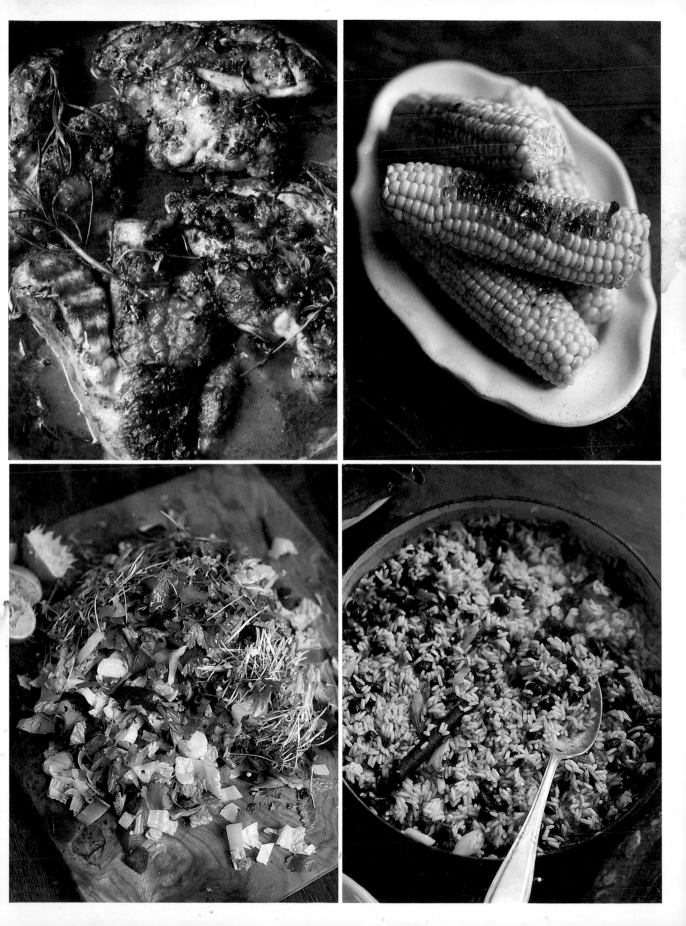

CHICKEN SKEWERS
AMAZING SATAY SAUCE
FIERY NOODLE SALAD
FRUIT & MINT SUGAR

SERVES 4

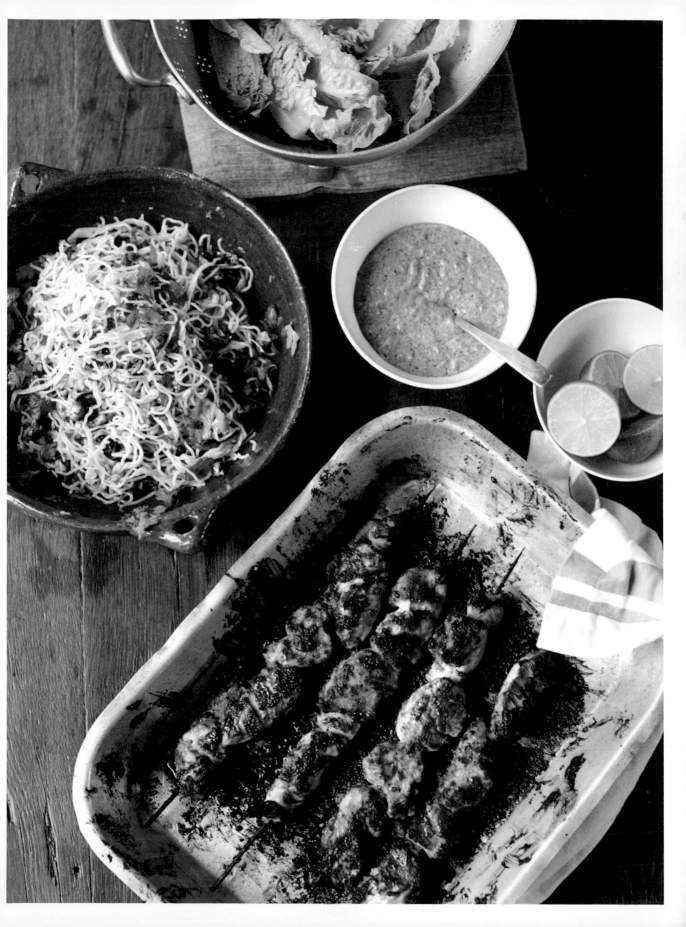

SATAY

½ a small bunch of fresh coriander
1 fresh red chilli
½ a clove of garlic
3 heaped tablespoons good-quality
 crunchy peanut butter
soy sauce
a 2cm piece of fresh ginger
2 limes

CHICKEN

4 x 180g skinless chicken breasts
runny honey, for drizzling

NOODLES

250g dried medium egg noodles
 (1 nest per person)

100g unsalted cashews
½ a medium-sized red onion
1 fresh red chilli
a small bunch of fresh coriander
1–2 tablespoons soy sauce
1 lime
1 teaspoon sesame oil
1 teaspoon fish sauce
1 teaspoon runny honey

GARNISHES

2 little gem lettuces
½ a small bunch of fresh coriander
optional: 1 fresh red chilli
soy sauce
1 lime

SEASONINGS

olive oil
extra virgin olive oil
sea salt & black pepper

FRUIT & MINT SUGAR

1 large pineapple
150g blueberries or other nice fresh
 berries or soft fruits
a small bunch of fresh mint
3 tablespoons golden caster sugar
1 lime
½ a 500g pot of Rachel's Organic
 Greek-style coconut yoghurt

TO START Get all your ingredients and equipment ready. Turn the grill on to full whack. Lay 4 wooden skewers in a tray of cold water to soak (if they float, use a plate to weight them down). Put the standard blade attachment into the food processor.

SATAY Put the coriander (stalks and all) into the food processor with the chilli (stalk removed), peeled garlic, 3 heaped tablespoons of peanut butter and a lug of soy sauce. Peel and roughly chop the ginger and add. Finely grate in the zest of both limes, then squeeze in the juice from 1 of them. Add a couple of splashes of water and whiz to a spoonable paste. Season to taste. Spoon half into a nice bowl and drizzle with extra virgin olive oil, put the rest aside.

CHICKEN Line the chicken breasts up on a plastic board, alternating ends, and close together. Gently and carefully push the skewers through the breasts. Slice between the skewers to give you 4 kebabs – see the picture on the opposite page (🍢). Thread any stray pieces on the ends of the skewers. To make the chicken crispier you can score it lightly on both sides. Scoop the rest of the satay mix from the processor into a roasting tray, add the chicken skewers and toss with your hands to coat, rubbing the flavour into the meat. Clear away the board and wash the knife and your hands. Drizzle the chicken with olive oil and season with salt. Put on the top shelf of the oven, under the grill, for about 8 to 10 minutes on each side, or until golden and cooked through.

GARNISHES Trim the bases off the little gem lettuces and get rid of any tatty outer leaves. Click the rest of the leaves off, halving the cores. Rinse in a colander, spin dry, then take straight to the table. Fill and boil the kettle.

NOODLES Put the nests of noodles in a large bowl, cover with boiling water and a plate, then leave to soak for 6 minutes. Put a medium frying pan on a low heat. Bash the cashew nuts with a rolling pin or against a work surface in a clean tea towel. Add to the warm pan and leave to toast, tossing occasionally and keeping an eye on them as you do other jobs.

Peel the red onion half and put in the processor with the chilli (stalk removed) and the stalks from the bunch of coriander. Pulse until finely chopped, then put into a large serving bowl with 1 or 2 tablespoons of soy sauce and a few lugs of extra virgin olive oil. Squeeze in the juice of 1 lime, and stir in 1 teaspoon each of sesame oil and fish sauce. Mix well, then taste and correct the seasoning. Drain the noodles in a colander, refresh quickly under cold water, drain again, then add to the bowl.

Toss your cashews and turn the heat under them up to high. Add 1 teaspoon of honey, mixing and tossing the nuts in the pan. Once dark golden, tip them into the serving bowl and add the coriander leaves. Toss everything together and take to the table with the bowl of satay sauce.

CHICKEN Turn the skewers over, drizzle with a little runny honey and put back under the grill for 8 to 10 minutes.

FRUIT & MINT SUGAR Peel and slice the pineapple and arrange on a large platter with the blueberries. Rip the leaves off the mint and pound in a pestle & mortar till you have a paste. Add the caster sugar and pound again. Scatter 1 tablespoon of this mint sugar over the pineapple (keep the rest in a small jar in the fridge for another time). Halve a lime for squeezing over, then take to the table with the pot of coconut yoghurt and a spoon.

GARNISHES Roughly chop the coriander leaves and finely slice the chilli, if using. Put into little side bowls, take both to the table and put next to the lettuce.

TO SERVE Take the chicken to the table with a bottle of soy sauce and a few wedges of lime for squeezing over. Let everyone build parcels of lettuce, noodles, chicken, a sprinkle of coriander and chilli and a squeeze of lime.

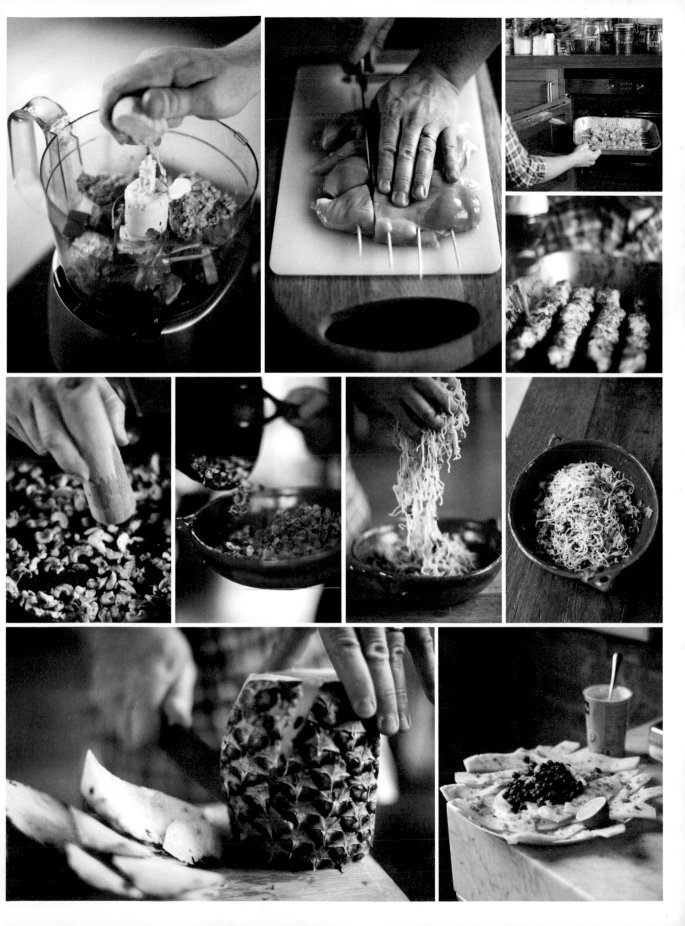

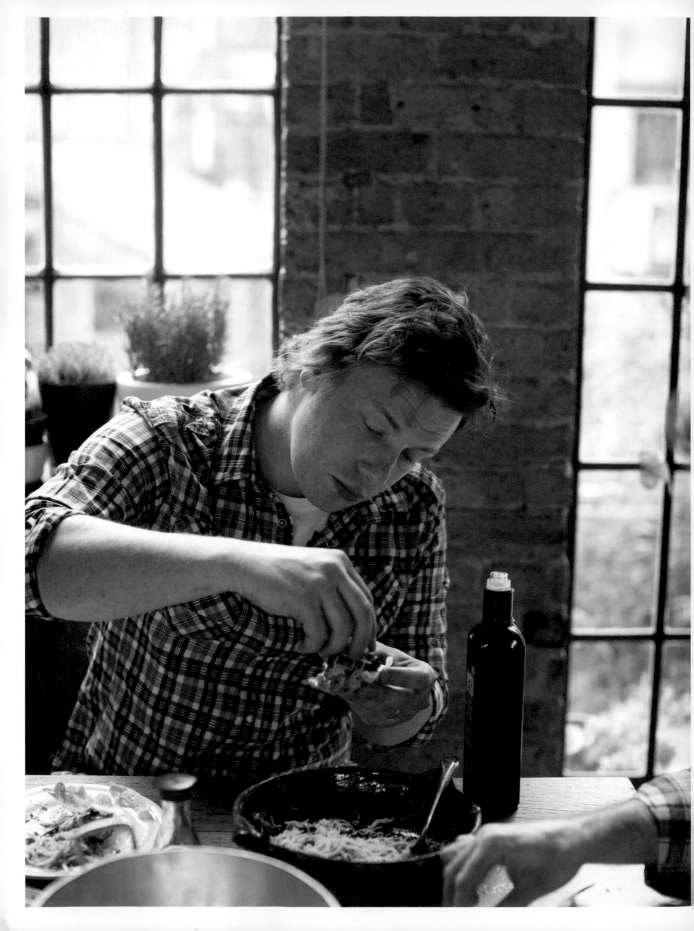

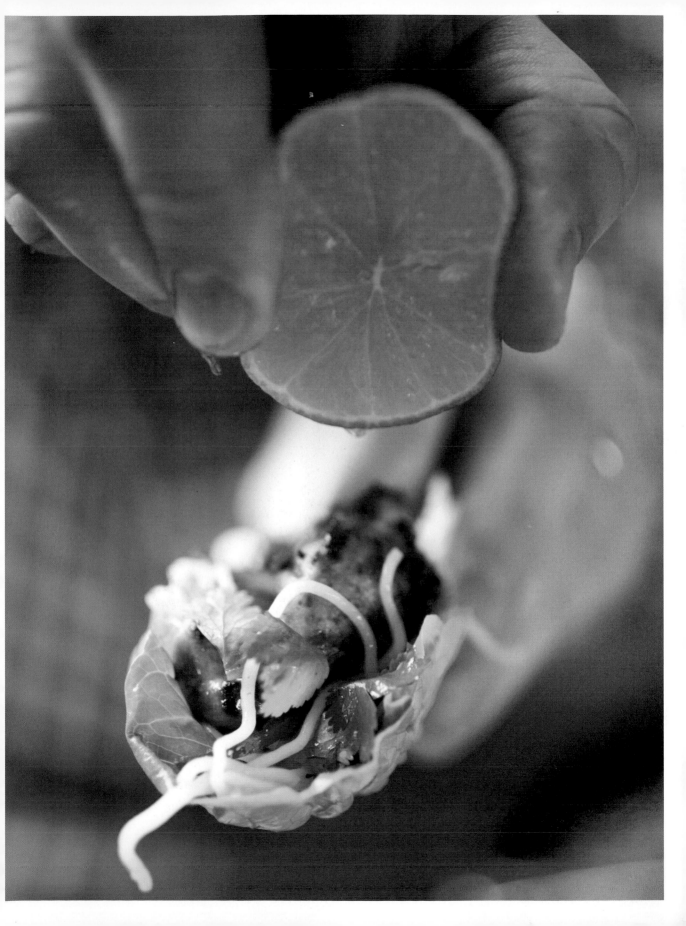

STUFFED CYPRIOT CHICKEN

PAN-FRIED ASPARAGUS & VINE TOMATOES

CABBAGE SALAD

ST CLEMENT'S DRINK

VANILLA ICE CREAM FLOAT

SERVES 4

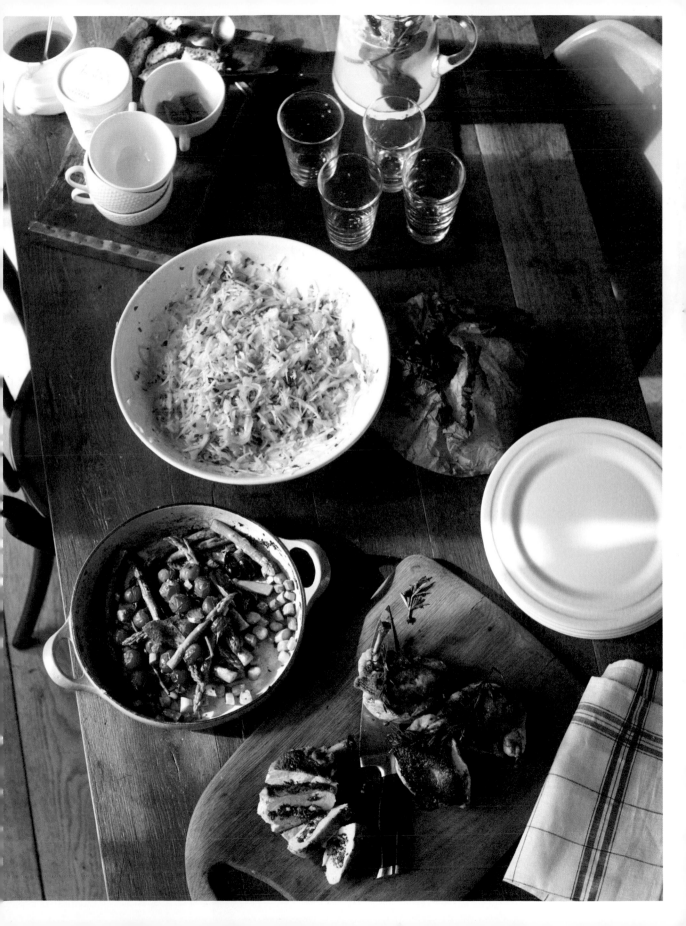

CHICKEN
a small bunch of fresh flat-leaf parsley
a small bunch of fresh basil
8 jarred sun-dried tomatoes in oil
2–3 cloves of garlic
100g feta cheese
zest of 1 lemon
4 x 180g chicken breasts, skin on and
 bone in, if possible
4 sprigs of fresh rosemary

VEG
5–6 cloves of garlic
200g cherry tomatoes on the vine
a small bunch of fresh herbs, such as
 thyme, rosemary and bay
250g asparagus
8–10 jarred black olives, stoned

FLATBREADS
1 teaspoon dried oregano
2 cloves of garlic
6 flatbreads

CABBAGE SALAD
½ a small white cabbage
1 onion
a few sprigs of fresh flat-leaf parsley
a few sprigs of fresh Greek basil or
 basil
½ a fresh red chilli
2 lemons

SEASONINGS
olive oil
extra virgin olive oil
sea salt & black pepper

DRINK
ice cubes
5–6 sprigs of fresh mint
1 lemon
2 oranges
1 bottle of sparkling water

ICE CREAM FLOAT
1 x 500ml tub of good-quality vanilla
 ice cream
a few teaspoons instant coffee (or
 shots of espresso, if you prefer)
2 sugar cubes
a handful of cantucci biscuits

TO START Get all your ingredients and equipment ready. Turn the oven on to 220°C/425°F/gas 7 and put 2 large frying pans on a medium heat. Put the thick slicing disc attachment into the food processor.

CHICKEN Pile the parsley, basil and sun-dried tomatoes, with a drizzle of their oil and a pinch of pepper, on to a chopping board. Crush over 2 or 3 unpeeled cloves of garlic, then finely chop everything together, mixing with the knife as you go. Crumble over the feta, finely grate over the lemon zest and mix again.

VEG Drizzle olive oil into one .of the frying pans and squash and add the unpeeled cloves of garlic. Add the vine tomatoes and the herb sprigs. Reduce to a low heat.

CHICKEN Tear off a big sheet of greaseproof paper and line up the chicken breasts, skin side down, on top. Use a small knife to carefully fold back the fillets and cut a little pocket in each one, slitting and cutting down until you can open each breast out like a book. Divide the filling from the board into the middle of each chicken breast, pat it down, then fold the chicken back over to cover (🍳). Wash your hands.

Add 2 lugs of olive oil to the empty frying pan. Using tongs, lay the chicken skin side down. Scrunch up a sheet of greaseproof under the tap. Flatten out and tuck over the chicken, then leave to cook, shaking the pan every now and again.

FLATBREADS Sprinkle salt & pepper over the messy chopping board, add 1 teaspoon of oregano and a good couple of lugs of olive oil. Crush over 2 unpeeled cloves of garlic. Wipe and roll the flatbreads in these flavours. Scrunch up another large piece of greaseproof under the tap, flatten, then stack the breads up on it and wrap. Put in the oven. Fill and boil the kettle.

VEG Flip the chopping board over and trim the ends of the asparagus, throwing the tips into the pan whole. Mix and toss, then add 8 to 10 black olives.

CABBAGE SALAD Remove the outer leaves of the cabbage half, then quarter and shred in the food processor. Tip into a large bowl. Peel and halve the onion, shred in the processor with the parsley, basil and chilli (stalk removed) and add to the bowl.

Squeeze the juice of 2 lemons into the bowl, add a few lugs of extra virgin olive oil and a good pinch of salt. Toss and scrunch everything with your hands, tasting and tweaking as necessary. Take to the table.

CHICKEN By now the chicken should be golden underneath, so carefully turn each breast over and add 4 small sprigs of rosemary to the pan. Re-cover with the greaseproof. Put a medium frying pan on top of the chicken to push it down a bit and help it crisp up.

DRINK Fill a large jug halfway with ice. Scrunch up the mint sprigs and add to the jug along with the juice from the lemon and the oranges. Chuck in 2 orange halves, top up with sparkling water and stir. Take to the table.

ICE CREAM FLOAT Take the ice cream out of the freezer. Make a jug of instant coffee using 200ml of boiled water. Stir in the sugar cubes. Pile the cantucci biscuits on a board with teacups to serve. Put at the end of the table or nearby, with the ice cream.

CHICKEN Transfer the golden chicken to a wooden serving board and slice a chicken breast to check it's cooked through. Pour over the juices from the pan and take to the table so everyone can help themselves.

TO SERVE Take the pan of vegetables and the stack of flatbreads straight to the table.

ICE CREAM FLOAT When ready, put a scoop of ice cream into each teacup and top with a shot of coffee (or espresso) and a biscuit. Lovely!

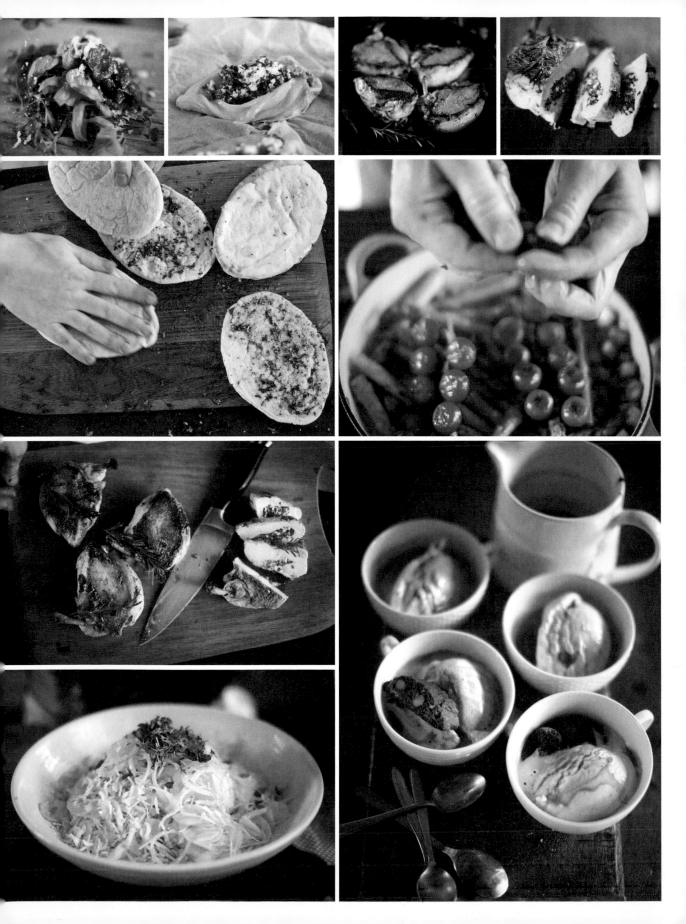

PIRI PIRI CHICKEN
DRESSED POTATOES
ROCKET SALAD
QUICK PORTUGUESE TARTS

SERVES 4

(with 2 tarts left over)

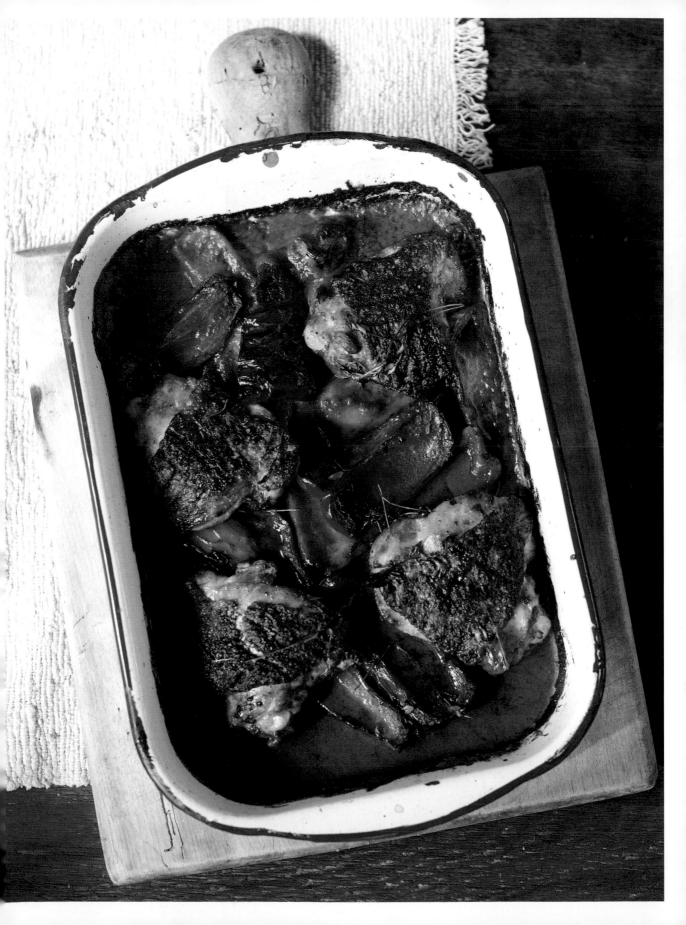

CHICKEN
4 large chicken thighs, skin on and
  bone in
1 red pepper
1 yellow pepper
6 sprigs of fresh thyme

POTATOES
1 medium potato
2 sweet potatoes
½ a lemon
1 fresh red chilli
a bunch of fresh coriander
50g feta cheese

PIRI PIRI SAUCE
½ a red onion
2 cloves of garlic
1–2 bird's-eye chillies
1 tablespoon sweet smoked paprika
1 lemon
2 tablespoons white wine vinegar
1 tablespoon Worcestershire sauce
a bunch of fresh basil

SALAD
1 x 100g bag of prewashed wild
  rocket
½ a lemon

SEASONINGS
olive oil
extra virgin olive oil
sea salt & black pepper

TARTS (makes 6 tarts)
plain flour, for dusting
1 x 375g pack of pre-rolled puff pastry
ground cinnamon
125g crème fraîche
1 egg
1 teaspoon vanilla paste or vanilla
  extract
5 tablespoons golden caster sugar
1 orange

TO START Get all your ingredients and equipment ready. Turn the oven on to 200°C/400°F/gas 6. Put a large griddle pan on a high heat.

CHICKEN Put the chicken thighs on a plastic chopping board, skin side down, and slash the meat on each one a few times. Drizzle with olive oil and season, then put on the griddle pan that is heating up, skin side down. Cook until golden underneath, then turn over. Wash your hands.

TARTS Dust a clean surface with flour. Unroll the sheet of pastry, then cut it in half so you end up with two 20 x 20cm squares of pastry (put one in the fridge for another day). Sprinkle over a few good pinches of ground cinnamon, then roll the pastry into a Swiss roll shape and cut into 6 rounds. Put these into 6 of the holes in a muffin tin, and use your thumbs to stretch and mould the pastry into the holes (just like in the picture) so the bottom is flat and the pastry comes up to the top. Put on the top shelf of the oven and cook for around 8 to 10 minutes (set the timer), or until lightly golden.

POTATOES Wash the potato and sweet potatoes and halve lengthways. Put them into a large microwave-safe bowl with ½ a lemon. Cover with clingfilm and put into the microwave on full power for 15 minutes.

CHICKEN Turn the chicken over.

TARTS Spoon the crème fraîche into a small bowl. Add the egg, vanilla paste or extract, 1 tablespoon of golden caster sugar and the zest of 1 orange. Mix well.

PIRI PIRI SAUCE Peel and roughly chop the red onion half and add to the liquidizer with 2 peeled cloves of garlic. Add the chillies (stalks removed), 1 tablespoon of paprika, the zest of 1 lemon and juice of ½ a lemon. Add 2 tablespoons of white wine vinegar, 1 tablespoon of Worcestershire sauce, a good pinch of salt & pepper, the bunch of basil and a swig of water. Blitz until smooth.

CHICKEN Slice the peppers into strips and add to the griddle pan. Turn the heat down to medium and keep moving the peppers around.

TARTS Take the muffin tin out of the oven, and use a teaspoon to press the puffed up pastry back to the sides and make room for the filling. Spoon the crème fraîche mixture into the tart cases, and return to the top shelf of the oven. Set the timer for 8 minutes.

CHICKEN Pour the piri piri sauce into a snug-fitting roasting tray. Lay the peppers on top and put aside. Add the chicken to the roasting tray with the sauce. Scatter over the sprigs of thyme, then put the tray into the middle of the oven.

TARTS Put a small saucepan on a high heat. Squeeze in the juice from the zested orange and add 4 tablespoons of golden caster sugar. Stir and keep a good eye on it, but remember caramel can burn badly so don't touch or taste.

POTATOES Finely chop the red chilli and most of the coriander on a board, mixing as you go. Add the feta and keep chopping and mixing.

CHICKEN Take the tarts out of the oven and move the chicken up to the top shelf to cook for around 10 minutes, or until cooked through.

TARTS Pour some caramel over each tart (they'll still be wobbly, but that's good). Put aside to set.

SALAD Quickly dress the rocket, still in its bag, with extra virgin olive oil, a good pinch of salt & pepper and the juice of ½ a lemon. Tip into a bowl and take to the table.

POTATOES Check the potatoes are cooked through, then use tongs to squeeze over the cooked lemon. Add the coriander mixture from the chopping board and mix everything together. Season, then take to the table.

TO SERVE Get the tray of chicken out of the oven, sprinkle over a few coriander leaves and take straight to the table.

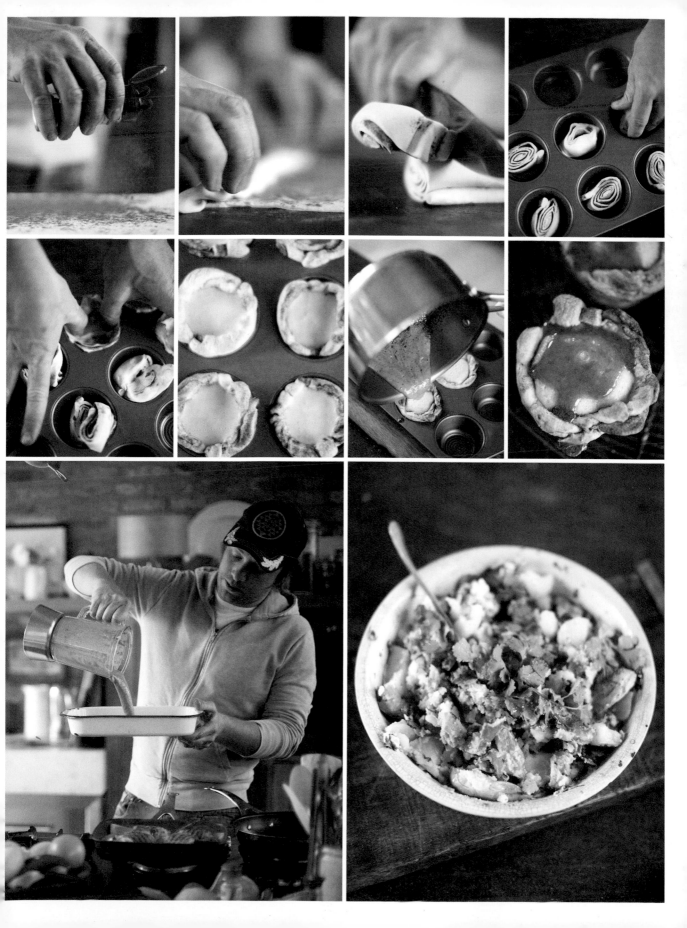

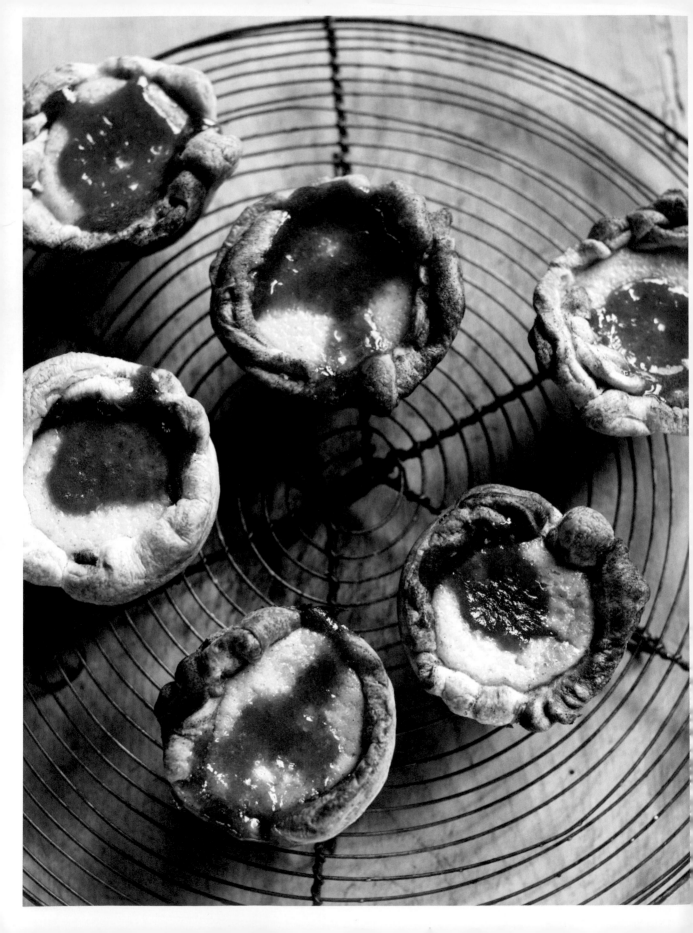

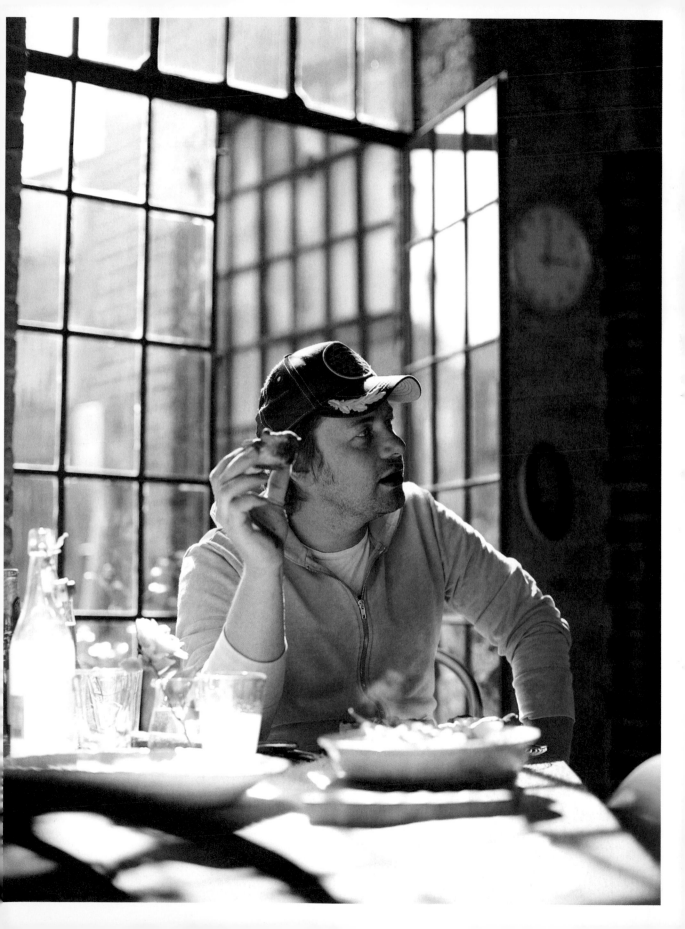

DUCK SALAD

SERVES 4

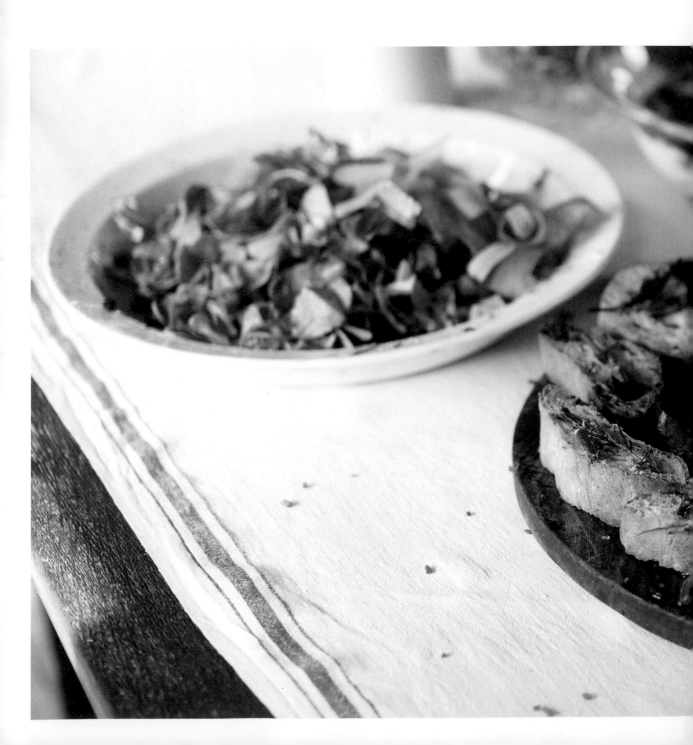

GIANT CROUTONS
CHEAT'S RICE PUDDING
WITH STEWED FRUIT

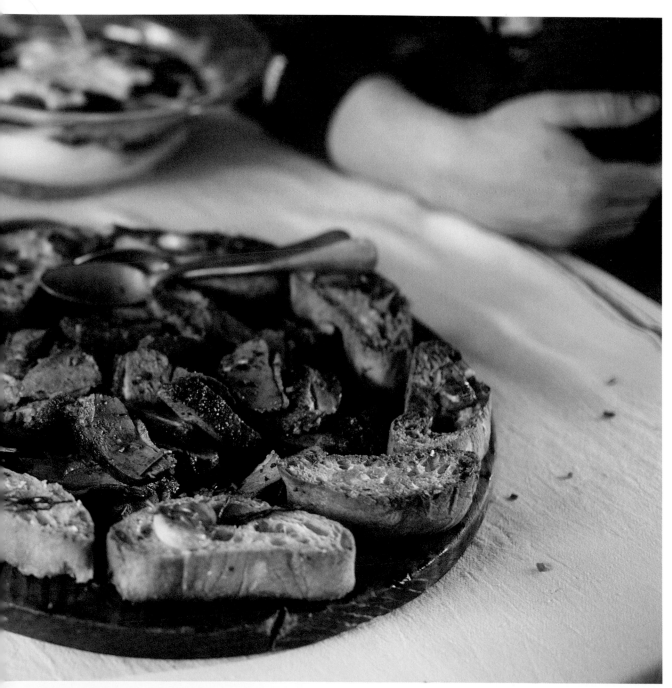

DUCK

4 x 200g duck breasts, skin on
Chinese five-spice
dried thyme
1 fresh red chilli
a small bunch of fresh mint
½ a lemon
1 teaspoon runny honey

CROUTONS

1 ciabatta loaf
a small bunch of fresh rosemary
5 cloves of garlic
1 teaspoon fennel seeds

SALAD

1 pomegranate
1 x 100g bag of prewashed lamb's
    lettuce or rocket
2 carrots
a small bunch of radishes
1 punnet of cress
a small bunch of fresh mint
balsamic vinegar
½ a lemon

SEASONINGS

olive oil
extra virgin olive oil
sea salt & black pepper

RICE PUDDING & FRUIT

a handful of flaked almonds
5 heaped tablespoons icing sugar
2 oranges
12 ripe plums, mixed colours if you
    can get them
optional: 1 teaspoon vanilla paste or
    extract
4 x 150g tubs of good-quality rice
    pudding (from the chilled section)

TO SERVE

a bottle of chilled rosé wine

TO START Get all your ingredients and equipment ready. Put a large (approx. 30cm) frying pan on a medium heat and a large saucepan on a low heat. Turn the oven on to 200°C/400°F/gas 6.

DUCK Score the fat on the duck breasts in a crisscross fashion, season with salt and a good pinch each of Chinese five-spice and dried thyme, then rub all over with a drizzle of olive oil. Put into the large hot frying pan, fat side down, and cook for around 16 to 18 minutes, turning every few minutes for blushing meat, or until done to your liking. Get a lid slightly smaller than the pan and press down on the breasts to help them get nice and crispy. Leave the lid on.

RICE PUDDING & FRUIT Quickly rinse the almonds in a sieve, then sprinkle over 2 heaped tablespoons of icing sugar. Lay them in a baking tray and pop on the top shelf of the oven for about 10 minutes to get golden and gorgeous.

CROUTONS Cut the ciabatta into 2cm thick slices. Put them into a roasting tray and drizzle over some olive oil. Tear in a few sprigs of rosemary and quickly bash or crush 5 unpeeled cloves of garlic over the bread. Add a good pinch of salt & pepper and the fennel seeds, then toss and mix together and put on the middle shelf of the oven to cook for around 16 minutes.

DUCK Don't forget to keep coming back and turning the duck every few minutes.

RICE PUDDING & FRUIT Quickly peel the zest of 1 orange into strips and add to the large saucepan, squeeze in the juice of both oranges and add 3 heaped tablespoons of icing sugar. Halve and quarter the plums, discarding their stones, then add to the pan with the vanilla paste or extract and mix well. Turn the heat up to high and put the lid on. Leave to cook for around 15 minutes or until soft and delicious. Check on the almonds and move them around with a wooden spoon. Cook for a few more minutes until golden, then take out of the oven and put aside.

SALAD Halve the pomegranate, then hold it cut side down over a large serving bowl and bash the back with a spoon to release the seeds. Pick out and discard any skin or pith. Empty the lamb's lettuce or rocket on top. Top and tail the carrots and speed-peel them in. Halve or slice the radishes and add to the bowl. Snip over the cress, then pick and finely chop the mint leaves. Get a small jug for the dressing and add a good drizzle of extra virgin olive oil, a good splash of balsamic, a pinch of salt & pepper and the juice of ½ a lemon. Take to the table, so you can toss and dress the salad at the last minute.

RICE PUDDING & FRUIT If you haven't already done so, take the almonds out of the oven. Stir the fruit gently, put the lid back on and reduce to a low heat. Tip the cold rice pudding into a large serving bowl or on to a platter.

CROUTONS By now your croutons should be golden and crisp, so take them out of the oven and put aside.

DUCK Once the duck is cooked to your liking (I like mine blushing to medium), get a nice big wooden chopping board. Deseed the chilli and finely chop with the rest of the mint. Move a little to one side for garnish later, then hit the rest of the mixture with a pinch of salt & pepper, a good drizzle of extra virgin olive oil, the juice of ½ a lemon and 1 teaspoon of honey. Mix and chop everything together on the board. Move the duck breasts to the dressed board with tongs. Cut at an angle into 1cm slices, then toss everything together. Arrange the croutons around the meat to catch and suck up any tasty juices. Drizzle with extra virgin olive oil, scatter over the reserved chilli and mint and take to the table. Take the stewed fruit off the heat and put aside until ready to serve.

TO SERVE Quickly dress your salad, then let everyone help themselves. Serve with a nice glass of chilled rosé. After dinner, taste the stewed fruit and add more icing sugar if necessary. Spoon over the rice pudding and take to the table with the toasted nuts for sprinkling over.

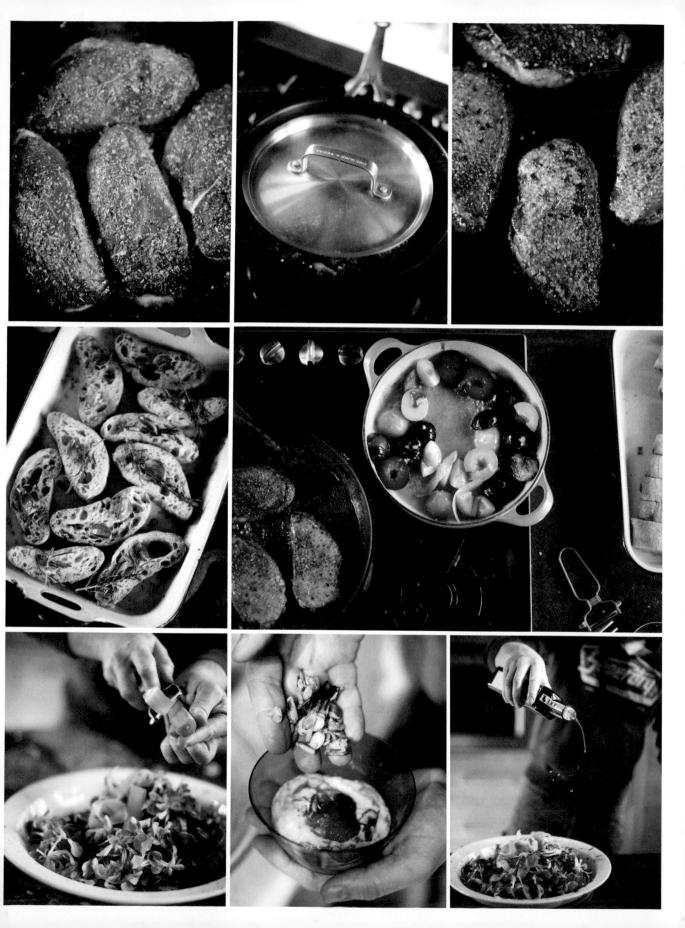

THAI RED PRAWN CURRY
JASMINE RICE
CUCUMBER SALAD
PAPAYA PLATTER

SERVES 4

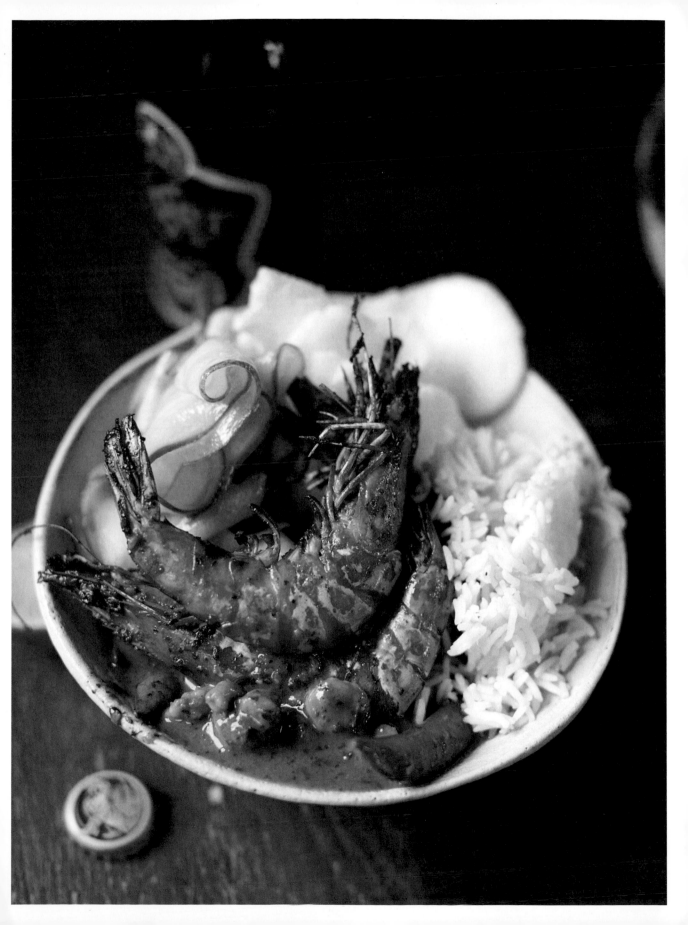

CUCUMBER SALAD
a 2cm piece of fresh ginger
1 tablespoon soy sauce
1 teaspoon sesame oil
1 lime
1 cucumber
a small handful of fresh coriander
½ a fresh red chilli

JASMINE RICE
1 mug of basmati rice
2 jasmine tea bags or 1 jasmine
 flower

RED CURRY
2 stalks of lemongrass
1 fresh red chilli
2 cloves of garlic
optional: 4 kaffir lime leaves, fresh,
 dried or frozen
a bunch of fresh coriander
2 jarred red peppers in oil
1 heaped teaspoon tomato purée
1 tablespoon fish sauce
2 tablespoons soy sauce
1 teaspoon sesame oil
a 2cm piece of fresh ginger
8 large unpeeled raw tiger prawns
200g sugar snap peas
220g small cooked prawns
1 x 400g tin of coconut milk
2 limes, to serve
1 bag of prawn crackers, to serve

SEASONINGS
olive oil
extra virgin olive oil
sea salt & black pepper

PAPAYA PLATTER
2 papayas
Greek yoghurt
1 lime
2 bananas
a few sprigs of fresh mint
optional: some biscuits or
 macaroons, to serve

TO START Get all your ingredients and equipment ready. Turn the oven on to 200°C/400°F/gas 6. Fill and boil the kettle. Put the standard blade attachment into the food processor.

CUCUMBER SALAD Peel and grate 2cm of fresh ginger on to a serving platter and add 1 tablespoon of soy sauce, 3 tablespoons of extra virgin olive oil and 1 teaspoon of sesame oil. Squeeze in the juice of 1 lime, then check the seasoning. Use a speed-peeler to peel the cucumber in long ribbons over the platter. Discard the watery core. Take a small handful of coriander and finely chop the stalks, putting the leaves aside. Sprinkle the stalks over the cucumber. Finely chop ½ a chilli and sprinkle over. Take to the table but don't toss and dress until you're ready to eat.

JASMINE RICE Put a medium saucepan on a medium heat. Add the mug of rice, a pinch of salt, a splash of olive oil, the 2 jasmine teabags or flower, and cover with 2 mugs of boiling water (use the same mug you used for the rice). Cover with a lid and cook for 7 minutes, then take off the heat and leave to steam with the lid on for 7 minutes.

RED CURRY Put a large frying pan on a medium heat. Trim the ends and tough outer leaves of the lemongrass stalks, bash up the stalks with the side of a knife, then put into a food processor with 1 fresh red chilli (stalk removed), 2 peeled cloves of garlic, 4 lime leaves, a bunch of coriander, 2 jarred red peppers, 1 heaped teaspoon of tomato purée, 1 tablespoon of fish sauce, 2 tablespoons of soy sauce and 1 teaspoon of sesame oil. Peel and add 2cm of fresh ginger. Blitz to a paste – you might need to stop and use a spatula to scrape down the sides so it all gets whizzed up.

Drizzle some olive oil into the hot frying pan and add the unpeeled raw tiger prawns. Let them fry for around 1 minute, then add a tablespoon of the curry paste and fry for 1 more minute. Tip into an ovenproof dish and put into the oven on the top shelf for about 8 to 10 minutes. Put the pan you cooked the prawns in back over a medium heat. Drizzle in a little olive oil, then add the sugar snap peas followed by the small prawns. Spoon in the rest of the curry paste, and stir and fry for a minute or two before adding the coconut milk. Stir as it melts down, then leave to simmer on a medium to low heat.

PAPAYA PLATTER Halve the papayas and scoop out their seeds. Fill a small bowl or teacup with Greek yoghurt and grate over some lime zest. Halve the bananas lengthways with their skins still on and place on a platter. Halve a lime and squeeze over the whole platter, then tear over a few mint leaves and take to the table with some biscuits or macaroons if you like.

TO SERVE Taste the curry and correct the seasoning with a few drops of soy sauce if needed. Scatter over the reserved coriander leaves, then take to the table with the dish of prawns from the oven. Cut the remaining limes into wedges for squeezing over. Put the prawn crackers into a serving bowl, and take to the table. Fluff up the rice with a fork, then take to the table. Toss and dress the cucumber salad. Dish up the rice, ladle over the curry and divide the large prawns between everyone.

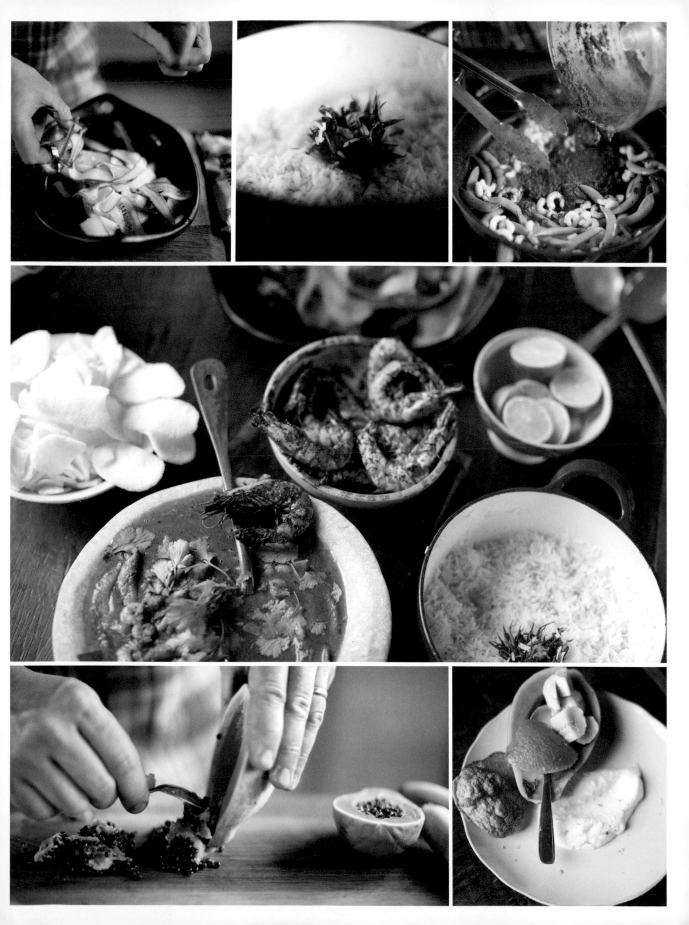

GRILLED SARDINES
CRISPY HALLOUMI
WATERCRESS SALAD & FIGS
THICK CHOCOLATE MOUSSE

SERVES 4

(makes enough mousse for 8)

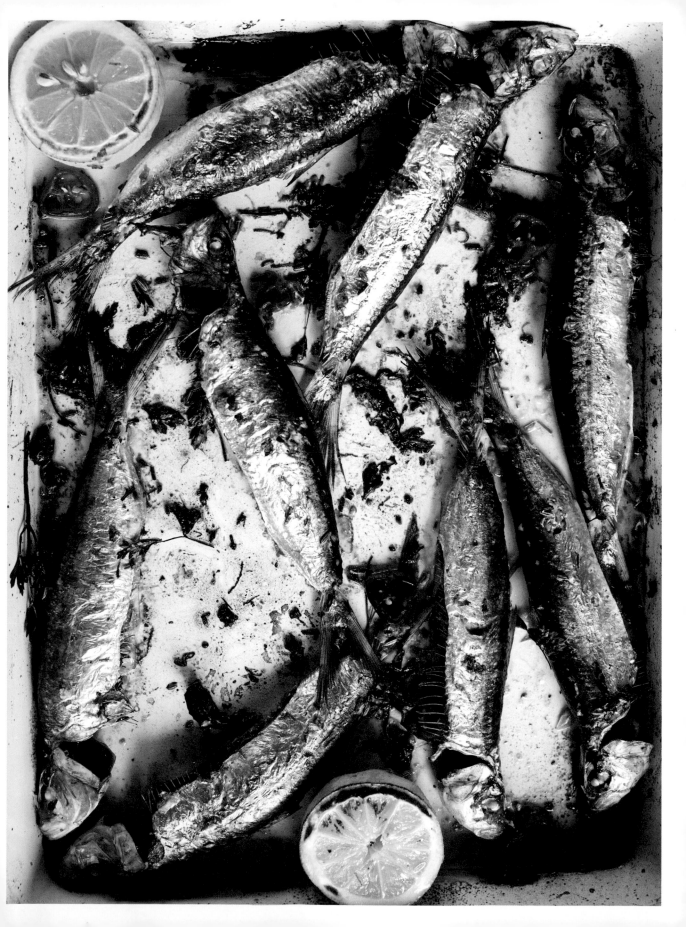

SARDINES

8 whole sardines (approx. 85g
   each), scaled and gutted
4 cloves of garlic
1 lemon
1 fresh red chilli
a small bunch of fresh flat-leaf parsley
1 teaspoon fennel seeds

SALAD

2 tablespoons flaked almonds
1 x 100g mixed bag of prewashed
   rocket and watercress
1 x 50g pack of alfalfa shoots
5 or 6 sprigs of fresh mint
1 pomegranate
1 tablespoon white wine vinegar

HALLOUMI

1 x 250g pack of halloumi
2 tablespoons sesame seeds
3 cloves of garlic

FIGS

4 figs
runny honey
2 sprigs of fresh mint

SEASONINGS

olive oil
extra virgin olive oil
sea salt & black pepper

MOUSSE (serves 8)

2 x 100g bars of good-quality dark
   chocolate (70% cocoa solids)
a small knob of butter
2 tablespoons golden caster sugar
300ml double cream
1 teaspoon vanilla paste or extract
2 large eggs
a splash of brandy, Baileys, Grand
   Marnier or Armagnac
cocoa powder, for dusting
1 orange, clementine or a handful of
   strawberries

TO SERVE

1 x 6-pack of wholemeal pitta breads
1 lemon
a bottle of chilled rosé wine

TO START Get all your ingredients and equipment ready. Turn the oven on to 220°C/425°F/gas 7. Put a medium saucepan on a medium heat and fill halfway with hot water.

MOUSSE Leave the chocolate bars in their wrappers and smash them against the counter. Get a large serving bowl and 2 mixing bowls out. Tip the chocolate chunks into a heatproof mixing bowl with the butter, then place over the pan of simmering water and leave to melt, stirring occasionally. Meanwhile, add 2 tablespoons of sugar to the nice serving bowl with 300ml of cream and 1 teaspoon of vanilla paste or extract and whip until silky with soft peaks.

Separate the eggs, adding the yolks to the whipped cream and the whites to the empty mixing bowl. Gently mix through, then put aside. Add a pinch of salt to the whites and whisk really well until stiff. By now the chocolate should be melted, so spoon it into the bowl of whipped cream with a swig of your favourite liqueur and stir through. Gently fold the egg whites through with a spatula, then put into the freezer to set.

SALAD Put a medium frying pan on a medium heat. Add 2 tablespoons of almonds and toast, tossing occasionally until golden, then tip into a small bowl and put the frying pan back on a low heat.

SARDINES Put the sardines into a large roasting tray. Crush over the 4 unpeeled cloves of garlic. Sprinkle over a pinch of salt & pepper. Finely grate over the zest of 1 lemon, then squeeze in all the juice and add the halves to the tray, cut side up. Drizzle over a little olive oil. Finely slice 1 fresh red chilli and sprinkle over the top. Finely chop the parsley stalks and scatter them over, along with 1 teaspoon of fennel seeds. Roughly chop the parsley leaves and put aside. Toss with your hands. Put the roasting tray on the top shelf of the oven for around 10 minutes, or until golden and crisp. Wash your hands.

HALLOUMI Cut the halloumi into 8 chunks. Scatter over the sesame seeds and press them into the halloumi. Put a lug of olive oil into the hot frying pan. Squash a few unpeeled cloves of garlic and add to the oil. Turn the heat up to medium. As soon as the garlic starts sizzling, add the halloumi to the pan. Leave to cook for 2 minutes, until golden, then flip over and turn the heat down. Tip any seeds left behind on the board into the pan.

PITTAS Splash all the pitta breads on both sides with cold water and stack them on the bottom shelf of the oven to warm through.

SALAD Tip the salad leaves and alfalfa on to a platter. Finely slice the leaves from 5 or 6 sprigs of mint and scatter over, along with the toasted almonds. Halve a pomegranate, then hold 1 half cut side down in your hand and bash the back with a spoon so the seeds fall over the salad. Pour 3 tablespoons of extra virgin olive oil into a small jug. Squeeze in the juice from the remaining pomegranate half. Add 1 tablespoon of white wine vinegar, mix, then take to the table with the salad to dress at the last minute.

FIGS Cut a cross in the top of each fig, then pinch the bottoms so they burst open. Pop them on a little serving board with a small bowl of runny honey in the centre. Pick over the leaves from a couple of sprigs of mint. Drizzle over a little extra virgin olive oil and add a pinch of salt. Cut the lemon into wedges, pop 1 wedge alongside the figs and take to the table.

TO SERVE Take the tray of sardines to the table with the warm pitta breads and the pan of golden halloumi. Scatter the chopped parsley over the the halloumi and serve with wedges of lemon for squeezing over and some chilled rosé. When you're ready, take the mousse out of the freezer, quickly dust with cocoa powder and serve with wedges of orange, clementine or some strawberries on the side.

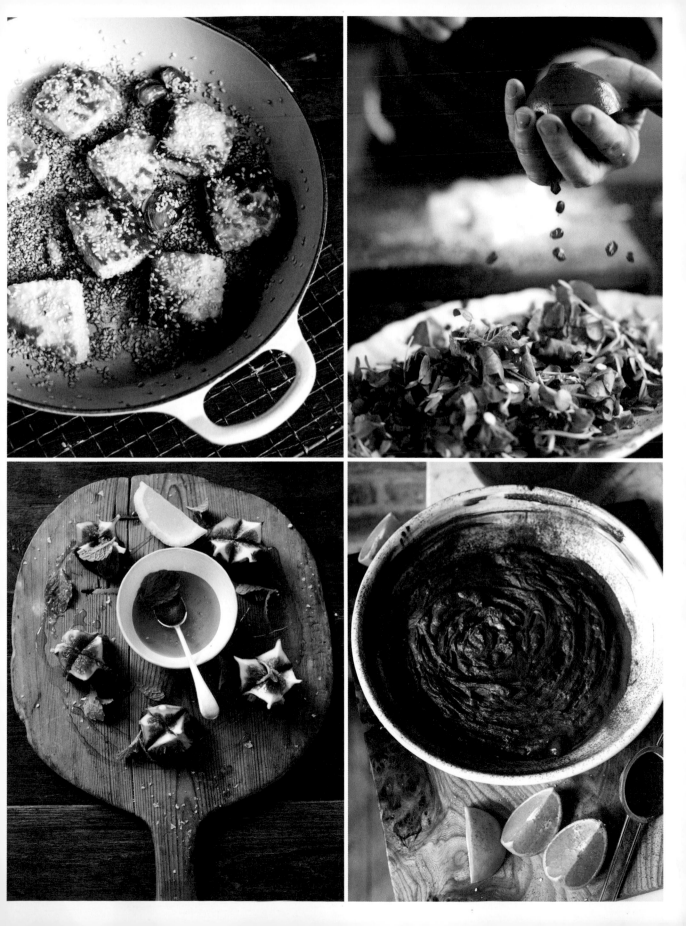

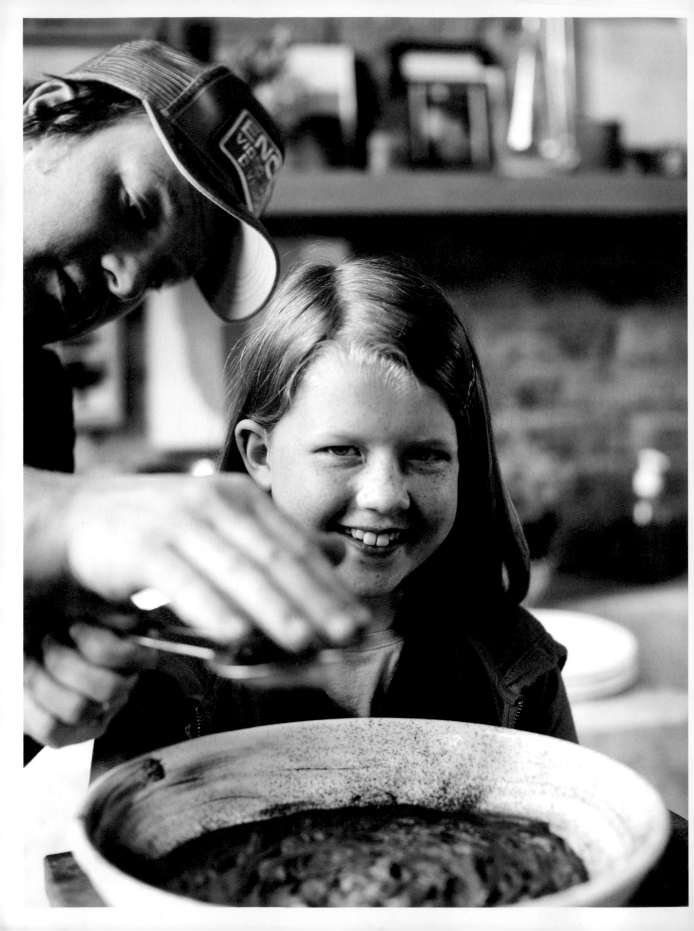

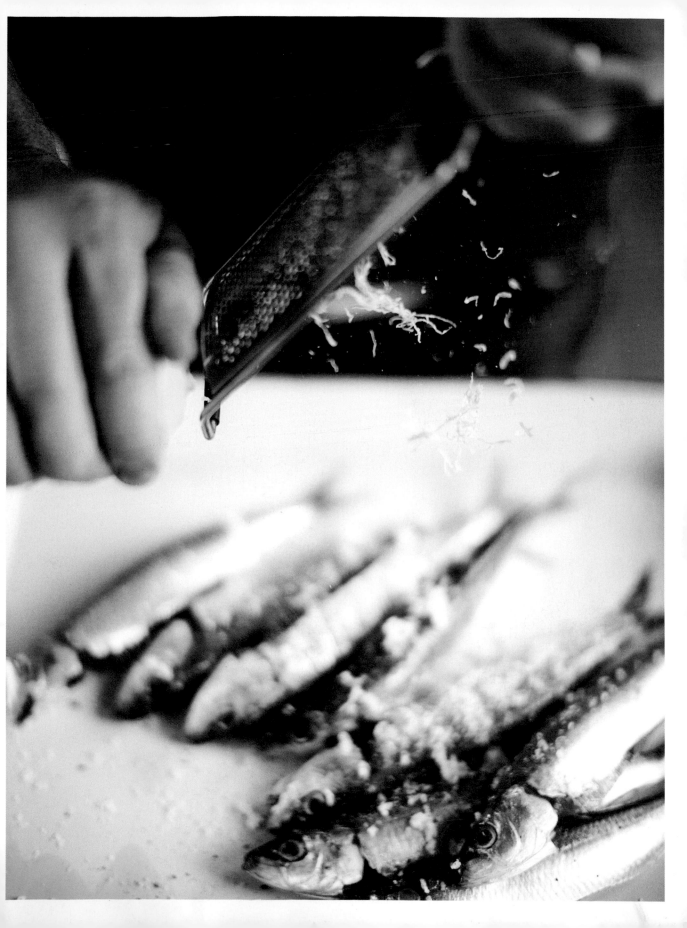

TASTY CRUSTED COD

MY MASHY PEAS

TARTARE SAUCE

WARM GARDEN SALAD

SERVES 6–8

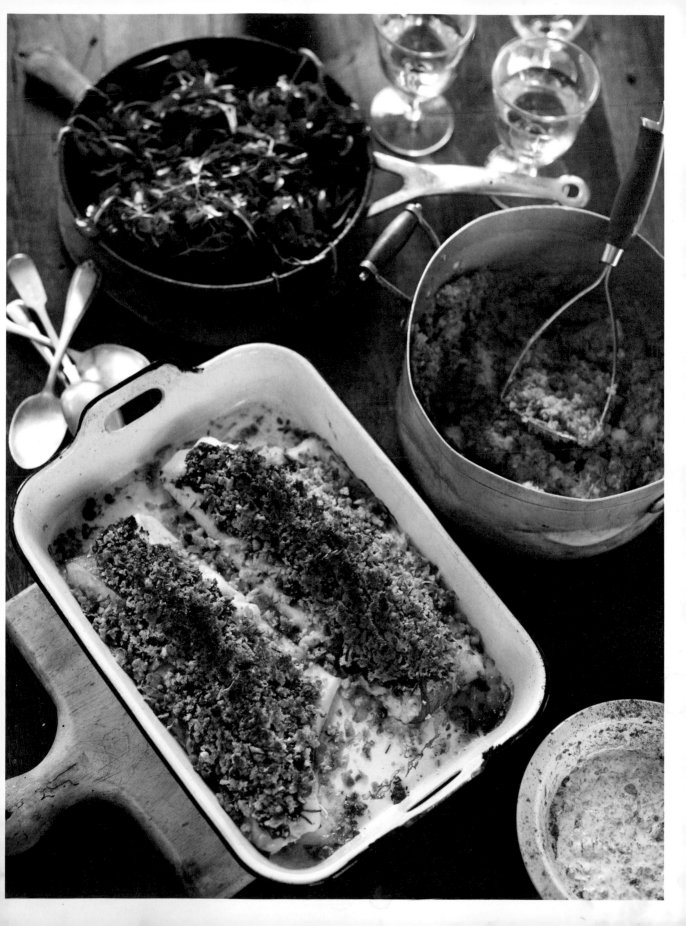

MASHY PEAS

4 medium baking potatoes
1 head of broccoli
500g frozen peas
a large knob of butter
1–2 dessertspoons mint sauce

TARTARE SAUCE

3 cornichons
1 heaped teaspoon small capers
a small bunch of fresh flat-leaf parsley
½ a 30g tin of anchovy fillets in oil
1 lemon
½ a 400g jar of good-quality
  mayonnaise
sweet paprika, for dusting

COD

1 teaspoon fennel seeds
2 x 600g (or 6 x 180g) fillets of cod,
  skin on, scaled and pin-boned
200g chunk of white crusty bread
4 cloves of garlic
½ a 30g tin of anchovy fillets in oil
½ a 280g jar of sun-dried tomatoes
  in oil
a small bunch of fresh basil
½–1 fresh red chilli
40g Parmesan cheese
1 lemon
balsamic vinegar
a couple of sprigs of fresh rosemary
a couple of sprigs of fresh thyme

SEASONINGS

olive oil
extra virgin olive oil
sea salt & black pepper

SALAD

6 rashers of pancetta
4 cloves of garlic
5 tablespoons balsamic vinegar
1 x 100g bag of prewashed watercress
1 x 100g bag of prewashed rocket

TO SERVE

a bottle of chilled white wine

TO START Get all your ingredients and equipment ready. Fill and boil the kettle. Turn the grill on to full whack. Put a large saucepan on a low heat. Put the standard blade attachment into the food processor.

MASHY PEAS Quickly peel the potatoes (or leave the skins on if you prefer) and chop into 2cm chunks, add to the saucepan with a pinch of salt and cover with boiled water. Put a lid on the pan and turn the heat to medium. Trim and discard the bare end of the broccoli stalk. Slice the rest up and add to the potatoes. Break the florets into even-sized pieces and set aside.

COD Put a few good lugs of olive oil into a large roasting tray, sprinkle with salt & pepper and scatter over a teaspoon of fennel seeds. Rub and toss the fish fillets in the flavours, then place skin side down. Drizzle with olive oil, then put under the grill in the middle of the oven for 5 minutes while you make the topping.

Roughly chop the bread and add to the food processor. Whiz, adding 2 peeled cloves of garlic with a drizzle of oil from the tin of anchovies as it's whizzing, then tip the breadcrumb mixture into a bowl.

Put half the tin of anchovy fillets into the empty food processor with the drained sun-dried tomatoes, 2 cloves of peeled garlic, basil, chilli (stalk removed) and the chunk of Parmesan. Finely grate in the zest from the lemon, then squeeze in the juice. Add a couple of splashes of balsamic vinegar and whiz to a paste. You may need to scrape round the sides between whizzes. Get the fish out of the oven. Spoon and spread this paste over each fillet in a thick even layer, then scatter over the breadcrumbs. Drizzle a little olive oil over the thyme and rosemary sprigs, then lay on top of the two fillets and put back under the grill on the middle shelf for 10 minutes, or until golden and crisp.

MASHY PEAS Add the peas and the broccoli florets to the potatoes, and put the lid back on.

SALAD Put a medium frying pan on a medium heat and add the pancetta. Leave to crisp up, tossing occasionally.

TARTARE SAUCE Quickly rinse out the food processor and add 3 cornichons, a heaped teaspoon of capers, a small bunch of fresh parsley and half the tin of anchovies and their oil. Pulse a few times with a drizzle of extra virgin olive oil and the zest and juice of ½ a lemon. Whiz until fairly smooth, then transfer to a small bowl and add ½ the jar of mayo. Mix well, adding the juice of the rest of the lemon, tasting and tweaking as necessary. Sprinkle with the sweet paprika, drizzle over a little extra virgin olive oil and take to the table.

SALAD Once the rashers of pancetta are crispy and golden, turn the heat to low, then crush 2 unpeeled cloves of garlic into the frying pan. Take the pan off the heat and add 5 tablespoons of balsamic vinegar. Add a little bit of extra virgin olive oil and shake the pan about. Use a wooden spoon to break the crispy pancetta into pieces in the pan.

MASHY PEAS Drain the veg, let it steam dry for a few minutes, then tip back into the pan. Add the butter, a good drizzle of extra virgin olive oil, a pinch of salt & pepper, 1 to 2 dessertspoons of mint sauce and roughly mash about ten times. Put in a serving bowl.

COD Check the fish, and when the crust is golden and crisp take it out of the oven and straight to the table along with your bowl of mashy peas.

SALAD At the very last minute tip the salad leaves into the pan of warm dressing and toss quickly with your hands. Take to the table in the pan and serve with chilled white wine.

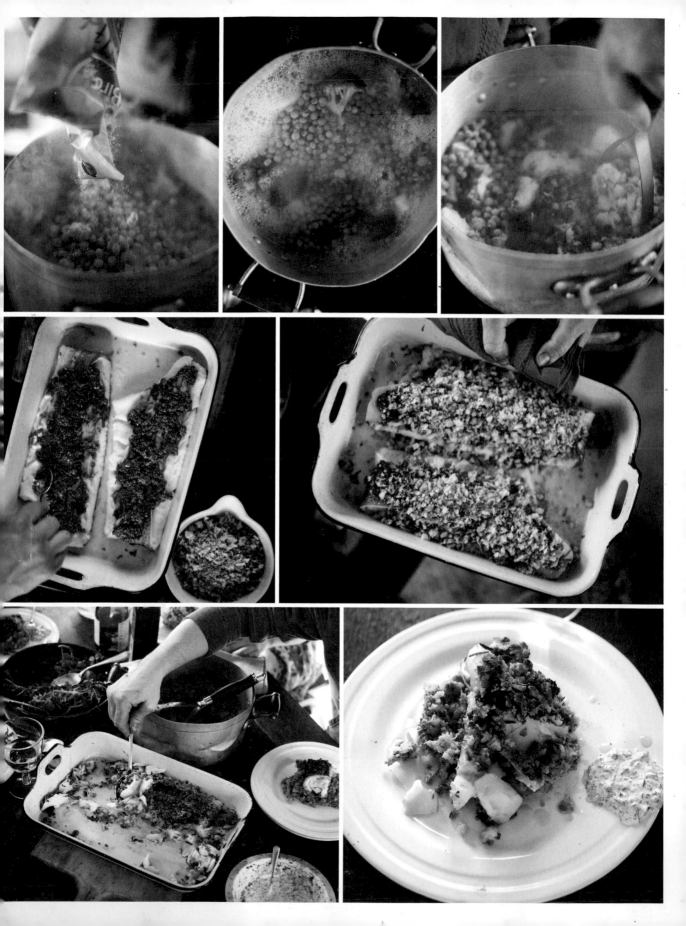

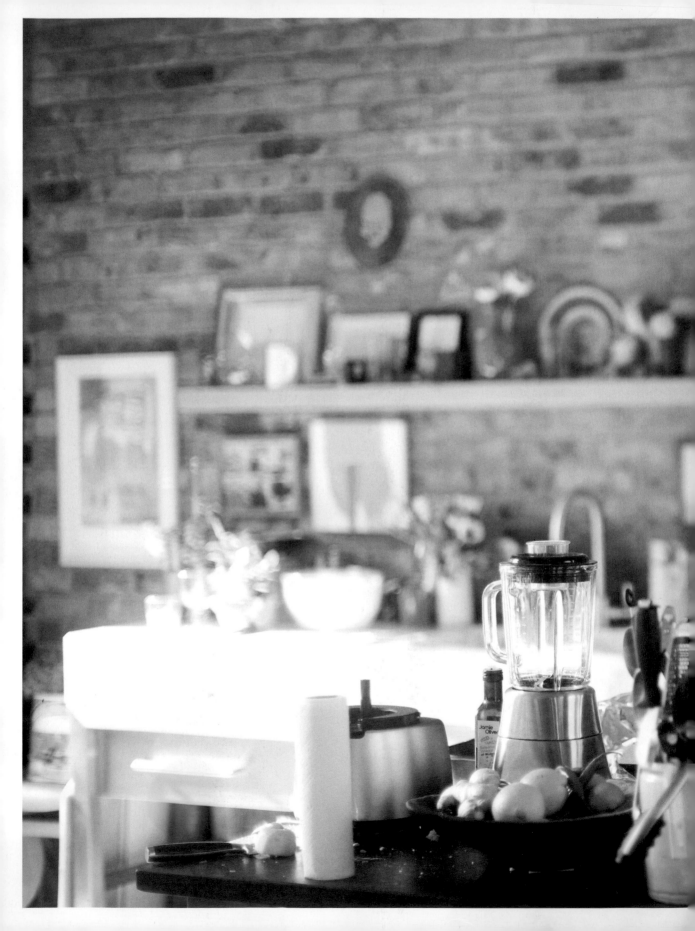

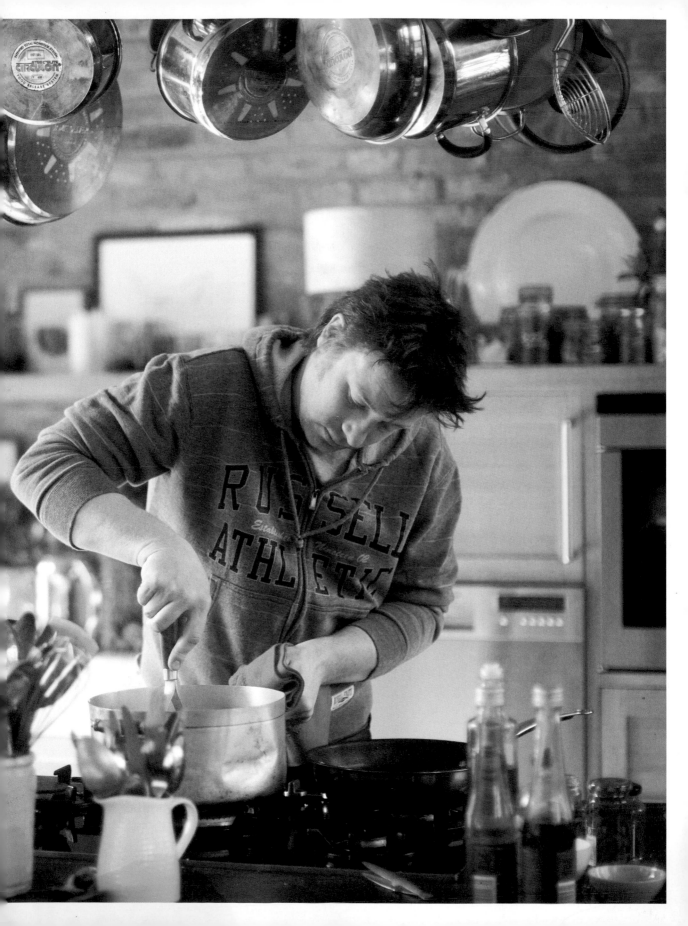

SWEDISH-STYLE FISHCAKES

ROASTED BABY NEW POTATOES

SPROUT SALAD

FRESH ZINGY SALSA

SERVES 4

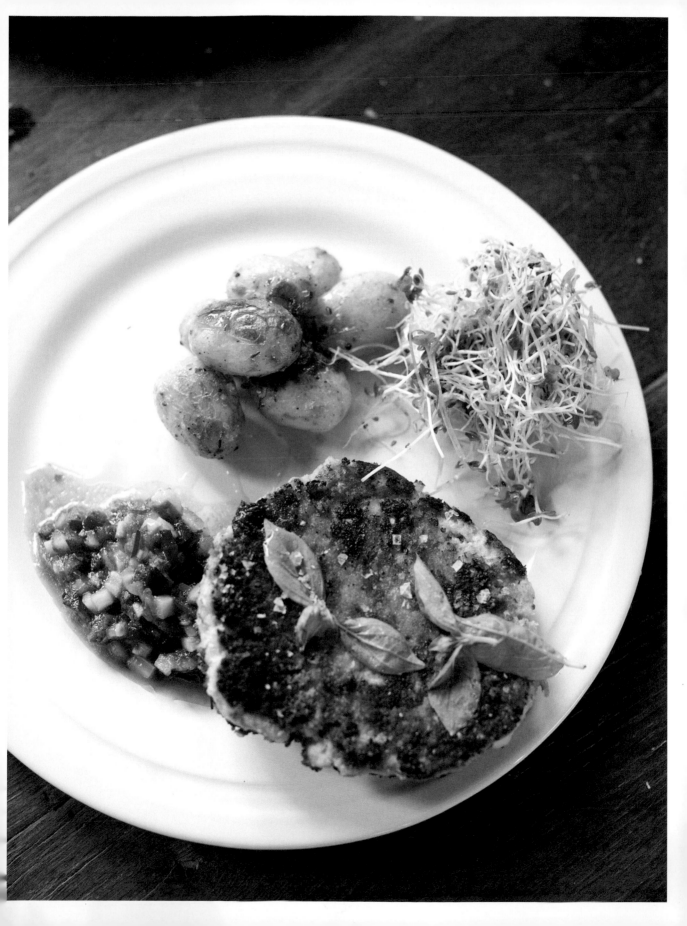

POTATOES

500g baby new potatoes
½ a lemon
a small bunch of mixed fresh herbs,
  such as thyme and rosemary

FISHCAKES

2 slices of stale or crusty bread
2 x 150g salmon fillets, skin off and
  pin-boned
1 x 300g haddock fillet, skin off and
  pin-boned
1 x 200g tuna steak
1 lemon
a small bunch of fresh flat-leaf parsley
1 clove of garlic

SALSA

1 fresh red chilli
1 fresh green chilli
4 spring onions
4 ripe red or yellow tomatoes
red wine vinegar
½ a cucumber
1 yellow pepper
1 red pepper
2 limes
a small bunch of fresh basil

SALAD

100g alfalfa and/or radish sprouts
1 pack of crisp breads or
  carta di musica
a small bunch of fresh mint
2 ripe avocados
1 punnet of cress
1 lemon

SEASONINGS

olive oil
extra virgin olive oil
sea salt & black pepper

TO SERVE

a bottle of chilled white wine

TO START Get all your ingredients and equipment ready. Fill and boil the kettle. Turn the oven on to 220°C/425°F/gas 7. Put the standard blade attachment into the food processor.

POTATOES Pop the potatoes into a large microwave-safe bowl with ½ a lemon and cover with a double layer of clingfilm. Put into the microwave and cook on full power for 7 to 10 minutes, or until cooked through.

FISHCAKES Whiz the bread in a food processor until fine. Meanwhile, tear off a large sheet of tin foil. Put the breadcrumbs on top, then put to one side. Add all the fish to the processor. Finely grate in the zest of 1 lemon and rip in the parsley leaves, discarding the stalks. Add a really good pinch of salt & pepper and pulse a few times until coarsely mixed.

POTATOES Quickly pick the leaves from your herbs and finely chop them. Get the potatoes out of the microwave, use a knife to check they are cooked, then carefully remove the clingfilm. Add the chopped herbs, a good pinch of salt & pepper and a good lug of olive oil. Mix well. Tip into a heatproof serving dish then place on the top shelf until golden and crisp.

FISHCAKES Tip the fish mix on to a platter and add 2 heaped tablespoons of the breadcrumbs. Scrunch and mix with your clean hands, then divide into 4 patties. If you've got a round pastry cutter (approx. 10cm diameter) use that as a mould. If not, use your hands to roll them into 4 balls then push, squeeze and pat them into fishcakes. Place on top of the breadcrumbs, making sure the cakes are of even thicknesses, then sprinkle the breadcrumbs on top to evenly coat them (🍴).

Put a large frying pan on a medium heat and add a good couple of lugs of olive oil. Bash a clove of garlic with the heel of your hand and add to the pan. When the garlic sizzles, use a fish slice to carefully transfer the fishcakes to the pan. Cook for about 7 minutes while you make the salsa, once golden underneath flip over and cook for another 7 minutes or so until golden on the other side.

SALSA Quickly wash your processor bowl. Deseed the chillies and remove the stalks, trim the spring onions, and add both to the food processor with the whole tomatoes and a pinch of salt & pepper. Add a swig of red wine vinegar and pulse until very finely chopped. Have a taste and adjust the flavours if needed and when you're happy pour on to a platter.

Halve the cucumber half lengthways then finely chop into smaller pieces. Halve, deseed and finely chop the peppers. Mix with the rest of the salsa on the platter and the juice of 2 limes. Pick the baby basil leaves and put aside for garnish, then roughly chop the rest of the leaves and add.

FISHCAKES By now the fishcakes should be lovely and golden brown, so use a fish slice to carefully flip them over.

SALAD Scatter the alfalfa over another platter and break over some crisp breads or carta di musica. Finely slice the mint leaves, discarding the stalks, and scatter over. Halve the avocados and spoon big chunks of the flesh over the platter. Snip over the punnet of cress, sprinkle with salt & pepper, and take to the table with a bottle of extra virgin olive oil for drizzling over and 1 lemon, cut in half, for squeezing over.

POTATOES Take the potatoes out of the oven and put them on the table.

FISHCAKES Use a fish slice to put the fishcakes on top of the salsa. Sprinkle over the reserved baby basil leaves and a pinch of salt. Take to the table with a bottle of cold white wine.

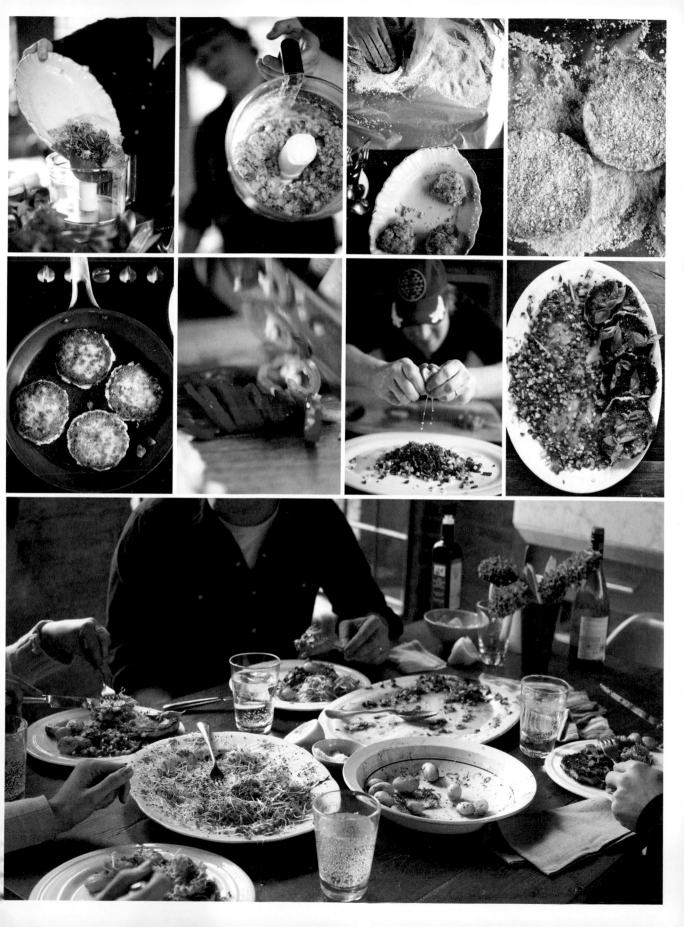

STICKY PAN-FRIED SCALLOPS

SERVES 4 (with lots of brownies left over)

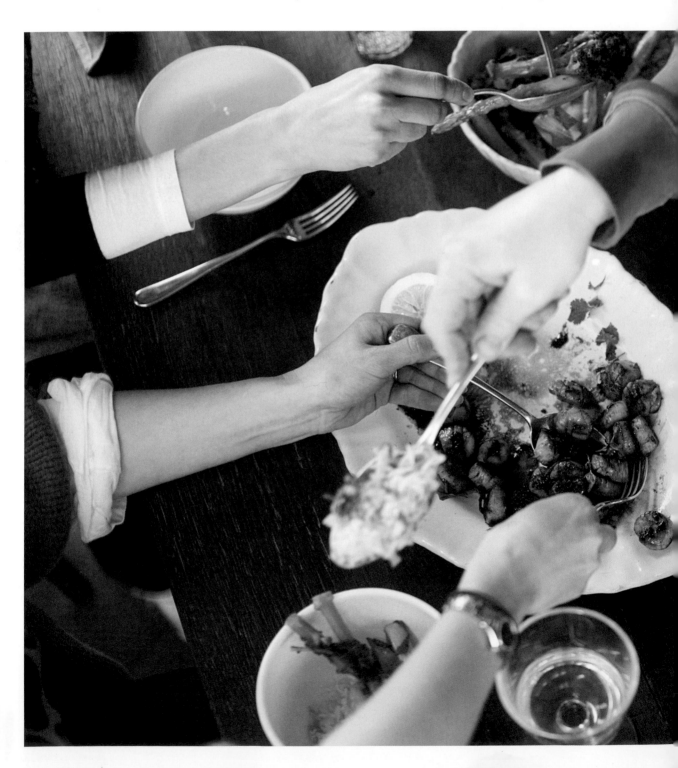

SWEET CHILLI RICE, DRESSED GREENS
QUICK BROWNIES

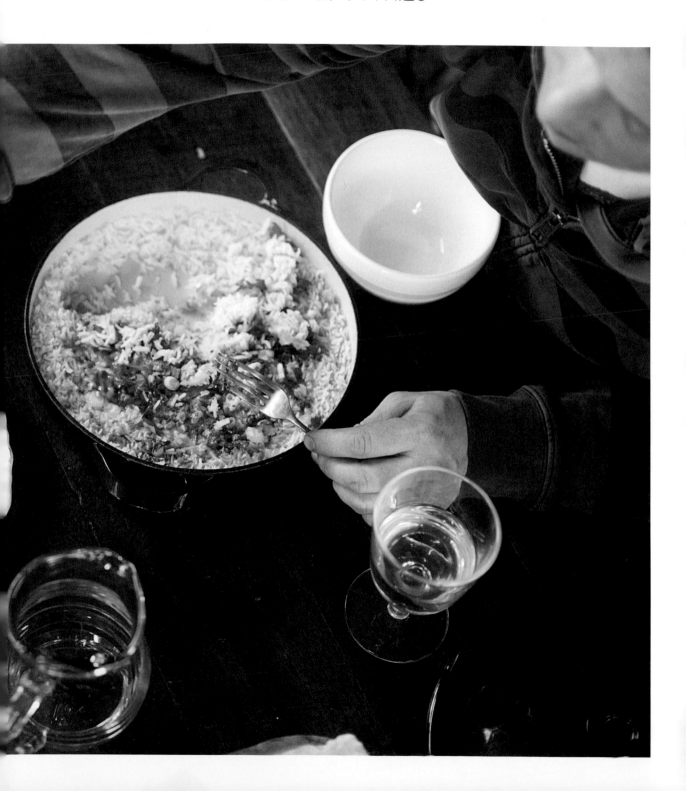

RICE

1 large mug of basmati rice
a small bunch of spring onions
3 eggs
1 tablespoon soy sauce
1 tablespoon sesame oil
½ a lemon
a small bunch of fresh coriander
sweet chilli sauce

GREENS

4 pak choi
200g purple sprouting broccoli
200g asparagus
½ a lime

SCALLOPS

400g fresh scallops, shelled and
  trimmed
1 lemon
Chinese five-spice
sesame oil
optional: ½ a fresh red chilli
1 clove of garlic
runny honey
2 small knobs of butter
a small bunch of fresh coriander

SEASONINGS

olive oil
extra virgin olive oil
sea salt & black pepper

BROWNIES (serves 12)

2 x 100g bars of good-quality dark
  chocolate (70% cocoa solids)
250g unsalted butter, at room
  temperature
200g golden caster sugar
6 level tablespoons cocoa powder
4 heaped tablespoons self-raising flour
a handful of crystallized or stem ginger
4 eggs
a handful of pecans
a handful of sour dried cherries
1 clementine
créme fraîche, to serve

TO START Get all your ingredients and equipment ready. Fill and boil the kettle. Turn the oven on to 180°C/375°F/gas 4 and put a shallow casserole-type pan (approx. 26cm diameter) on a medium heat. Put the standard blade attachment into the food processor.

RICE Put the rice into the shallow pan with 2 pinches of salt. Cover with 2 mugs' worth of boiled water (use the same mug you measured the rice in). Pop a lid on and leave to cook for 7 minutes. Fill and reboil the kettle.

BROWNIES Smash the chocolate and chop the butter into rough chunks, then put both into the food processor and add 200g of caster sugar, 6 level tablespoons of cocoa powder, 4 heaped tablespoons of self-raising flour, a pinch of salt and the crystallized or stem ginger. Whiz together. While the processor is running, crack in the eggs. Scrunch up a large piece of greaseproof paper under a tap. Flatten it, lay it in a baking tray (approx. 32 x 26cm) and drizzle it with olive oil, then rub in. Use a spatula to spoon and spread the brownie mixture evenly into the tray, about 2.5cm thick. Sprinkle over the pecans and sour cherries and press them down a bit. Finely grate over the zest of the clementine. Put the tray in the oven on the top shelf and cook for 12 to 14 minutes.

SCALLOPS Lay the scallops on a piece of greaseproof paper. Score crisscrosses on top, only going halfway through. Drizzle over some olive oil, season with salt & pepper, finely grate over some lemon zest and dust with Chinese five-spice. Drizzle with sesame oil and toss together to coat in the flavours.

RICE Trim and finely slice the spring onions and put into a mixing bowl. Crack in the eggs, and add 1 tablespoon each of soy sauce and sesame oil and a drizzle of olive oil, then whisk. Take the lid off the rice and use a fork to fluff it up. Pour the egg mixture all over. Squeeze in the juice of ½ a

lemon and add a pinch of pepper. Put the lid back on and turn down to the lowest heat for another 4 to 5 minutes.

SCALLOPS Get a large frying pan on the highest heat.

GREENS Half-fill a large saucepan with boiled water and put it on a medium heat. Halve each pak choi lengthways, trim the broccoli and asparagus, then put in a large colander or sieve and cover tightly with tin foil. Put over the saucepan of water to steam for a few minutes until tender, then take off the heat.

RICE Finely slice the leaves and stalks of a small bunch of coriander and sprinkle over the rice. Drizzle a good lug of sweet chilli sauce on top, then put the lid on and take to the table.

SCALLOPS Put a good lug of olive oil into the empty frying pan. Quickly add the scallops, scored side down. Finely chop the fresh chilli, if using. You can jiggle the pan but don't turn the scallops until they've had 2 to 3 minutes, or are golden underneath. Quickly turn them all over and cook for 30 seconds, then crush over 1 unpeeled clove of garlic and sprinkle over the chilli. Squeeze in the juice of ½ a lemon and add a tiny drizzle of honey and 2 small knobs of butter. Take off the heat, and when melted and sticky put on a plate and sprinkle over the leaves from a small bunch of coriander.

GREENS Once tender, tip on to a platter. Drizzle with soy sauce and extra virgin olive oil. Squeeze over the juice of ½ a lime. Taste, tweaking if needed.

TO SERVE Take the rice, scallops and greens to the table. Divide everything between bowls and tuck in. Remove the brownies from the oven to cool while you enjoy the scallops. When ready, serve the warm brownies with a wedge of zested clementine and a dollop of créme fraîche.

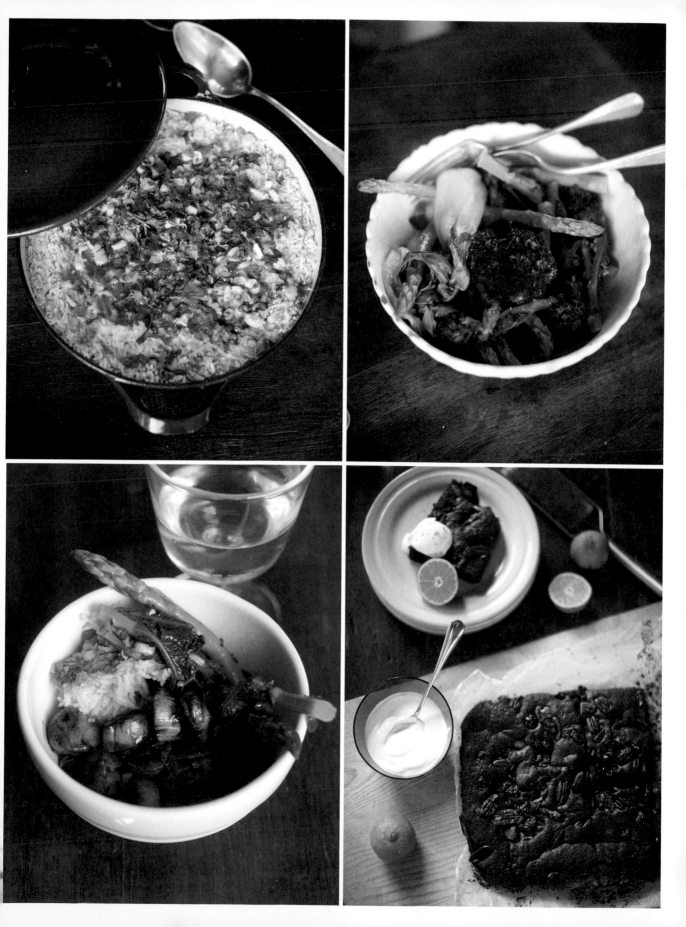

SERIOUSLY GOOD

FISH TAGINE

FENNEL & LEMON SALAD

COUSCOUS

ORANGE & MINT TEA

SERVES 4

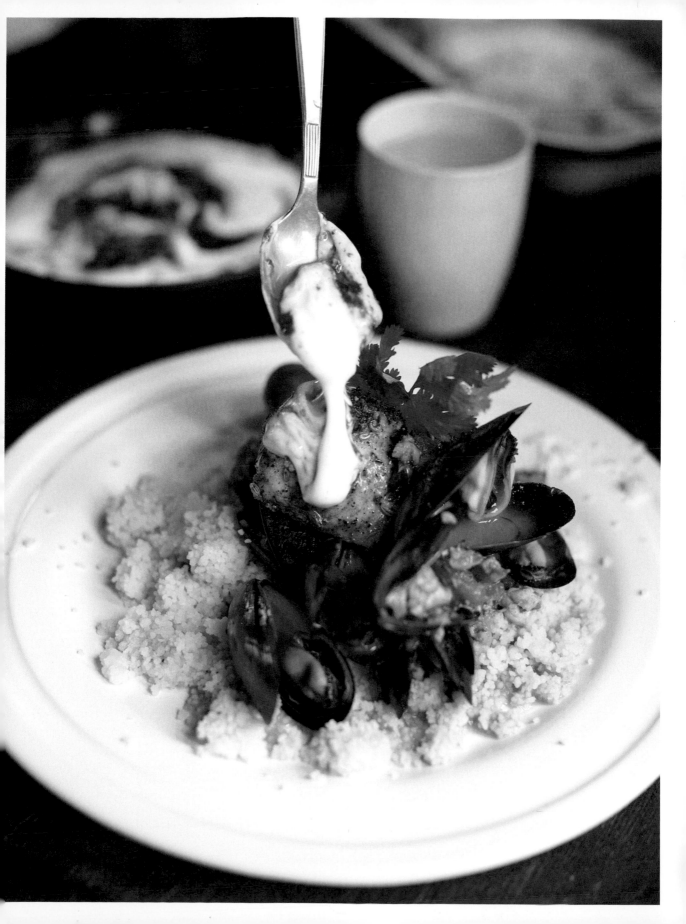

TAGINE
fennel seeds
1 cinnamon stick
1 small red onion
½ a fresh red chilli
12 mixed jarred olives, stoned
4 tomatoes
1 small preserved lemon
1 heaped teaspoon ras el hanout
  spice mixture or garam masala
saffron
4 sprigs of fresh coriander
400g mussels, cleaned and
  debearded (ask your fishmonger
  to do this for you)

COUSCOUS
250g couscous

MONKFISH
4 x 150g monkfish fillets,
  skin off and pin-boned
2 cloves of garlic
fennel seeds
ras el hanout spice mixture or
  garam masala
dried oregano

SALAD
2 bulbs of fennel
1 lemon
a small bunch of fresh coriander

YOGHURT
250g natural yoghurt
1 tablespoon harissa

SEASONINGS
olive oil
extra virgin olive oil
sea salt & black pepper

TEA
a bunch of fresh mint
½ an orange
optional: runny honey
optional: ice cubes

TO START Get all your ingredients and equipment ready. Turn the grill to full whack. Put a large tagine or casserole-type pan on a medium heat. Put the fine slicer disc attachment into the food processor. Fill and boil the kettle.

TAGINE Put a lug of olive oil, a pinch of fennel seeds and 1 cinnamon stick into the large pan. On a plastic chopping board, line up the 4 monkfish fillets and trim 1cm or so off the ends of each fillet so they're all the same size. Put the fillets into a snug-fitting roasting tray or earthenware dish. Roughly chop the trimmings and add to the large pan, stirring frequently. Peel and finely slice the onion, finely slice ½ a red chilli and add both to the pan. Tear in the olives, mix well and leave to cool.

COUSCOUS Put the 250g of couscous into a serving dish or pan and season with a pinch of salt & pepper. Just cover with boiling water, drizzle over some extra virgin olive oil, then cover with a lid or plate.

MONKFISH Drizzle olive oil over the fillets in the roasting tray. Crush in 2 unpeeled cloves of garlic. Scatter over a pinch each of fennel seeds, ras el hanout or garam masala, dried oregano and salt & pepper. Toss, then whack under the hot grill on the top shelf for 14 minutes, or until cooked through.

TAGINE Roughly chop half the tomatoes, finely chop the rest and add to the pan. Finely chop 1 small preserved lemon and add to the pan with 1 heaped teaspoon of ras el hanout and a pinch of saffron. Give it a good stir, then pour in 250ml water. If you've got a tagine, put the lid on. If not, make a mock lid by tearing off a large sheet of tin foil (about arm's length) and folding it into a cone shape. There's no right or wrong way. Scrunch the edges together and make sure it fits just inside the pan. Finely chop 4 sprigs of coriander and add to the pan. Shake the mussels. If any are open, throw them away. Add the mussels to the pan. Put your foil lid on top, sitting it just inside the edges of the pan. Leave to tick away for around 8 minutes, or until the mussels have opened.

SALAD Trim the base and ends of the fennel bulbs, discarding the outer leaves if necessary and reserving the herb ends if you have them. Halve the bulb, then shred in a food processor, using the fine slicer disc attachment. Squash the lemon with the heel of your hand, then shred in the food processor too. Tip into a large serving bowl. Pick out and discard any end chunks of lemon or fennel. Roughly chop the coriander leaves, then finely slice the stalks, discarding the very ends. Put the stalks into a bowl with a good lug of extra virgin olive oil and a pinch of salt & pepper. Mix and toss with your hands. Scatter most of the coriander leaves over the salad and take to the table.

MONKFISH Check the monkfish. If it's cooked through when you cut into it, turn the grill off, cover the fish with foil and leave it in the oven until you're ready to eat. Refill and boil the kettle.

YOGHURT Put the yoghurt into a bowl. Spoon 1 tablespoon of harissa and a good lug of extra virgin olive oil into the centre, then gently swirl it through the yoghurt. Sprinkle with a pinch of salt and take to the table.

TEA Rip the mint leaves into a jug or teapot. Speed-peel in strips of zest from ½ an orange. Top up with boiling water, sweeten with a little honey if you like, and take to the table. (Or, if you want, serve it cold poured over ice cubes.)

TO SERVE Take the tagine and couscous straight to the table with the monkfish. Remove the foil from the tagine. The mussels should all be open, so discard any that aren't. Scatter over the reserved coriander leaves. Fluff up the couscous with a fork, have a quick taste to check the seasoning, then serve with some of the lovely monkfish and tagine.

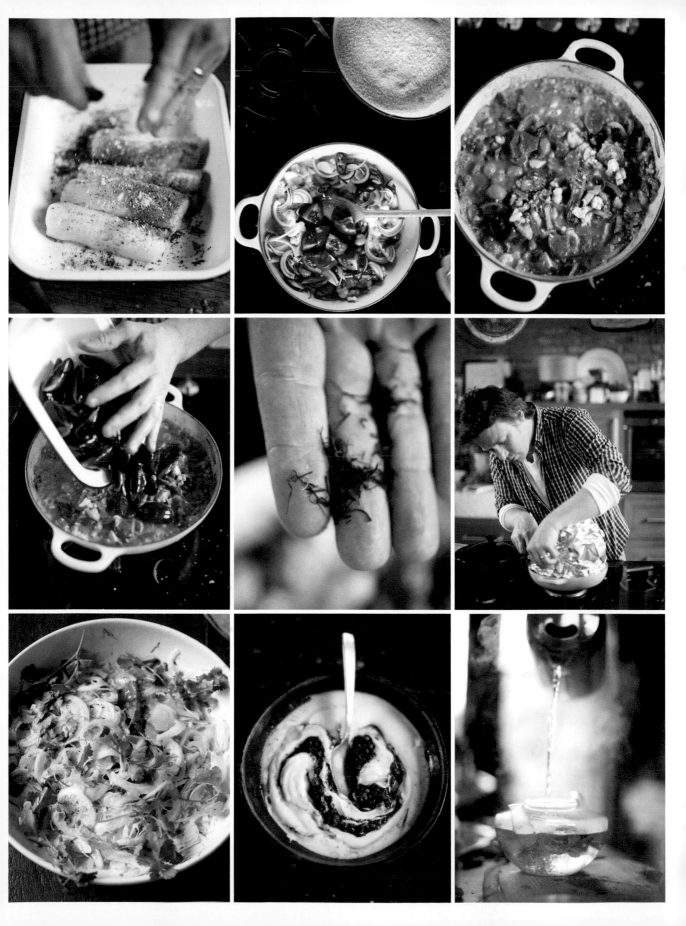

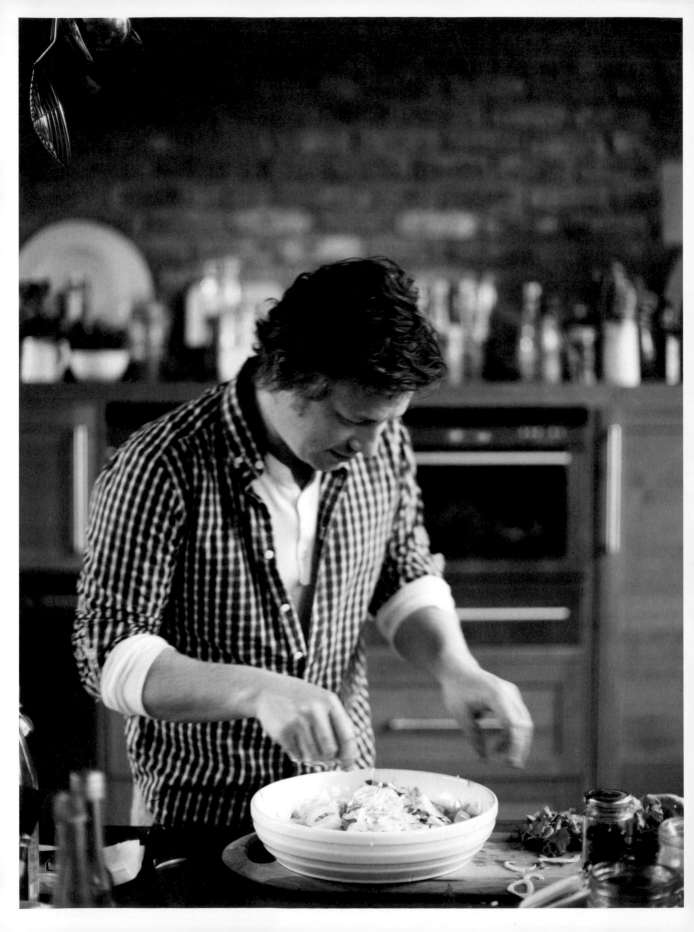

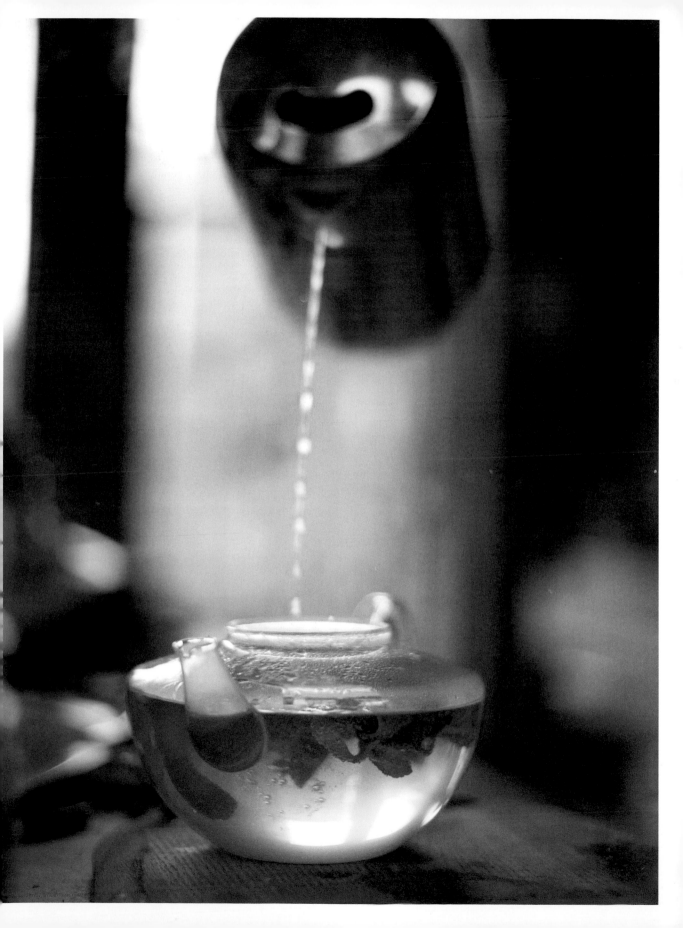

SMOKED SALMON

SERVES 4

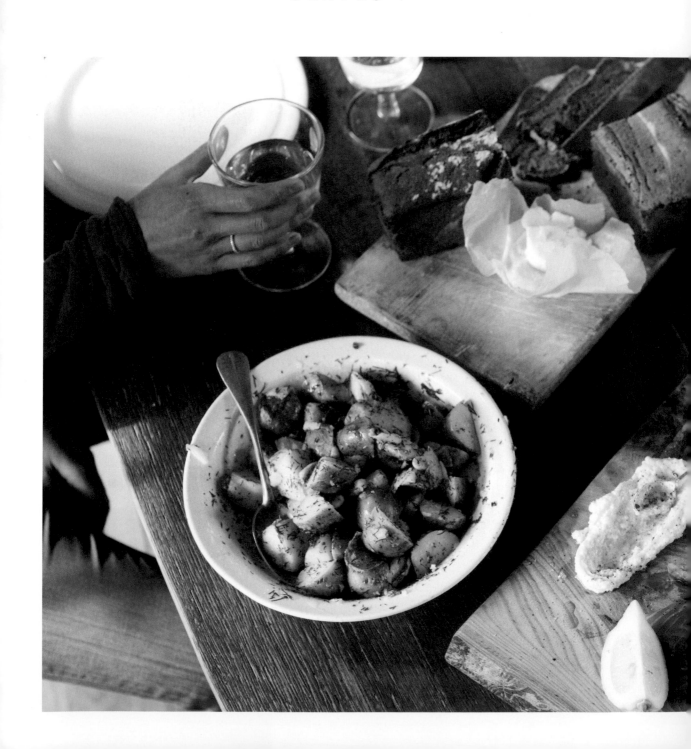

POTATO SALAD
BEETS & COTTAGE CHEESE
RYE BREAD & HOMEMADE BUTTER

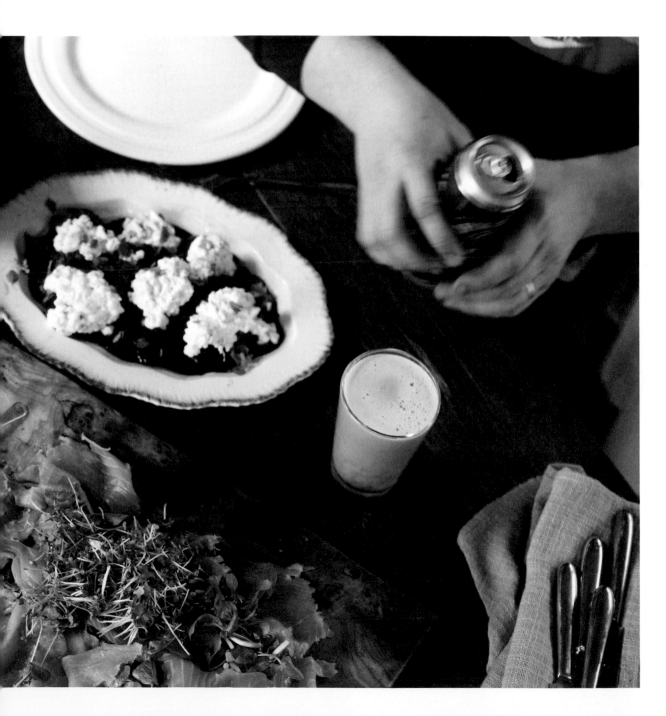

POTATO SALAD
500g red-skinned potatoes, skin on
1 lemon
2 sprigs of fresh thyme
a small bunch of fresh dill

SALMON
1 x 100g bag of prewashed
  watercress
400g good-quality smoked salmon
1 lemon
3 heaped teaspoons creamed
  horseradish
1 punnet of cress

BUTTER
300ml double cream

BEETS
1 x 250g pack of cooked vac-packed
  beetroots
balsamic vinegar
a small handful of fresh Greek basil
  or basil
1 x 250g tub of cottage cheese
a few sprigs of fresh thyme
1 lemon

SEASONINGS
olive oil
extra virgin olive oil
sea salt & black pepper

TO SERVE
a loaf of rye bread
a bottle of chilled white wine
  or bitter

TO START Get all your ingredients and equipment ready. Fill and boil the kettle. Put a saucepan with a lid on a medium heat. Put the rye bread on a board and take to the table with a bread knife. Put the beater attachment into the food processor.

POTATO SALAD Wash the potatoes, then roughly quarter them and cut into 3cm chunks, removing any gnarly bits. Pour boiled water into the saucepan and add a pinch of salt. Add the potatoes, then speed-peel in a few strips of lemon zest and add the thyme. Put a lid on and cook for around 10 minutes, or until soft when stabbed with a knife.

SALMON Tip the watercress on to a serving board. Lay the salmon slices over the leaves in rustic waves. Quarter the lemon. Smear 3 heaped teaspoonfuls of creamed horseradish on one end of the board, season with salt & pepper, squeeze over 2 of the lemon wedges and drizzle with extra virgin olive oil. Take to the table.

BUTTER Pour the double cream into the food processor. Leave to beat away – the whole point is to over-beat it.

BEETS Put the beets on a board and cut into erratic chunks. Move them to a serving platter and add 2 splashes of good balsamic vinegar, a good drizzle of extra virgin olive oil and a pinch of salt & pepper. Quickly pick the Greek basil leaves and sprinkle most of them over. Toss and mix to dress, tasting and tweaking as necessary.

BUTTER By now the cream should be thick and coming together into one big clump. When ready, it will look like butter and the sound coming from the food processor will change. Put it into a sieve over the sink, then use your clean hands to quickly scrunch and shape it so that any excess water drains away. Put it on some greaseproof paper; try not to handle it too much or it will melt. Sprinkle over a pinch of salt, then put it beside the bread.

BEETS Open the cottage cheese and drizzle a little extra virgin olive oil straight into the tub. Rip over the thyme tips and add a pinch of salt & pepper. Finely grate in the zest of ½ your lemon and stir. Arrange the beets on a platter, dollop over the flavoured cottage cheese, sprinkle over some pepper, drizzle with extra virgin olive oil and scatter with the remaining Greek basil leaves. Take to the table.

POTATO SALAD Drain the potatoes and leave them to steam dry for 2 minutes while you finely chop the dill. Tip the potatoes into a bowl and add the dill and a knob of your homemade butter, plus a good drizzle of extra virgin olive oil, a pinch of salt & pepper and the juice of ½ a lemon. Toss and take to the table.

TO SERVE Snip the cress on top of the salmon. Serve with chilled white wine or bitter and any leftover wedges of lemon.

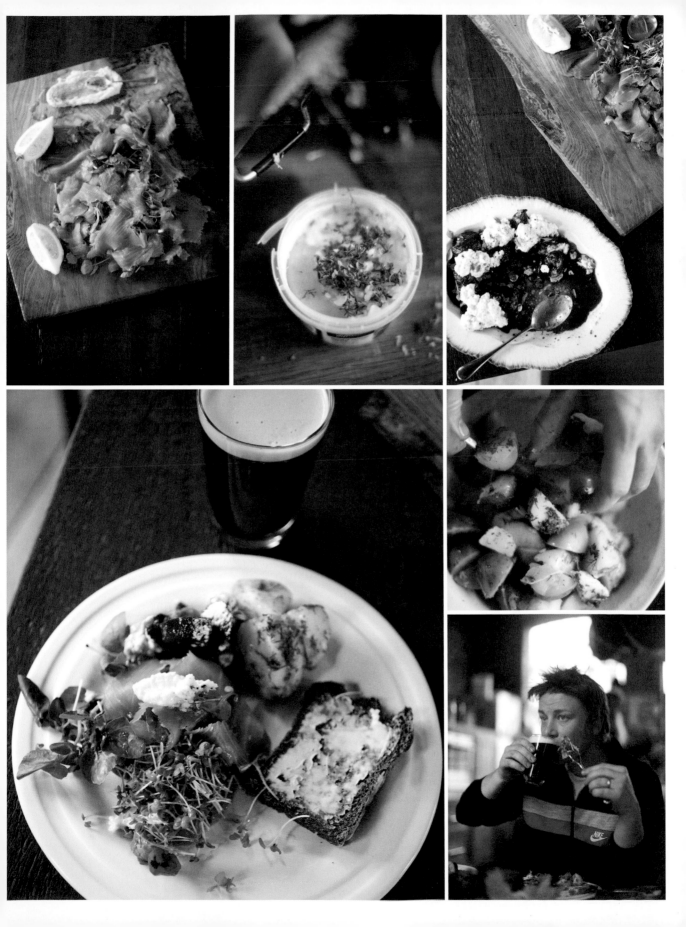

SMOKY HADDOCK CORN CHOWDER

SPICED TIGER PRAWNS

RAINBOW SALAD

RASPBERRY & ELDERFLOWER SLUSHIE

SERVES 4

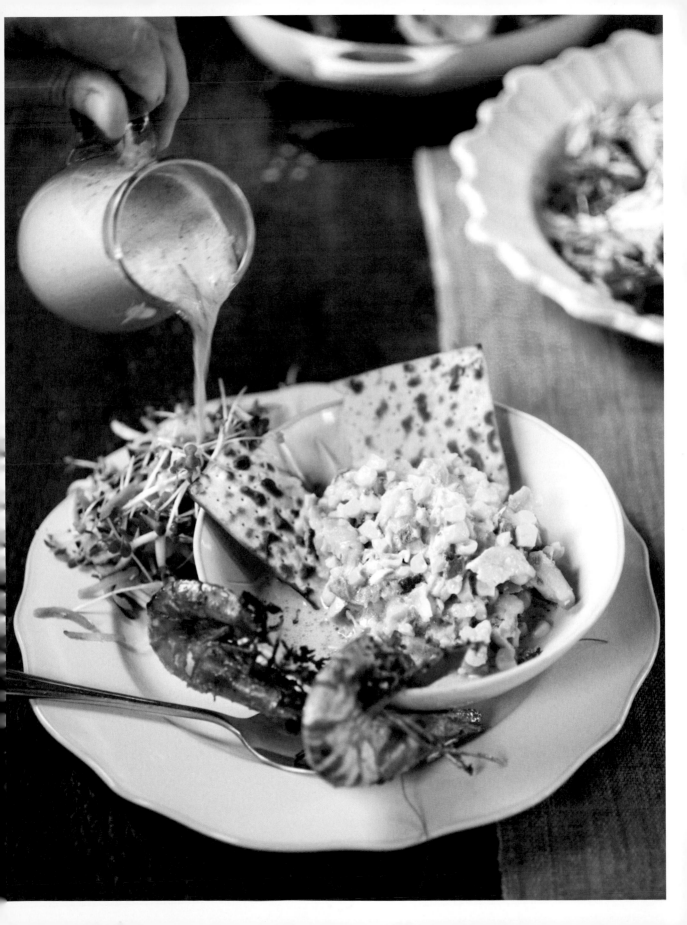

CHOWDER

4 rashers of smoked streaky bacon
a small bunch of spring onions
250g red-skinned potatoes
4 corn on the cob
1 x 300g fillet of smoked haddock,
 skin off and pin-boned
3 fresh bay leaves
3 sprigs of fresh thyme
1 litre organic chicken stock
150ml single cream
200g peeled cooked prawns
1 x 150g pack of large matzo crackers
 or similar (look in your supermarket)

SPICED PRAWNS

8 large unpeeled raw tiger prawns
a knob of butter
a few sprigs of fresh thyme
1 level teaspoon cayenne pepper
ground cinnamon
4 cloves of garlic
½ a fresh red chilli
½ a lemon

SEASONINGS

olive oil
extra virgin olive oil
sea salt & pepper

SALAD

½ a fresh red chilli
1 clove of garlic
a small bunch of fresh tarragon
2 tablespoons red wine vinegar
3 tablespoons low-fat natural yoghurt
1 large courgette
2 carrots
1 fresh red or golden beetroot
1 punnet of cress

BERRY SLUSHIE

ice cubes
2 sprigs of fresh mint
elderflower cordial
150g raspberries
1 litre bottle of soda water

TO START Get all your ingredients and equipment ready. Fit the coarse grater attachment into the food processor. Put a large deep saucepan on a high heat. Turn the grill to full whack.

CHOWDER Finely slice the bacon and put it into the saucepan with a good lug of olive oil. Stir until golden. Trim and finely slice the spring onions, add to the pan and stir. Wash the potatoes and chop into 2cm chunks. Add to the pan and mix well. Keep an eye on the pan, stirring often. Meanwhile, put a clean tea towel over a board and ruffle up the edges to catch the corn. Hold a corn cob upright on the board and run a knife gently down to the base of the kernels, all the way round. Repeat with the rest of the cobs, discarding the cores. Tip the kernels directly from the tea towel into the pan. Add the smoked haddock to the pan with 3 bay leaves and the leaves from 3 sprigs of thyme. Cover with the chicken stock, then put the lid on and cook for 12 minutes.

SPICED PRAWNS Put the tiger prawns into an ovenproof pan with a few lugs of olive oil, a knob of butter, a pinch of salt & pepper, a few sprigs of thyme, 1 level teaspoon of cayenne pepper and a small pinch of cinnamon. Crush in 4 unpeeled cloves of garlic, then deseed ½ a chilli, slice and add to the pan with ½ a lemon. Toss and mix well, then put under the grill on the top shelf for 8 to 10 minutes, or until dark pink and golden on the tips. Once ready, take out of the oven and leave to sit until ready to serve.

SALAD To make the dressing put ½ a red chilli, 1 peeled clove of garlic, a small bunch of tarragon, a pinch of salt & pepper, 2 tablespoons of red wine vinegar, 6 tablespoons of extra virgin olive oil and 3 tablespoons of low-fat natural yoghurt into a liquidizer. Whiz until combined. Have a taste – you want the salt and acid to be slightly over the top, so tweak if needed and whiz again. Pour into a small jug and take to the table.

CHOWDER Stir well, then put the lid back on.

SALAD Wash and trim the courgette and carrots. Quickly peel the beetroot. Using the coarse grater attachment, grate the vegetables one at a time, all in the food processor. Tip out on to a platter so it looks like a rainbow and snip cress over the top. Put on the table next to the jug of dressing and dress at the last minute.

CHOWDER Add the 150ml of single cream and the peeled prawns to the chowder and stir well. Put the lid back on and turn the heat down to low. Put the matzo crackers in a pile on the table.

BERRY SLUSHIE Rinse the food processor bowl and fit the standard blade attachment. Add a pint glass or 2 large handfuls of ice cubes and the leaves from 2 sprigs of mint and blitz to a slush. Leave the processor running and add 50ml of elderflower cordial and the raspberries. Pour in 500ml of soda water and leave to whiz until combined. Taste, adding another little splash of elderflower cordial to sweeten if needed. Pour into a large jug, top up with soda water and stir again right before serving.

CHOWDER Take the saucepan off the heat. You can leave it coarse and chunky, or use a potato masher to mash it up a little bit and make it silky, or purée the lot – it's up to you. I like to roughly mash one side of it, then mix it through.

TO SERVE Take the tiger prawns to the table with the saucepan of chowder. Roughly break a few crackers into each bowl, ladle the chowder on top and finish off with a couple of tiger prawns on the side. Toss the salad in the dressing, taste and season, then tuck in.

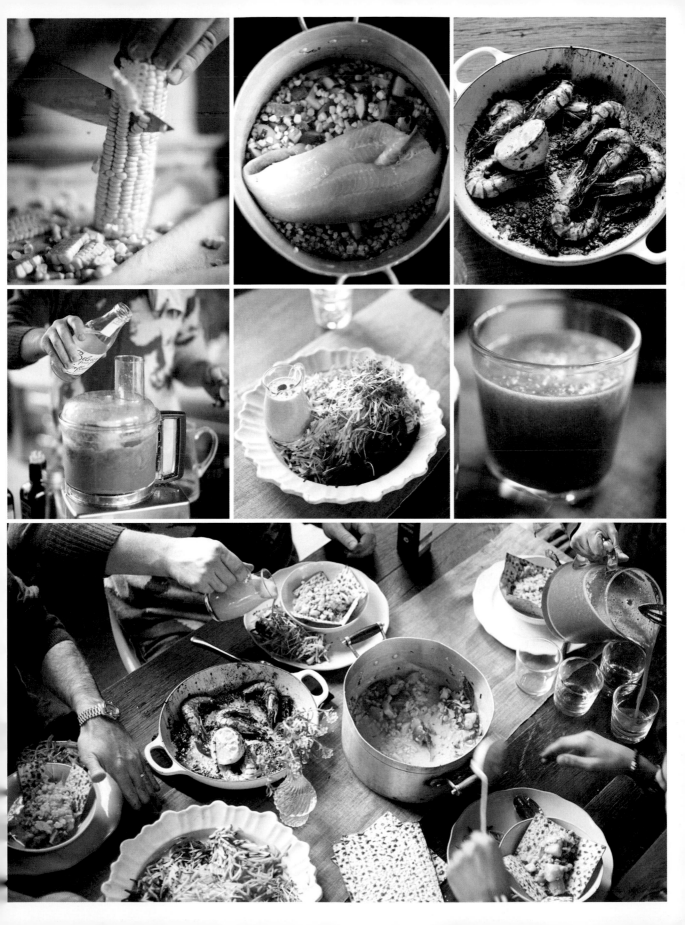

FISH TRAY-BAKE

SERVES 4 (makes enough banoffee pie for 10)

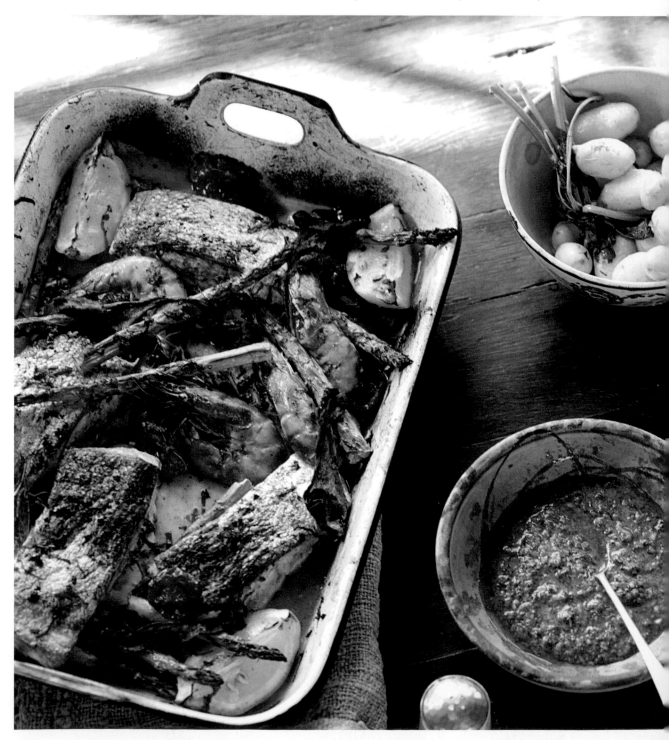

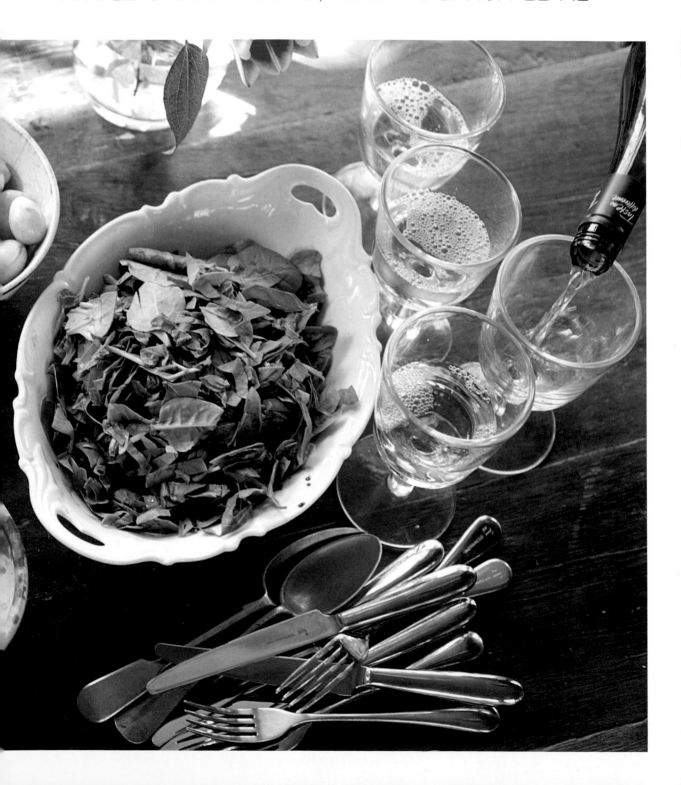

POTATOES

500g baby Jersey Royals or new
  potatoes
stalks from a large bunch of fresh
  mint
a squeeze of lemon juice

FISH

4 x 150g salmon fillets, skin on,
  scaled and pin-boned
8 large unpeeled raw tiger prawns
a bunch of asparagus
1 lemon
1 fresh red chilli
a small bunch of fresh basil
1 x 30g tin of anchovies in oil
4 cloves of garlic
3–4 tomatoes
4 slices of pancetta

SALSA VERDE

leaves from ½ a bunch of fresh
  mint (from the bunch used for
  the potatoes)
a small bunch of fresh flat-leaf parsley
1 clove of garlic
2 tablespoons red wine vinegar
1 heaped teaspoon Dijon mustard
1 heaped teaspoon capers
2 cornichons

SPINACH SALAD

balsamic vinegar
1 lemon
leaves from ½ a bunch of fresh mint
  (from the bunch used for the
  potatoes)
1 x 200g bag of prewashed baby
  spinach

SEASONINGS

olive oil
extra virgin olive oil
sea salt & black pepper

BANOFFEE PIE (serves 8–10)

4 heaped tablespoons golden caster
  sugar
4 ripe bananas
100ml semi-skimmed milk
1 pre-made sweet pastry case
  (approx. 200g)
300ml double cream
1 tablespoon Camp coffee
1 x 100g bar of good-quality dark
  chocolate (70% cocoa solids), to
  serve

TO START Get all your ingredients and equipment ready. Make a space in your freezer for a platter big enough to rest the pastry case on. Fill and boil the kettle. Put a saucepan on a high heat and turn the grill to full whack. Put the standard blade attachment into the food processor.

POTATOES Wash the potatoes and tip them into the saucepan. Rip the leafy tops off the bunch of mint and set aside. Leave the band on the mint then add the stalks to the saucepan with a pinch of salt. Just cover with boiled water and put the lid on.

BANOFFEE PIE Put a medium frying pan on a high heat. Put 4 heaped tablespoons of golden caster sugar into the frying pan and shake the pan to spread it around. Let it melt while you peel 2 of the bananas and blitz them with 100ml of milk in a liquidizer until you have a smoothie consistency. Carefully tilt the frying pan to help dissolve all the sugar. Once bubbling and golden, pour in the banana mixture. Do not touch anything in the pan – caramel is very hot and can burn badly. Keep stirring constantly, so it doesn't catch, for 1 to 2 minutes, until dark and golden, then pour into the pastry case (🎬). Spoon and spread it around evenly, then carefully slide the pastry case on to a platter and put it into the freezer to cool down for a few minutes.

FISH Lay the salmon fillets and prawns in a large roasting tray. Snap off the woody ends of the asparagus, then add the spears to the tray with a good pinch of salt & pepper. Quarter a lemon and add it to the tray. Finely chop the chilli and add to the tray with the basil leaves. Drizzle over the oil from the tin of anchovies and tear in 4 of the fillets. Crush in 4 unpeeled cloves of garlic and drizzle over some olive oil. Roughly chop the tomatoes and add.

Arrange everything nicely in the tray, so the lemons are facing up and the salmon is skin side up. Drape 4 slices of pancetta wherever you like in the tray, then whack under the grill on the middle shelf for about 10 minutes, or until the pancetta is lovely and crisp and the fish is cooked through.

POTATOES Check the potatoes are cooked through, then turn the heat off and drain them. Discard the mint stalks and tip the potatoes into a serving bowl and dress with a lug of extra virgin olive oil, a squeeze of lemon juice and a pinch of salt & pepper.

SALSA VERDE Put half of the reserved mint leaves into the food processor. Rip in all the parsley leaves, discarding the stalks. Peel a clove of garlic and add to the processor with the rest of the anchovy fillets, 2 tablespoons of red wine vinegar, 1 heaped teaspoon each of Dijon mustard and capers, the cornichons and 6 tablespoons of extra virgin olive oil. Blitz until combined, then taste and adjust the flavours if needed. Tip into a little bowl and take to the table.

SPINACH SALAD Pour a couple of lugs of extra virgin olive oil into a serving bowl. Add a pinch of salt & pepper, a couple of lugs of balsamic vinegar and a good squeeze of lemon juice. Finely slice the last of the mint leaves and add to the bowl. Tip the spinach on to a chopping board, scrunch it up and cut it into 1cm slices. Pile the spinach on top of the dressing and take to the table to dress at the last minute.

BANOFFEE PIE In a large bowl, whip the double cream with a balloon whisk until fairly thick. Lightly fold through 1 tablespoon of Camp coffee to get a marbled effect. Peel and finely slice your 2 remaining bananas at an angle. Get your filled base out of the freezer and top with slices of banana. Use a spatula to tip the cream on top of the pie. Scrape over a little dark chocolate (🎬) and pop back into the freezer until ready to serve.

FISH Take the tray straight from the oven to the table. Serve the fish and potatoes with a bottle of chilled white wine.

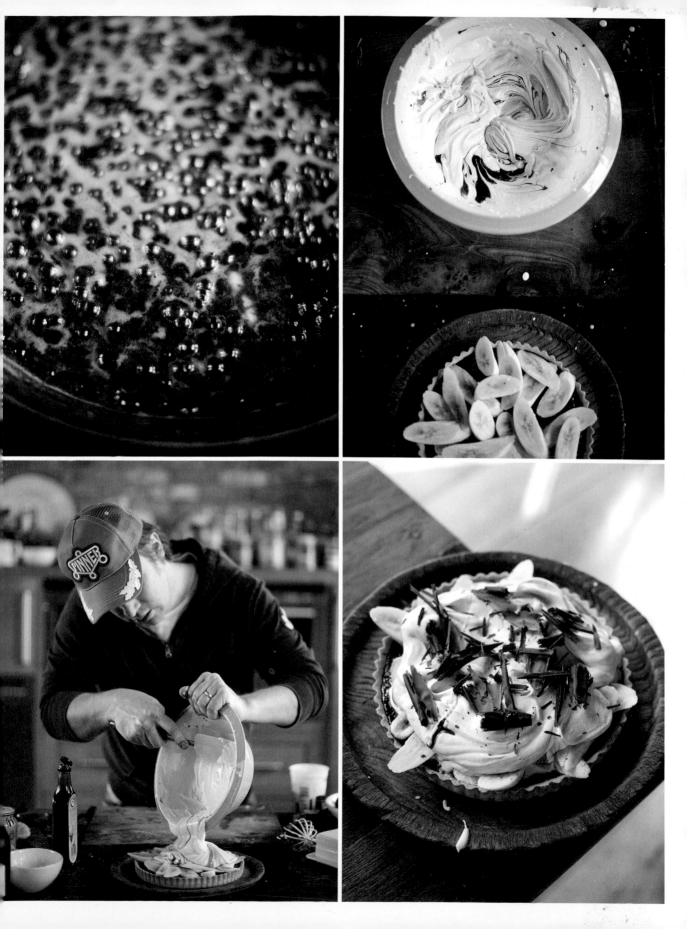

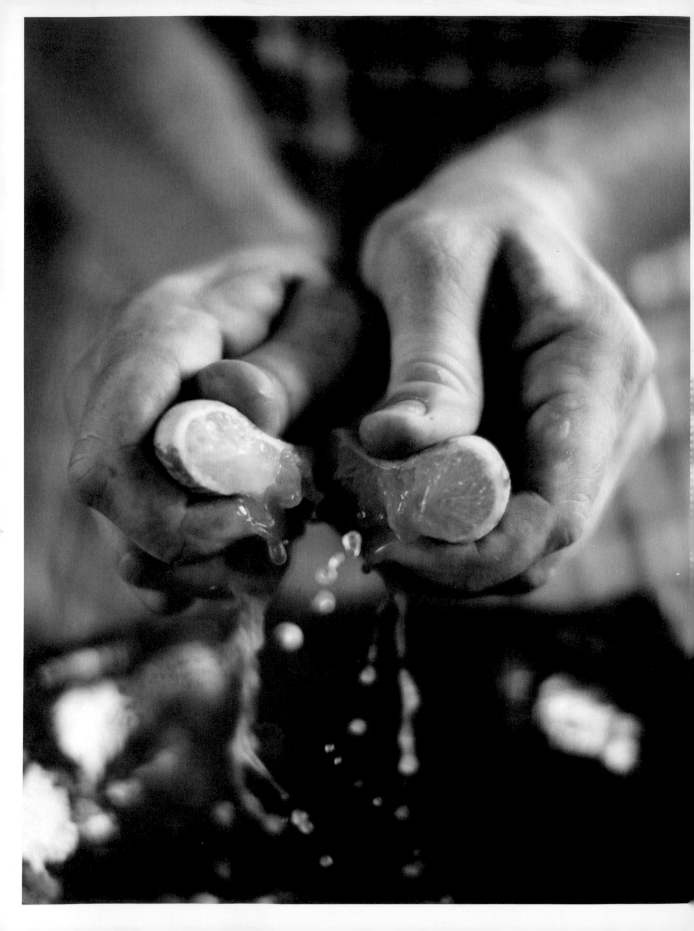

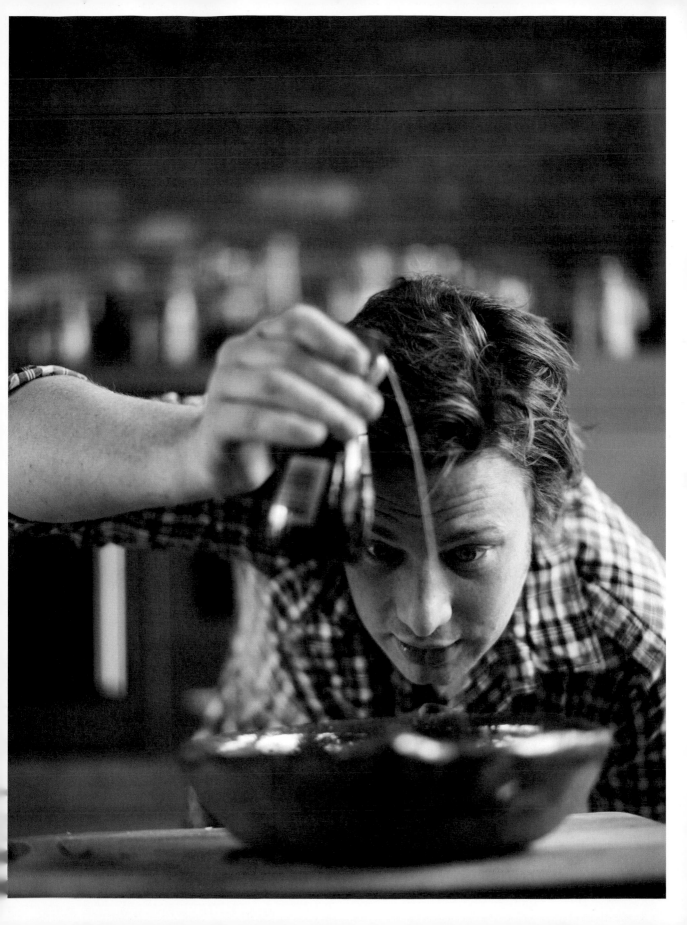

BLOODY MARY
MUSSELS
HERBY SALAD
GORGEOUS RHUBARB
MILLEFEUILLE

SERVES 4

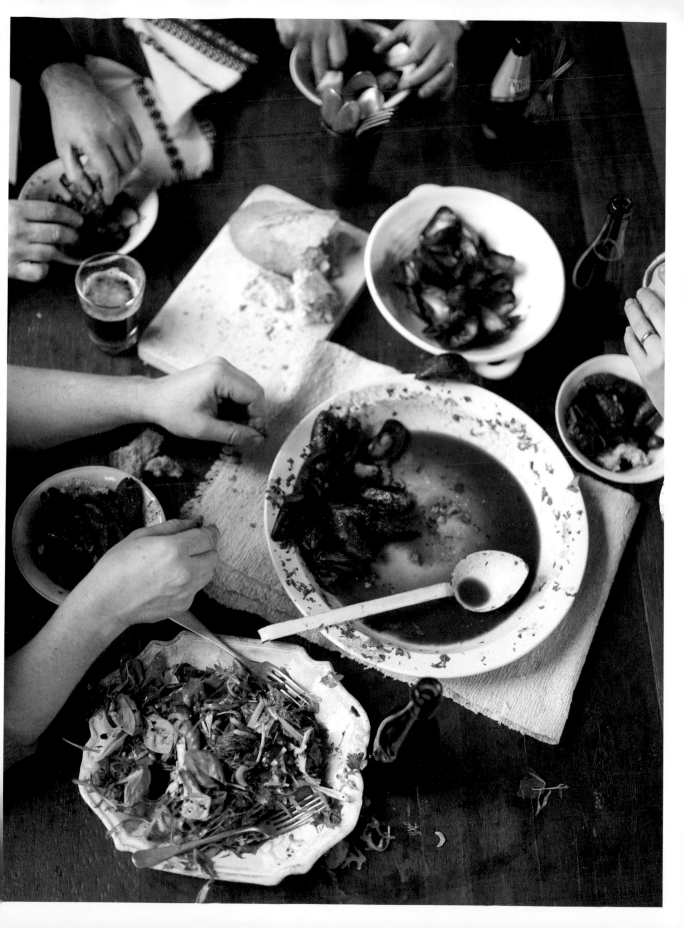

MUSSELS

300ml passata
1 tablespoon Worcestershire sauce
3 heaped teaspoons jarred horseradish
½–1 fresh red chilli, to taste
½ a head of celery
4 cloves of garlic
a splash of port
a good splash of vodka
1 lemon
2kg mussels, cleaned and debearded
  (ask your fishmonger to do this for you)
a small bunch of fresh flat-leaf
  parsley

HERBY SALAD

5 small tomatoes
balsamic vinegar
½ a lemon
5 sprigs each of fresh parsley,
  tarragon, dill, mint and basil
1 x 100g bag of prewashed rocket

SEASONINGS

olive oil
extra virgin olive oil
sea salt & black pepper

RHUBARB MILLEFEUILLE

plain flour, for dusting
1 x 375g pack of pre-rolled puff pastry
1 egg
200g rhubarb
2 heaped tablespoons golden caster
  sugar
1 orange
a 2cm piece of fresh ginger
1 teaspoon of vanilla paste or extract
125g crème fraîche
150g tub of good-quality custard

TO SERVE

a loaf of crusty bread
good ale or Belgian beer

TO START Get all your ingredients and equipment ready. Turn the oven on to 190°C/375°F/gas 5. Put a large saucepan with a lid and a smaller saucepan on a medium heat.

RHUBARB MILLEFEUILLE Dust a clean baking tray with flour. Unroll the sheet of puff pastry and cut in half so you end up with two 20 x 20cm squares of pastry. Put one half on the baking tray, freeze the rest for another time. Push down on each corner with your thumb, then score lightly all around the edges, about 1cm in, to create a border. Lightly run the knife over the pastry in a crisscross pattern. Beat the egg in a little bowl and use a pastry brush to paint it all over the pastry. Put into the oven on a high shelf for around 20 minutes.

Slice the rhubarb about 1cm thick and put it into the smaller saucepan with 2 heaped tablespoons of golden caster sugar. Finely grate over the zest of ½ an orange. Peel and finely grate 2cm of ginger and add to the pan. Add a teaspoon of vanilla paste or extract. Put the lid on. Check, stirring occasionally, as you get on with other things.

MUSSELS Put the loaf of bread in the oven on a low shelf to warm through. Pour the passata into a jug with 1 tablespoon of Worcestershire sauce and 3 heaped teaspoons of horseradish. Slice ½ a chilli very finely (or slice up more if you like it hot) and add to the jug. Pull the head of celery apart, wash the heart, then put the delicate yellow leaves on a serving platter. Trim the bottom off the celery stalks, then finely slice 2 or 3 stalks and add to the jug. Crush in 4 unpeeled cloves of garlic and add a swig of port and a generous swig of vodka. Stir really well. Squeeze in the juice of 1 lemon and season with a pinch of salt & pepper.

RHUBARB MILLEFEUILLE The rhubarb should have cooked down now, so turn the heat off and leave it to stand with the lid off so it thickens up.

HERBY SALAD Chop up the tomatoes and remaining celery and put on a serving platter. Scatter over a good pinch of salt & pepper and drizzle over some extra virgin olive oil and a little balsamic vinegar. Squeeze over the juice of ½ a lemon.

MUSSELS Pick through your cleaned mussels. If any are open, give them a tap; if they don't close, throw them away. Tip all the good mussels into the hot saucepan and pour in the bloody Mary mixture. Put the lid on, then shake the pan around and leave the mussels to steam open. Turn the heat up to high.

HERBY SALAD Pick the leaves from your herbs and add to the serving platter with the rocket. Add another lug of extra virgin olive oil and balsamic vinegar and season with a pinch of salt & pepper. Take to the table to toss and dress at the last minute.

MUSSELS Check on the mussels and give the saucepan another good shake.

RHUBARB MILLEFEUILLE By now, your puff pastry should be golden and beautiful, so take it out of the oven and use your hands or a fish slice to gently press the puffed-up middle back down. Leave to cool for a couple of minutes, then transfer to a serving board or platter. Take the warm bread out of the oven and take to the table.

MUSSELS Once all the mussels have popped open, remove them from the pan with a slotted spoon and put them on to a serving platter, leaving the cooking liquor in the pan over a high heat to thicken and reduce. If any of the mussels are still closed, throw them away. Finely chop the top of the small bunch of parsley. Pour the hot cooking juices all over the mussels. Drizzle with olive oil, scatter over the chopped parsley and take to the table. Divide between 4 serving bowls and let everyone mop up the juices with hunks of warm bread.

RHUBARB MILLEFEUILLE When ready for dessert, dollop and drizzle most of the crème fraîche and custard all over the pastry base. Top with spoonfuls of the stewed rhubarb, then the rest of the crème fraîche and custard, and take to the table so everyone can have a slice.

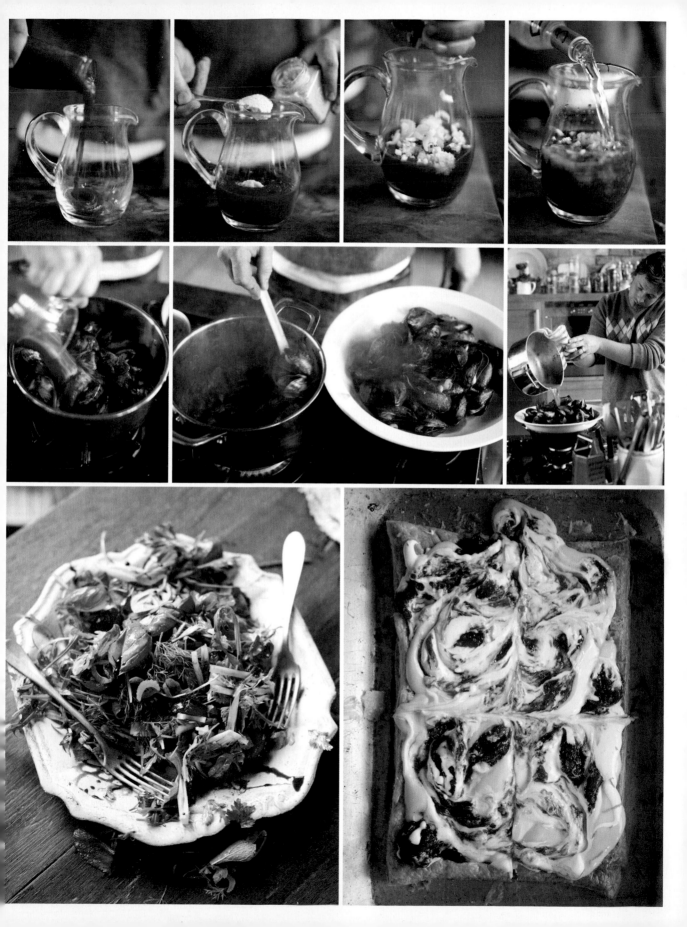

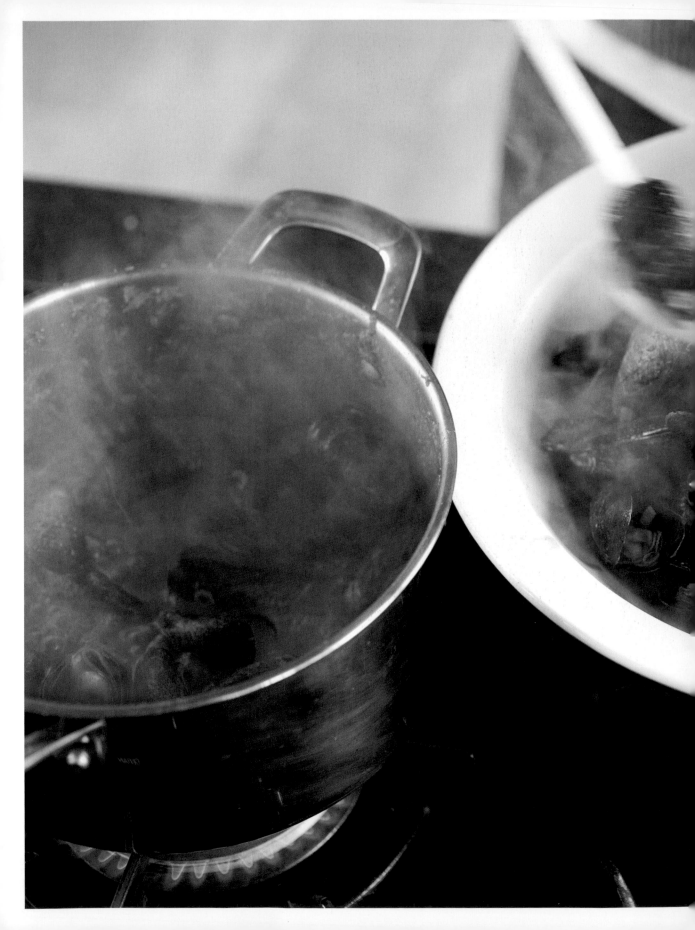

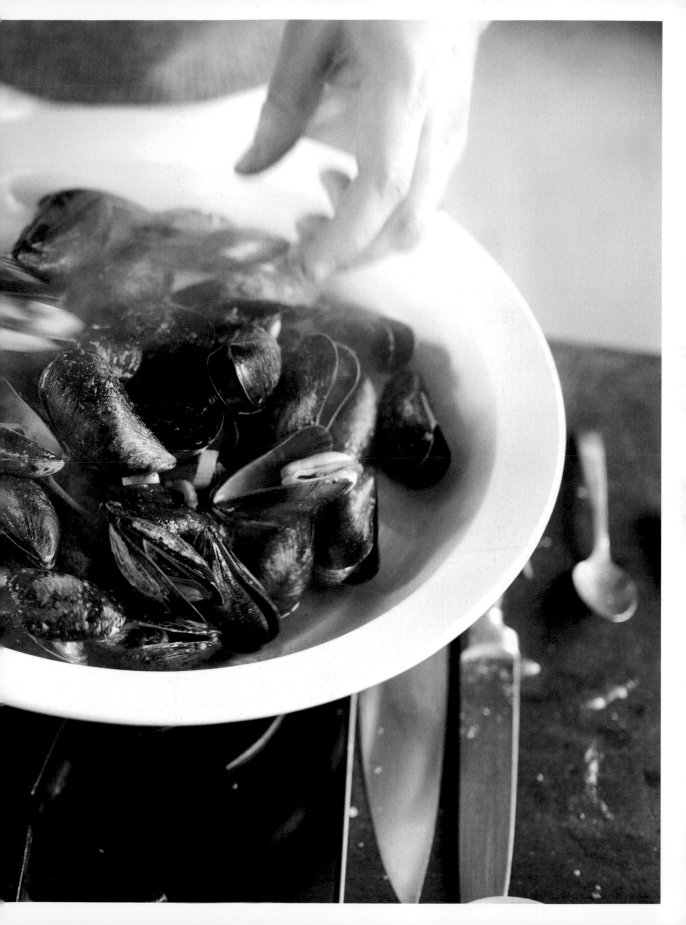

SEA BASS & CRISPY PANCETTA

SWEET POTATO MASH

ASIAN GREENS

1-MINUTE BERRY ICE CREAM

SPARKLING LEMON GINGER DRINK

SERVES 4

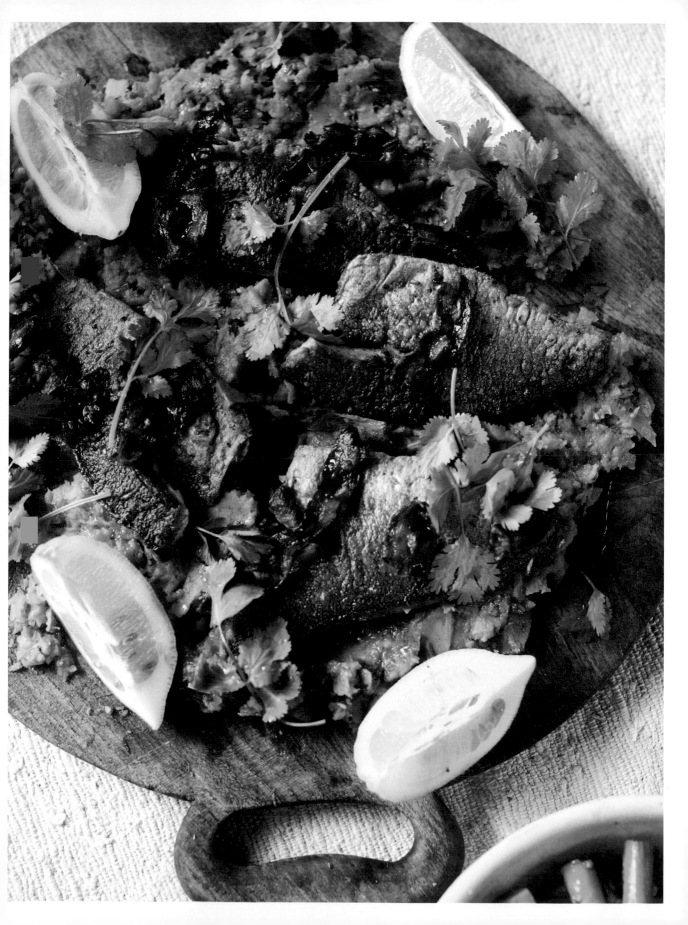

MASH
700g sweet potatoes
2 limes
a small bunch of fresh coriander
2 tablespoons mango chutney
soy sauce

GREENS
1 fresh red chilli
1 clove of garlic
soy sauce
1 lime
sesame oil
100g asparagus
1 head of broccoli

SEA BASS
8 thin slices of pancetta
4 x 150g fillets of sea bass, skin on,
  scaled and pin-boned
1 teaspoon fennel seeds
1 lemon

SEASONINGS
olive oil
extra virgin olive oil
sea salt & black pepper

LEMON GINGER DRINK
ice cubes
1 x 330ml can of fizzy lemonade
a few sprigs of fresh mint
a 2cm piece of fresh ginger
1 bottle of sparkling water

BERRY ICE CREAM
1 x 500g pack of mixed frozen berries
150g fresh blueberries
3–4 tablespoons runny honey
1 x 500g tub of natural yoghurt
a few sprigs of fresh mint

TO START Get all your ingredients and equipment ready. Fill and boil the kettle. Put a large saucepan with a lid and a large frying pan on a medium heat. Put 4 small glasses in the freezer for the dessert. Put the standard blade attachment into the food processor.

MASH Wash the sweet potatoes, trim off any gnarly bits, then stab them a few times with a knife. Put in a large microwave-safe bowl, halve one of the limes and add to the bowl, then cover with a double layer of clingfilm and microwave on full power for 12 minutes, or until cooked through.

GREENS Deseed and finely chop the chilli, adding half to a large serving bowl and setting the rest aside. Crush the unpeeled clove of garlic into the bowl and add 2 tablespoons of soy sauce and 4 to 6 tablespoons of extra virgin olive oil. Squeeze in the juice of 1 lime and add a splash of sesame oil. Mix, taste and tweak with the soy sauce if needed. Trim the asparagus stalks. Quarter the head of the broccoli lengthways from the head to the base of the stalk.

SEA BASS Put the pancetta into the frying pan with a drizzle of olive oil. Keep an eye on it, turning when crispy.

DRINK Fill a large jug halfway with ice. Add the lemonade and mint sprigs. Peel and finely grate in 2cm of ginger. Top up with sparkling water, mix with a wooden spoon and take to the table.

SEA BASS By now the pancetta should be golden so remove it to a plate, leaving the fat in the pan. Add the fish to the pan, skin side down. Shake the pan and use a spatula to press the fillets flat for a few seconds. Pound 1 teaspoon of fennel seeds in a pestle & mortar and scatter over the fish from a height with a pinch of salt & pepper. Finely grate over the zest of 1 lemon, then cut the lemon into quarters and set aside.

MASH Finely chop the coriander on a large wooden chopping board, setting a few leaves aside for the garnish.

Add the mango chutney, a good splash of soy sauce, a drizzle of extra virgin olive oil, the juice from ½ a lime and the reserved chopped chilli. Chop and mix everything together on the board.

GREENS Fill the large saucepan with boiling water and add a large pinch of salt. Add the broccoli and asparagus, making sure they are completely submerged. Put the lid on and turn the heat to high.

SEA BASS Check the fish – once the skin is golden and crispy, turn the heat down to low – but have confidence to let the skin become good and crispy before reducing the heat.

MASH Get the sweet potatoes out of the microwave and check they are cooked through, then use tongs to squeeze over the juice from the hot lime halves and discard them. Carefully tip the sweet potatoes on top of the mango chutney mixture and use a knife or masher to chop and mash everything together, including the skins. Season to taste, adding more fresh lime juice if needed.

SEA BASS Take the pan of fish off the heat and flip the fillets over so they gently finish cooking on the flesh side. Return the pancetta to the pan to warm through, then serve the fish and pancetta on top of the board of mash. Pop the lemon wedges on the side for squeezing and sprinkle over the reserved coriander. Take to the table.

GREENS Drain the broccoli and asparagus in a colander, then tip into the serving bowl with the dressing, quickly toss and take to the table.

BERRY ICE CREAM Get the glasses and the frozen berries out of the freezer. Divide the fresh blueberries between the glasses. Put the honey and yoghurt and leaves from the sprigs of mint into the food processor and whiz, then add the frozen berries and whiz again until combined. Spoon the frozen yoghurt over the fresh berries and serve. Yum.

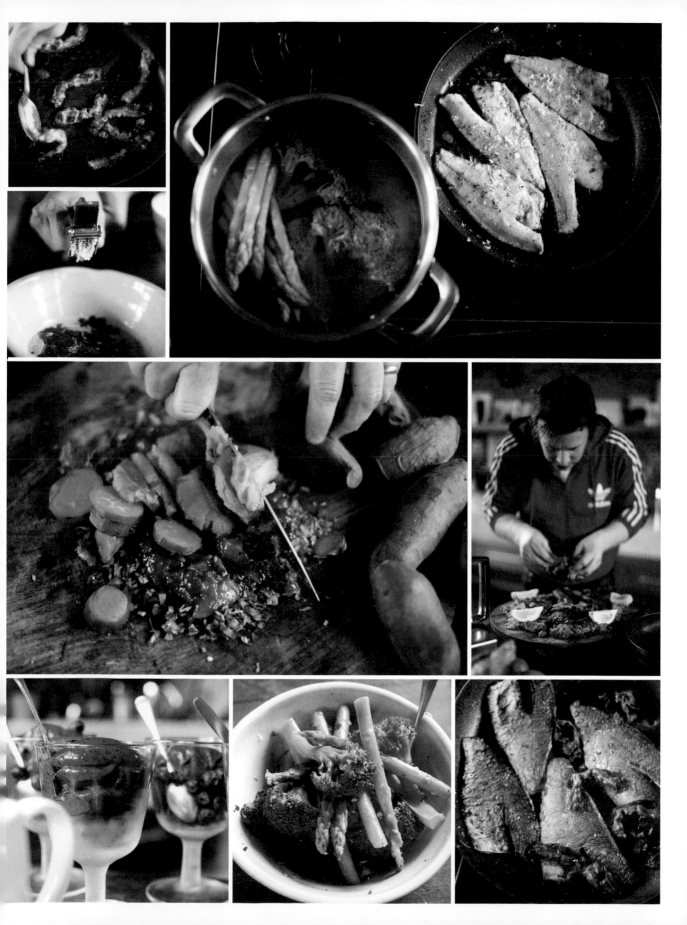

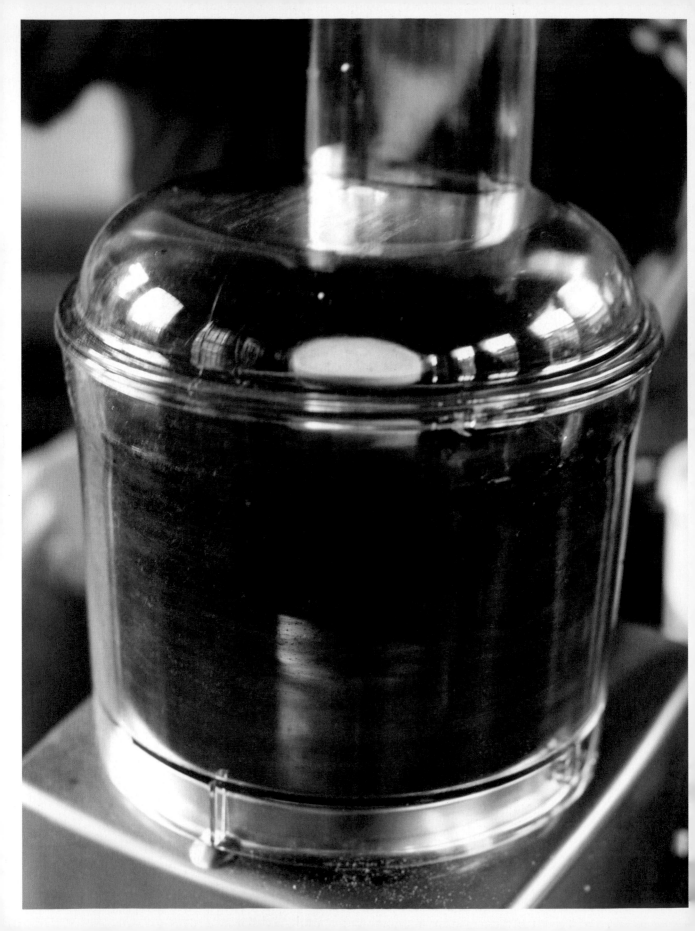

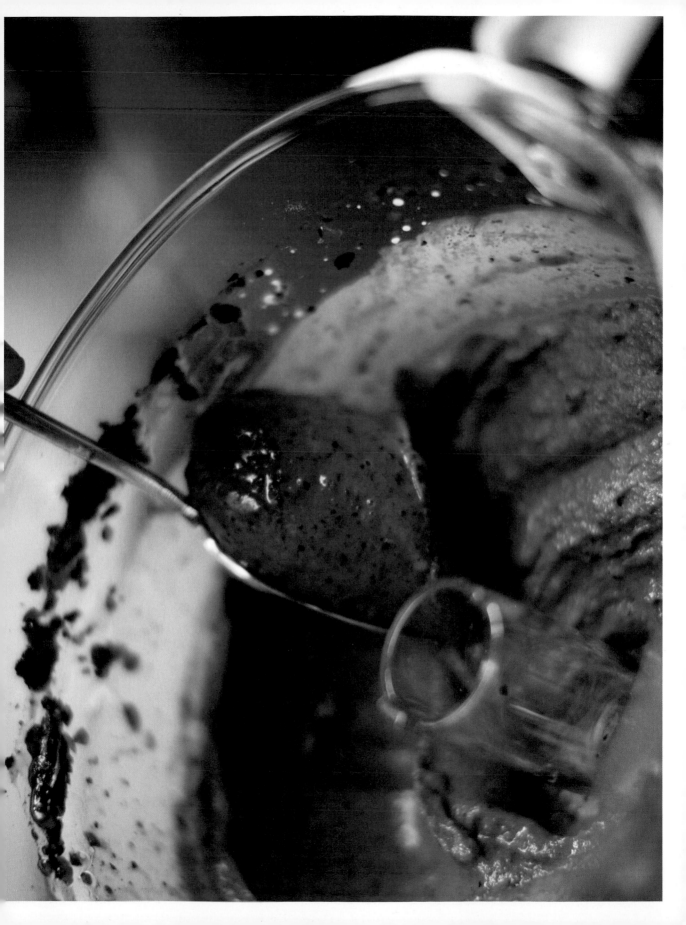

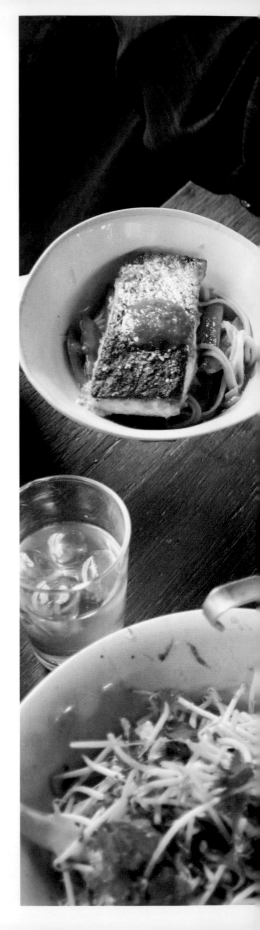

ASIAN-STYLE SALMON
NOODLE BROTH
BEANSPROUT SALAD
LYCHEE DESSERT

SERVES 4

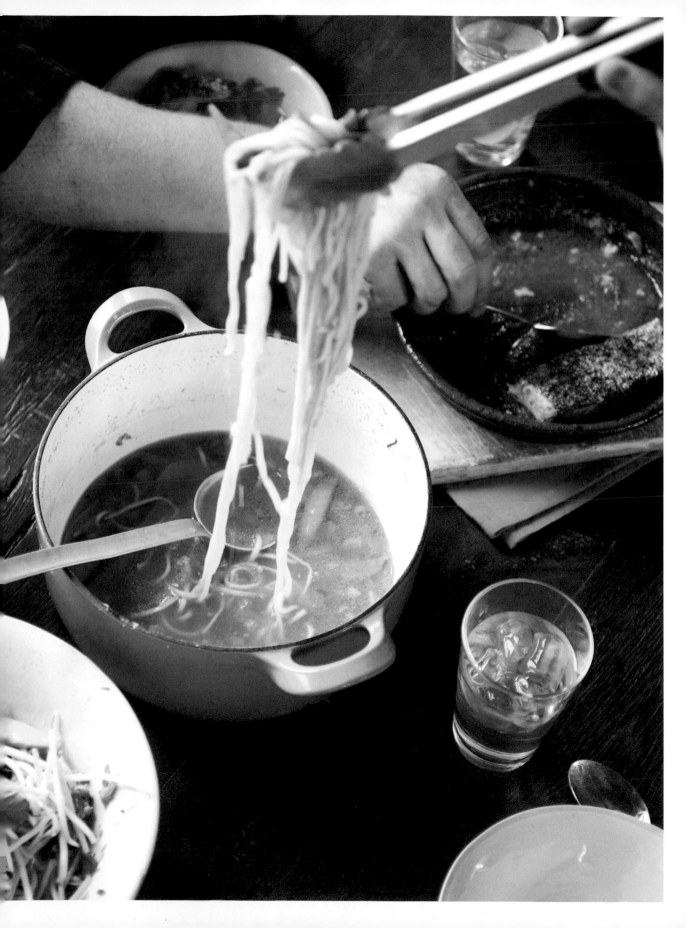

SALMON
a 2cm piece of fresh ginger
2 cloves of garlic
1 small red onion
½ a fresh red chilli
1 tablespoon soy sauce
2 limes
4 x 180g salmon fillets, skin on, scaled
  and pin-boned
Chinese five-spice

SALAD
a large bunch of fresh coriander
1 x 400g bag of beansprouts
100g cashew nuts
runny honey, for drizzling
½ a fresh red chilli
1 small ripe mango
soy sauce
sesame oil
1 lime or lemon

BROTH
4 spring onions
1–2 fresh red chillies
2 cloves of garlic
a 2cm piece of fresh ginger
1 teaspoon Chinese five-spice
3 teaspoons cornflour
1 organic chicken stock cube
200g sugar snap peas
soy sauce, to taste

200g dried fine egg noodles

SEASONINGS
olive oil
extra virgin olive oil
sea salt & black pepper

LYCHEE DESSERT
125g blueberries
1 x 425g tin of lychees in syrup
2 packs of sesame snaps
1 x 500ml tub of good-quality vanilla
  ice cream
a sprig of fresh mint

TO START Get all your ingredients and equipment ready. Fill and boil the kettle. Turn the oven on to 250°C/480°F/gas 9.

SALMON Peel a 2cm piece of fresh ginger, 2 cloves of garlic and a small red onion. Roughly chop and put into a liquidizer with ½ a red chilli and 1 tablespoon of soy sauce. Squeeze in the juice of 2 limes and blitz to a slurry. Taste to check the balance of sweet and salty, then put into an earthenware dish or a tin that will snugly fit the salmon. Add a couple of lugs of olive oil and put the salmon, skin side up, in the dish. Sprinkle a little five-spice and black pepper over the skin and whack into the oven on the top shelf for 18 minutes, or until beautifully cooked through.

SALAD Set aside a few coriander sprigs for garnish, then pick the leaves off the remainder and put them into a large bowl. Finely slice the stalks, then add to the bowl with the beansprouts and set aside. Put a large frying pan on a low heat.

BROTH Put a large saucepan on a medium heat. Trim and finely slice 4 spring onions, and put into the pan with a good lug of olive oil. Finely slice a red chilli and add to the pan, then stir and crush in 2 unpeeled cloves of garlic. Peel and finely grate in a 2cm piece of fresh ginger. Mix well.

SALAD Wrap the cashews in a clean tea towel and bash with a rolling pin or against the worktop, then put in the empty frying pan. Add a lug of olive oil, toss and leave to toast. Toss occasionally until golden.

BROTH Stir 1 teaspoon of five-spice and 3 teaspoons of cornflour into the pan of spring onions. Pour in 900ml of chicken stock and add 200g of sugar snaps. Turn the heat up to high, bring to the boil, then taste and correct the seasoning with soy sauce. Add the noodles and pop the lid on.

SALAD Check the cashews; they should be golden by now, so remove the pan from the heat, add a good drizzle of honey, then toss and set aside.

LYCHEE DESSERT Flip the chopping board over. Cut a small handful of blueberries in half and put into a large bowl with the rest of the whole blueberries. Tip the lychees into the bowl with some of their juices. Stir, then take to the table.

SALAD Finely slice the chilli half. Speed-peel the mango, then slice, clank and chip away at the flesh and add to the salad with the sliced chilli. Tip the honey-toasted cashews over the top. Dress with lugs of soy sauce, extra virgin olive oil and sesame oil, and the juice of 1 lime or lemon. Toss with your hands (but be careful in case the cashews are still hot).

LYCHEE DESSERT Wrap the sesame snap packs in a clean tea towel and whack them against a worktop to smash them to a powder. Tip out into a small bowl and take to the table with the ice cream.

TO SERVE Take the broth and the salad to the table. Remove the salmon from the oven, sprinkle over the reserved coriander and take straight to the table. Use tongs to divide the noodles and broth between the bowls. Top each one with a piece of salmon and some spoonfuls of the delicious sauce from the roasting tin.

LYCHEE DESSERT When ready, assemble the puds by layering up a couple of scoops of ice cream with the fruit in 4 little cups. Drizzle over the juices from the bowl, top each cup with a couple of fresh mint leaves and scatter over the crushed sesame snaps.

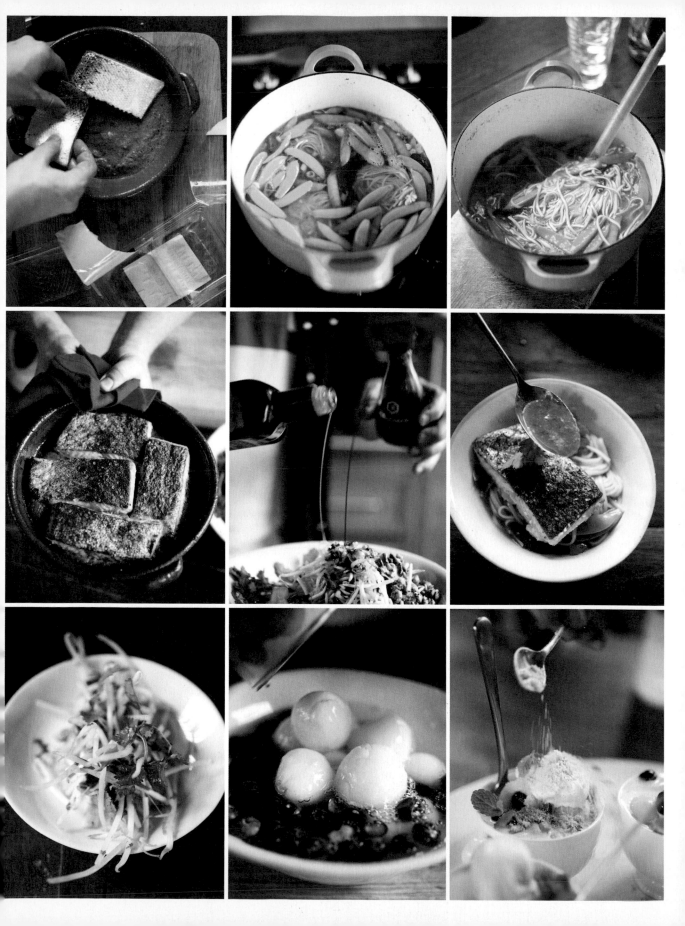

CRISPY SALMON

JAZZED-UP RICE

BABY COURGETTE SALAD

GORGEOUS GUACAMOLE

BERRY SPRITZER

SERVES 6

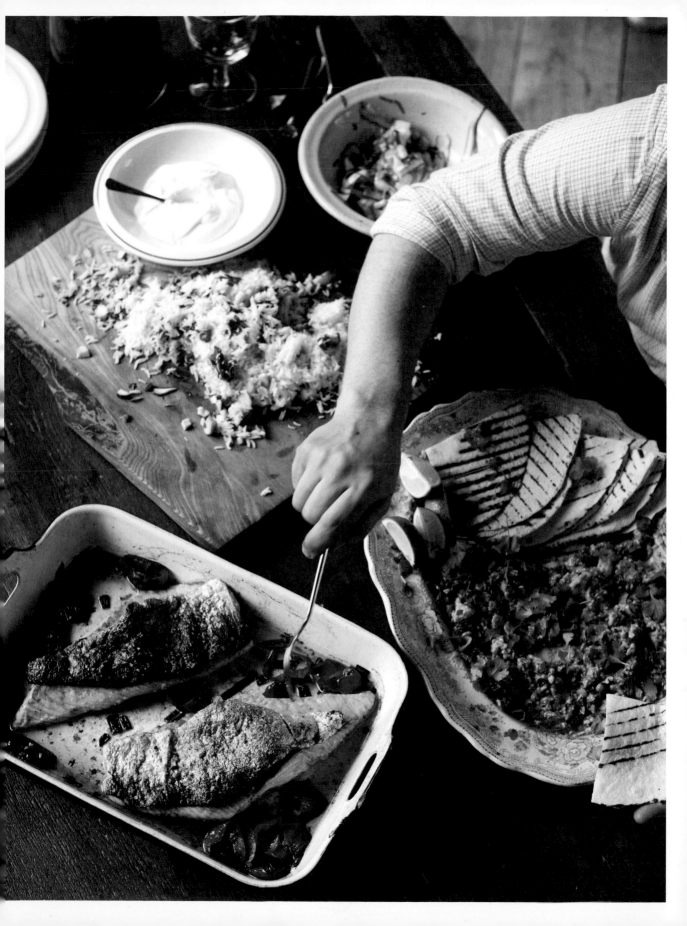

SALMON
2 long peppers, red and yellow
a bunch of spring onions
2 fresh red chillies
1 x 1kg fillet of salmon, skin on,
  scaled and pin-boned
1 lemon
fennel seeds

RICE
1 mug of basmati rice
½ a 450g jar of red peppers
a few sprigs of fresh basil
balsamic vinegar

SALAD
1 lemon
a couple of sprigs of fresh mint
1–2 fresh red chillies
400g baby courgettes

SEASONINGS
olive oil
extra virgin olive oil
sea salt & black pepper

GUACAMOLE
4 spring onions
a small bunch of fresh coriander
1 fresh red chilli
1 clove of garlic

2 limes
2–3 small ripe avocados
1 handful of cherry tomatoes

EXTRAS
1 pack of tortilla wraps
1 x 150ml tub of soured cream

SPRITZER
1 large punnet of blueberries,
  blackberries or strawberries
ice cubes
a few sprigs of fresh mint
a bottle of sparkling water

TO START Get all your ingredients and equipment ready. Fill and boil the kettle. Turn the grill on to full whack. Put a saucepan on a medium heat. Put the standard blade attachment into the food processor.

SALMON Pour a couple of lugs of olive oil into a large roasting tray. Halve and deseed the red pepper. Slice the pepper and the bunch of spring onions into 2cm pieces. Roughly chop the chillies. Drizzle olive oil over both sides of the salmon, season, and finely grate over some lemon zest. Rub these flavours all over the salmon, then wash your hands. If necessary, halve the salmon so it fits the roasting tray, then lay skin side up and arrange the sliced vegetables all around it. Whack under the grill on the middle shelf and set the timer for 14 minutes.

RICE Put the rice into a medium saucepan with a pinch of salt and cover by 1.5cm with boiling water. Put the lid on, then turn the heat right up and leave to cook for 7 minutes. Once cooked, take off the heat and leave to steam for 7 minutes, still covered with the lid.

SALAD Squeeze the juice of ½ a lemon into a large serving bowl and add a couple of lugs of extra virgin olive oil and a good pinch of salt & pepper. Finely chop the mint leaves and ½ a chilli and add to the bowl. Speed-peel as much of the baby courgettes as you can over the dressing and put whatever is left behind on a large wooden chopping board. Take the bowl of salad to the table but don't toss until right before you are ready to serve.

RICE Roughly chop and mix the jarred peppers and mint leaves on the chopping board with the remaining courgette. Add a pinch of salt & pepper, a good lug of extra virgin olive oil and a splash of balsamic.

SPRITZER Blitz the berries to a purée in the food processor. Half-fill a large jug with ice cubes and rip in the leaves from a few sprigs of mint. Put a sieve on top of the jug and quickly push the blitzed berries through, using the back of a spoon. Discard whatever is left behind, then top the jug up with sparkling water, stir and take to the table. Quickly rinse out the processor.

SALMON When the 14 minutes are up, take the tray out of the oven. Using a knife and your fingers, carefully peel the skin away from the flesh and flip it over. Add a pinch of salt and the fennel seeds. Turn the peppers over, then put the tray back under the grill and cook for a further 5 minutes, or until the skin is really crispy.

GUACAMOLE Trim the spring onions and put them into the processor with most of the coriander, the chilli (stalk removed), a peeled clove of garlic, the juice of 1 of your limes and a good drizzle of extra virgin olive oil. Whiz up while you stone the avocados and quarter the tomatoes. Stop whizzing, and squeeze the avocado flesh out of its skin into the processor. Add the tomatoes and pulse until chunky. Put into a bowl and add more seasoning or lime juice to taste if needed. Take to the table with a few wedges of lime for squeezing over.

RICE Quickly fluff up the rice with a fork, then tip over the board of chopped veg and gently mix together. Take to the table. Put a griddle pan on a high heat.

SALMON Use tongs to carefully turn the crispy salmon skin back over. Season with salt & pepper and cook for a further 5 minutes.

EXTRAS Warm the tortillas one at a time in the griddle pan for a few seconds on each side (or stack them up and put them into the microwave for 10 to 15 seconds). Tip the soured cream into a bowl, drizzle over a little extra virgin olive oil and take to the table.

TO SERVE Take the salmon straight to the table and serve with the lovely salad.

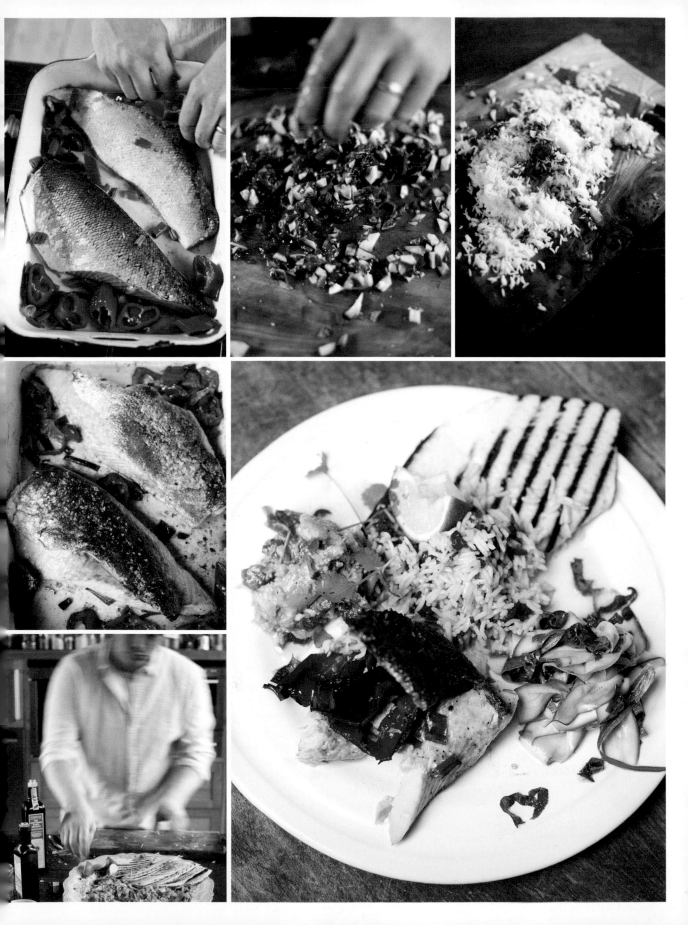

ROAST BEEF
BABY YORKIES
LITTLE CARROTS
CRISPY POTATOES
SUPER-QUICK GRAVY

SERVES 4

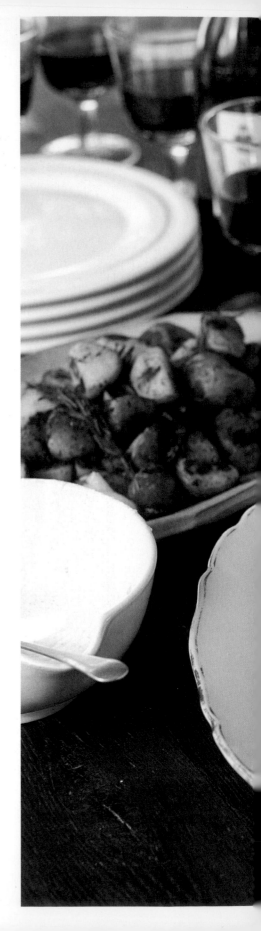

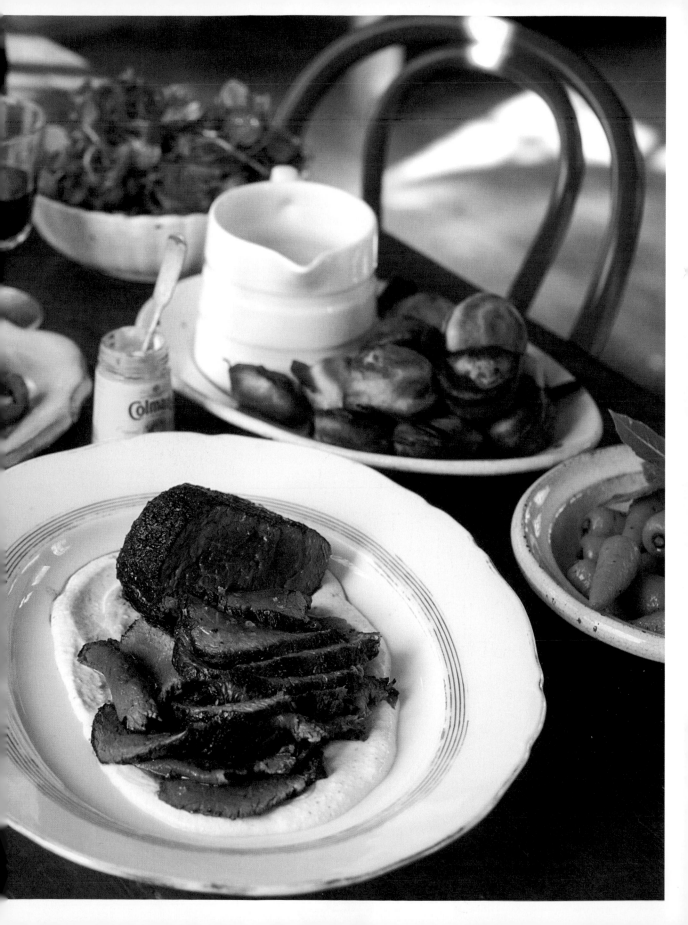

POTATOES
500g red-skinned potatoes
1 lemon
4 sprigs of fresh thyme or rosemary
1 bulb of garlic

BEEF
8 sprigs each of fresh rosemary, sage
 and thyme
700g fillet of beef

CARROTS
500g small carrots
2 sprigs of fresh thyme
2 fresh bay leaves
1 heaped tablespoon caster sugar
a knob of butter

YORKIES
just under 1 mug of plain flour
1 mug of milk
1 egg

WATERCRESS SALAD
½ a red onion
2 tablespoons red wine vinegar
1 tablespoon golden caster sugar
1 x 100g bag of prewashed
 watercress

GRAVY
½ a red onion
12 baby button mushrooms
1 heaped tablespoon plain flour
1 small wineglass of red wine
300ml organic chicken stock

SEASONINGS
olive oil
extra virgin olive oil
sea salt & black pepper

TO SERVE
creamed horseradish sauce
English mustard
a bottle of red wine

TO START Get all your ingredients and equipment ready. Fill and boil the kettle. Turn the oven on to 220°C/425°F/gas 7, and place a 12 hole shallow bun tin on the top shelf. Put 1 large saucepan and 2 large frying pans on a medium heat. Put the fine slicer disc attachment into the food processor.

POTATOES Wash the potatoes, leaving the skins on. Chop into 2cm chunks and throw into one of the large frying pans. Cover with boiling water, season with salt and cover with a lid. Turn the heat right up, and boil for 8 minutes, or until just cooked. Fill and reboil the kettle.

BEEF Quickly pick and finely chop the rosemary, sage and thyme leaves. Turn the heat under the empty frying pan up to full whack. Mix the herbs together and spread them around the chopping board with a good pinch of salt & pepper. Cut the fillet in half lengthways, then roll each piece back and forth so they are completely coated in herbs. Add the meat to the hot empty frying pan with a few good lugs of olive oil. You must turn it every minute while you get on with other jobs. Don't forget to seal the ends.

CARROTS Tip the carrots into the saucepan and just cover with boiling water. Add 2 sprigs of thyme, a couple of bay leaves, a good pinch of salt, a splash of olive oil and 1 heaped tablespoon of sugar. Cook with a lid on until tender.

YORKIES Put the flour, milk and egg into the liquidizer with a pinch of salt. Blitz, then quickly and confidently remove the bun tin from the oven and close the door. In one quick movement, back and forth, drizzle a little olive oil in each compartment, then do the same with the batter until each one is half full (any remaining batter can be used for pancakes another day). Place in the top of the oven, close the door and do not open for 14 minutes, until golden and risen.

POTATOES Check that the potatoes are cooked through, then drain and return to the same frying pan. Leave on a high heat and drizzle over some olive oil. Add a pinch of salt & pepper, speed-peel in strips of lemon zest and add 4 sprigs of thyme or rosemary. Halve the bulb of garlic widthways, squash each half with the back of a knife and add to the pan. Toss everything together, then roughly squash down with a masher. Toss every 3 minutes or so, until golden and crisp.

GRAVY Reduce the heat under the beef a little. Peel the red onion half. Finely slice in the food processor. Add half the onion to the beef pan with a splash of olive oil, the other half to a salad bowl. Rinse the mushrooms in a colander and slice in the processor, then add to the beef pan. Stir everything around and remember to keep turning the beef regularly for 5 minutes.

WATERCRESS SALAD Add 2 tablespoons of red wine vinegar, 1 tablespoon of caster sugar and a good pinch of salt & pepper to the onion bowl. Scrunch with one hand. Add 4 tablespoons of extra virgin olive oil. Empty the watercress on top and take to the table, but don't mix until serving.

GRAVY Remove the beef to a plate. Drizzle with a little olive oil, then cover with foil. Stir 1 heaped tablespoon of flour into the pan. Add a small glass of red wine and turn the heat up. Boil down to nearly nothing, then stir in 300ml of chicken stock and simmer until thick and shiny.

TO SERVE Drain the carrots, return to the pan, toss with butter and take to the table. Turn the potatoes out on to a platter. Smear 2 spoonfuls of horseradish sauce and 1 teaspoon of English mustard on to another platter. Quickly slice the beef 1cm thick, using long carving motions. Sprinkle over a pinch of salt & pepper from a height, then pile the beef on top of the horseradish sauce and mustard. Add any resting juices to the gravy and serve in a jug. Toss and dress the salad quickly, then get the Yorkies out of the oven, and take them to the table and tuck in with a glass of wine.

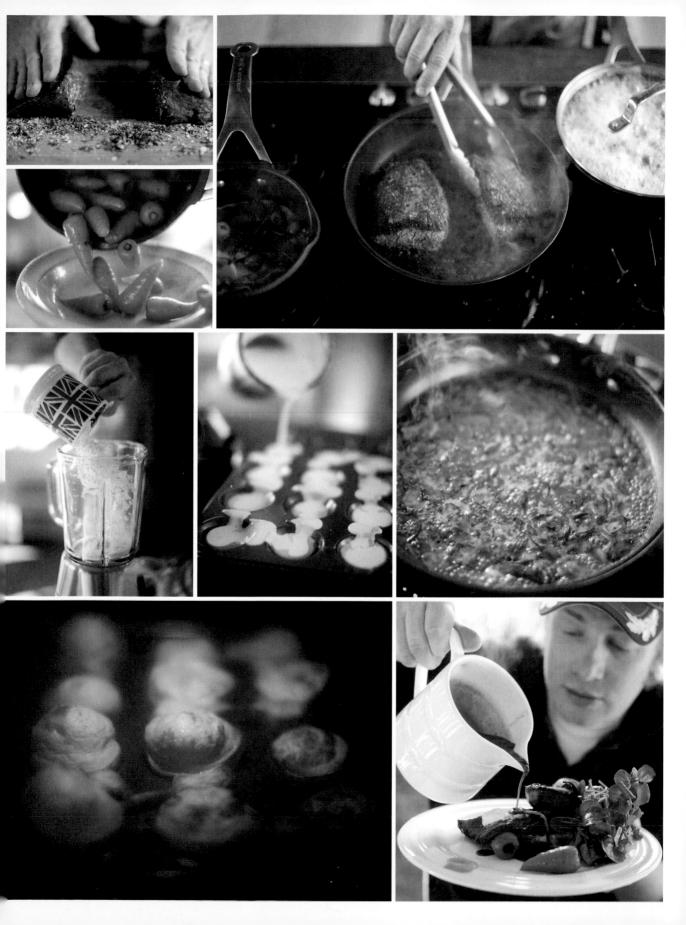

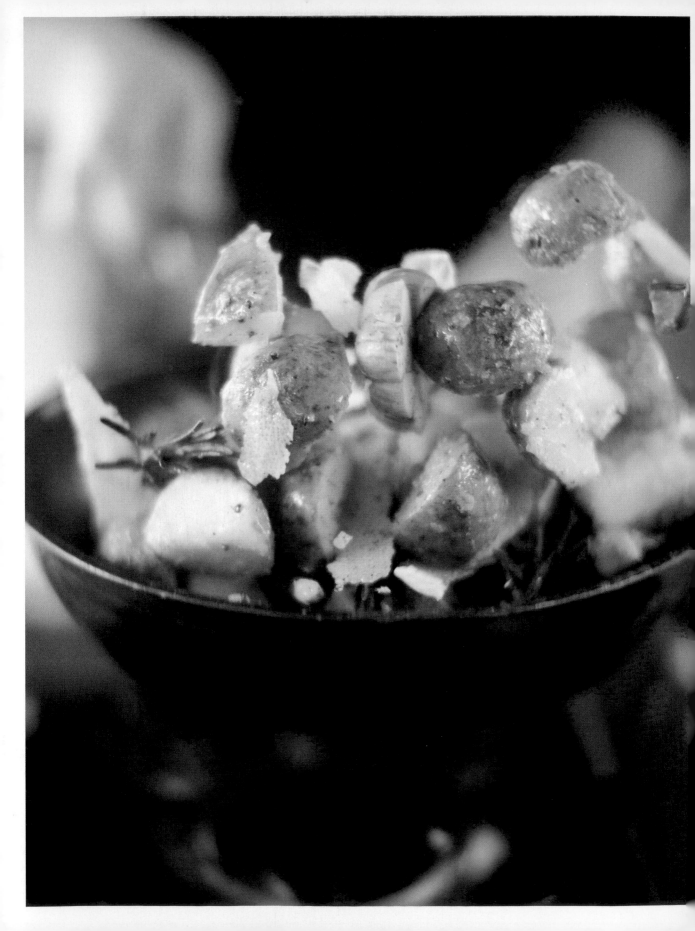

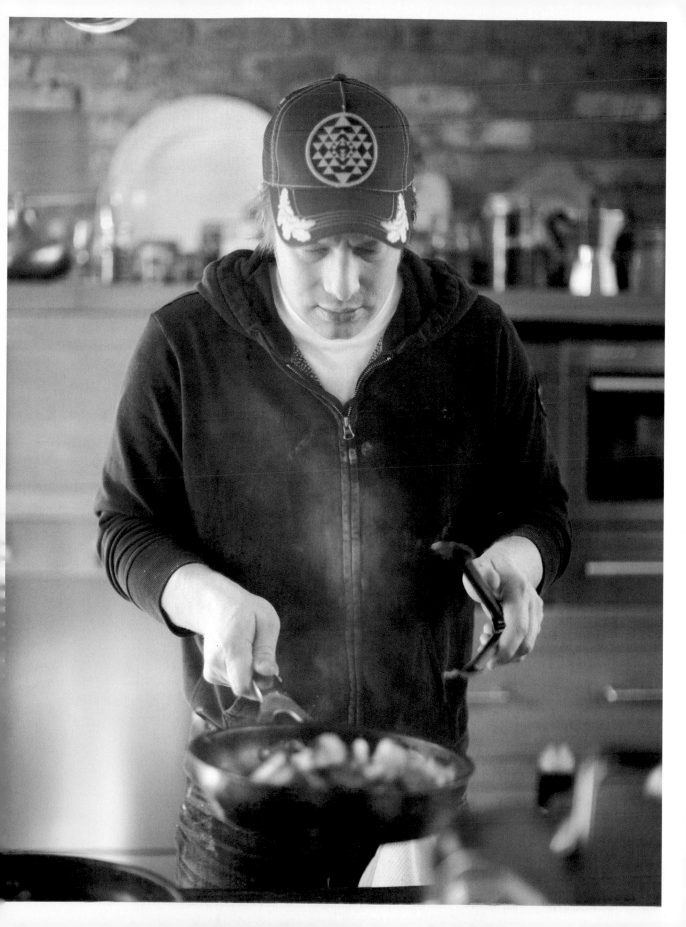

STEAK SARNIE
CRISPY NEW POTATOES
CHEESY MUSHROOMS
BEETROOT SALAD

SERVES 4

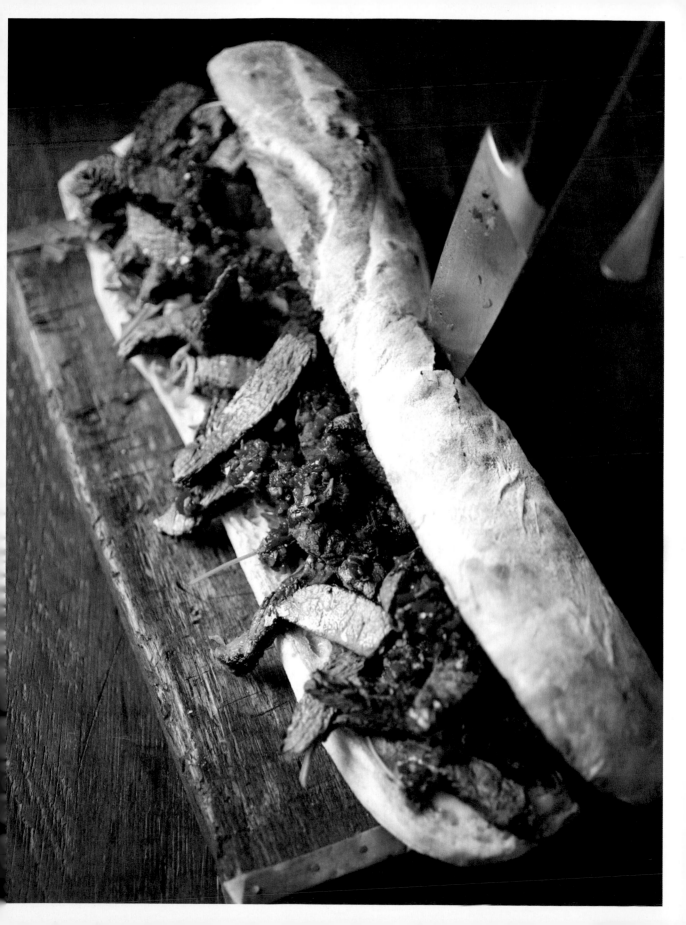

POTATOES
500g baby new potatoes
6 cloves of garlic
a few sprigs of fresh rosemary
½ a lemon

MUSHROOMS
4 large flat Portobello mushrooms
 (approx. 250g in total)
2 cloves of garlic
½ a fresh red chilli
2 sprigs of fresh flat-leaf parsley
½ a lemon
70g mature Cheddar cheese

BEETROOT SALAD
1 x 250g pack of cooked
 vac-packed beetroots
balsamic vinegar
½ a lemon
a bunch of fresh flat-leaf parsley
50g feta cheese

STEAK SARNIE
2 x 300g best-quality rump steaks
2 sprigs of fresh thyme
1 ciabatta loaf
a small handful of jarred peppers
a couple of sprigs of fresh flat-leaf
 parsley

horseradish sauce, to serve
a large handful of prewashed rocket,
 to serve

SEASONINGS
olive oil
extra virgin olive oil
sea salt & black pepper

TO START Get all your ingredients and equipment ready. Put a griddle pan on a medium heat and a large frying pan on a high heat. Turn the grill to full whack. Fill and boil the kettle. Put the coarse grater attachment into the food processor.

POTATOES Cut any larger new potatoes in half, then add all of them to the large empty frying pan with a good pinch of salt. Quickly squash 6 unpeeled cloves of garlic with the heel of your hand, then add to the pan. Pour in enough boiling water to cover, then cook for 12 to 15 minutes, or until cooked through.

MUSHROOMS Lay the mushrooms, stalk side up, on a chopping board. Trim the stalks and place the mushrooms stalk side up in a small earthenware dish that they fit into fairly snugly. Crush ½ an unpeeled clove of garlic over each mushroom. Finely chop ½ a red chilli and a couple of parsley sprigs, and divide between the mushrooms. Grate over the zest of ½ a lemon, drizzle well with olive oil and season. Cut the Cheddar into 4 chunks and pop 1 on each mushroom.

BEETROOT SALAD Grate the beetroot in the food processor. Remove the bowl from the processor, take out the grater attachment and pour in a couple of lugs of balsamic vinegar and a few lugs of extra virgin olive oil. Squeeze in the juice of ½ a lemon. Finely chop a bunch of parsley and add most of it. Stir to dress, then tip into a nice serving bowl. Scatter over the rest of the parsley. Crumble over the feta. Drizzle with extra virgin olive oil and take to the table.

MUSHROOMS Grill on the top shelf for 9 to 10 minutes, or until golden.

STEAK SARNIE Put the steaks on a board. Sprinkle with salt & pepper, pick and scatter over the thyme leaves, and drizzle with olive oil. Rub the flavours into the meat, then flip over and repeat on the other side. Pound the steaks once or twice with your fists to flatten them a little, then put them into the screaming hot griddle pan to cook for 1 to 2 minutes on each side for medium rare, or longer if you prefer. This depends on the thickness of your steaks of course, so use your instincts and cook them to your liking. Wash your hands.

POTATOES Check they are cooked through, and drain in a colander. Return the pan to a high heat, add a good lug of olive oil and tip the potatoes and garlic back in. Use a potato masher to lightly burst the skins open (don't mash them though). Add a few sprigs of rosemary and a pinch of salt. Toss every couple of minutes until golden and crisp.

STEAK SARNIE Put the ciabatta loaf into the bottom of the oven. Finely chop the peppers on a large clean board. Move the steaks to the board and drizzle with extra virgin olive oil. Finely chop a few parsley leaves, mixing them in with the peppers and all the steak juices. Scrape the pepper mix to one side of the board. Slice up the steaks at an angle.

MUSHROOMS Remove the mushrooms from the oven and turn the grill off. Take the mushrooms straight to the table.

STEAK SARNIE Get the ciabatta out of the oven and slice it open with a serrated knife. Drizzle with extra virgin olive oil from a height. Spread over as much horseradish as you like, then arrange the rocket leaves on one half. Lay the steak slices on top. Mix and scrape the peppers and juices from the board and scatter over the meat, then fold together and take to the table.

POTATOES Tip the potatoes on to a serving platter, and put ½ a lemon on the side for squeezing over. Take to the table.

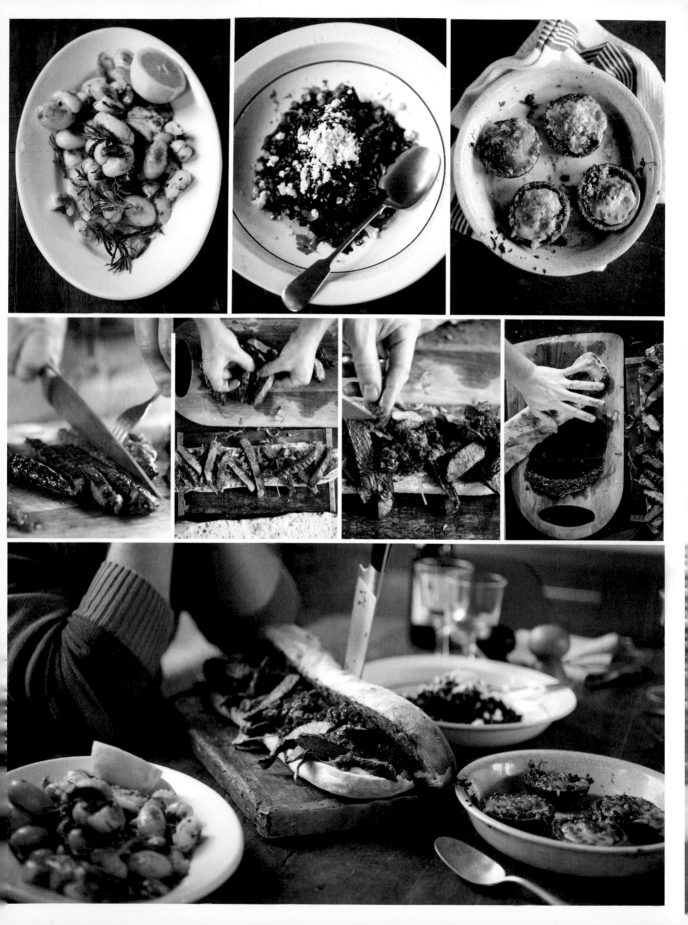

RIB-EYE STIR-FRY

DAN DAN NOODLES

CHILLED HIBISCUS TEA

SERVES 4

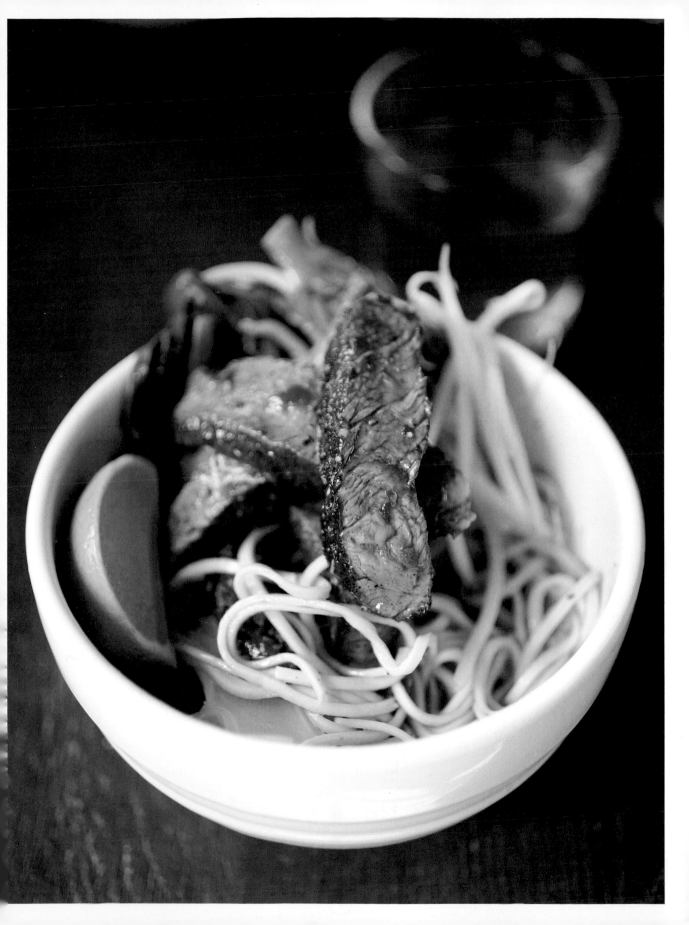

STEAKS
2 x 250g best-quality rib-eye steaks
1 heaped teaspoon Szechuan pepper
Chinese five-spice
a 2cm piece of fresh ginger
½ a red chilli
1 clove of garlic
1 lime
a few sprigs of fresh coriander

GREENS
150g sugar snap peas
2 bok choi
200g sprouting broccoli
1 heaped tablespoon black bean sauce
1 lemon or lime

DAN DAN NOODLES
6 tablespoons chilli oil
4 tablespoons soy sauce
1 clove of garlic
200g beansprouts
½ a bunch of fresh coriander
8 spring onions
400g dried medium egg noodles
  (1 nest per person)
1 organic beef stock cube
½ a lemon
runny honey
a squeeze of lime juice

SEASONINGS
olive oil
extra virgin olive oil
sea salt & black pepper

HIBISCUS TEA
2–3 hibiscus, mint or jasmine
  teabags
1 clementine
1 lime
1 heaped dessertspoon caster sugar
a few handfuls of ice
a few sprigs of fresh mint

TO START Get all your ingredients and equipment ready. Fill and boil the kettle. Put a griddle pan on a high heat and a large saucepan on a low heat. Get out 4 serving bowls.

STEAKS Put the meat on a wooden board and sprinkle salt & pepper from a height over the meat and board. Pound the Szechuan pepper using a pestle & mortar. Put a tiny pinch in each serving bowl, then sprinkle the rest over the meat along with a really good pinch of five-spice. Drizzle a little olive oil over the meat and board, then rub the meat all over the board so it picks up the flavours really well.

DAN DAN NOODLES Pour boiling water into the large saucepan. Turn the heat up to high and cover with a lid. Fill and reboil the kettle. Pour 1½ to 2 tablespoons of chilli oil and 1 tablespoon of soy sauce into each serving bowl. Crush 1 unpeeled clove of garlic and divide the pulped flesh between the bowls.

HIBISCUS TEA Put the teabags into a large jug, then use a speed-peeler to peel off the skin of the clementine and the lime into long strips. Add the peel to the jug along with the caster sugar. Fill the jug halfway with boiling water and leave to steep.

STEAKS Put the steaks on the hot griddle pan to cook for 2 minutes on each side for medium rare, or until cooked to your liking. Use tongs to turn them while you get on with other jobs.

DAN DAN NOODLES Get the garnishes ready. Put the beansprouts in a serving bowl with the coriander and take to the table.

GREENS Season the boiling water with a pinch of salt and add the sugar snap peas. Flip over the board you dressed the meat on, then halve the bok choi. Trim the ends off the broccoli lengthways, then add to the pan with the bok choi and sugar snap peas. Put the lid on.

DAN DAN NOODLES Trim and finely slice the spring onions and divide them between the serving bowls. (Don't forget to check the steaks – they should be perfect now.)

STEAKS Get a clean board, drizzle it with olive oil and lay your steaks on top. Take the griddle pan off the heat. Peel the ginger then finely grate it, with the chilli and garlic, over the steaks, just to flavour and perfume. Squeeze over the lime juice.

GREENS Spoon 1 heaped dessertspoon of black bean sauce into the middle of a platter and spread around. Squeeze over the lemon or lime juice and drizzle over a lug of olive oil. Use tongs and a slotted spoon to fish out all the peas and greens, holding them up for a minute to let some of the excess water drip away, then pile on top of the black bean sauce. Drizzle over a little extra virgin olive oil and take to the table to toss and dress at the last minute.

HIBISCUS TEA Remove the teabags. Add a few large handfuls of ice to the hibiscus tea, then halve the clementine and the lime and squeeze in all their juices. Add both halves of lime and the sprigs of mint to the jug.

DAN DAN NOODLES Add the nests of noodles to the water you used for the greens, with 1 stock cube. Squeeze a few drips of lemon juice and a thimble amount of honey into each serving bowl.

STEAKS Slice the steaks at an angle into 1cm strips, then toss so they mop up all the flavourful juices on the board. Tear over the coriander and take to the table.

DAN DAN NOODLES Use tongs to divide the noodles between the bowls. Ladle over a little broth and take to the table. Get everyone to toss their noodles, then assemble their own bowl by pimping it with garnishes and adding a pinch of beansprouts, some coriander leaves, some greens, a few strips of steak and a squeeze or two of lime juice.

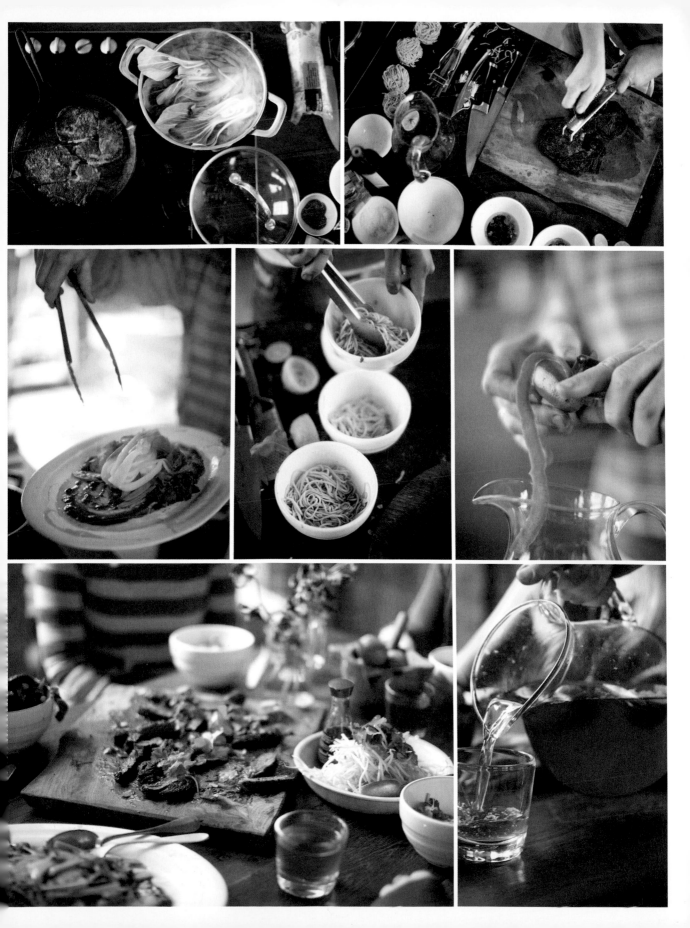

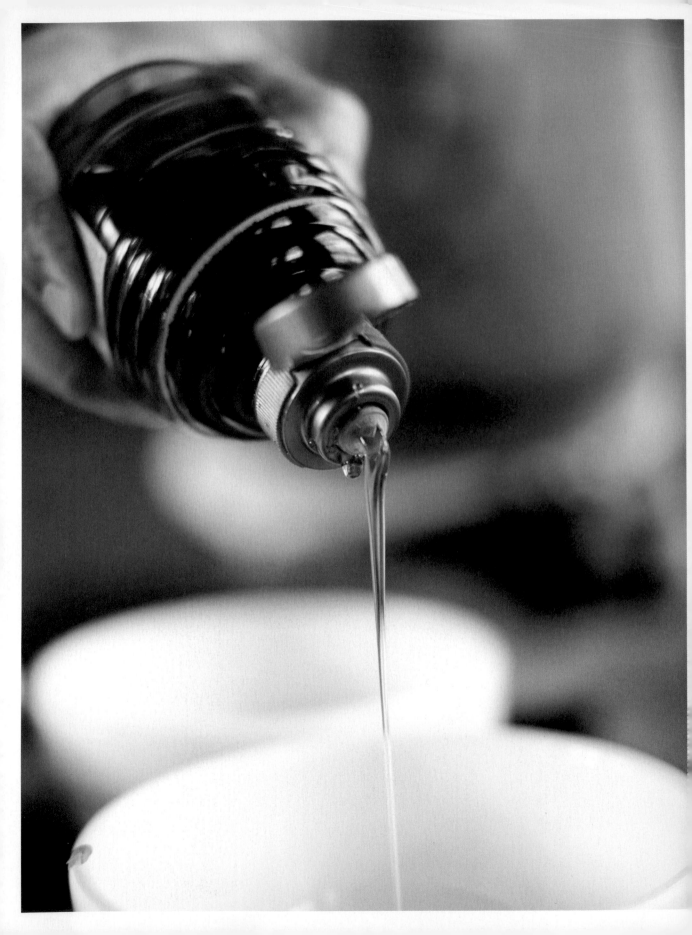

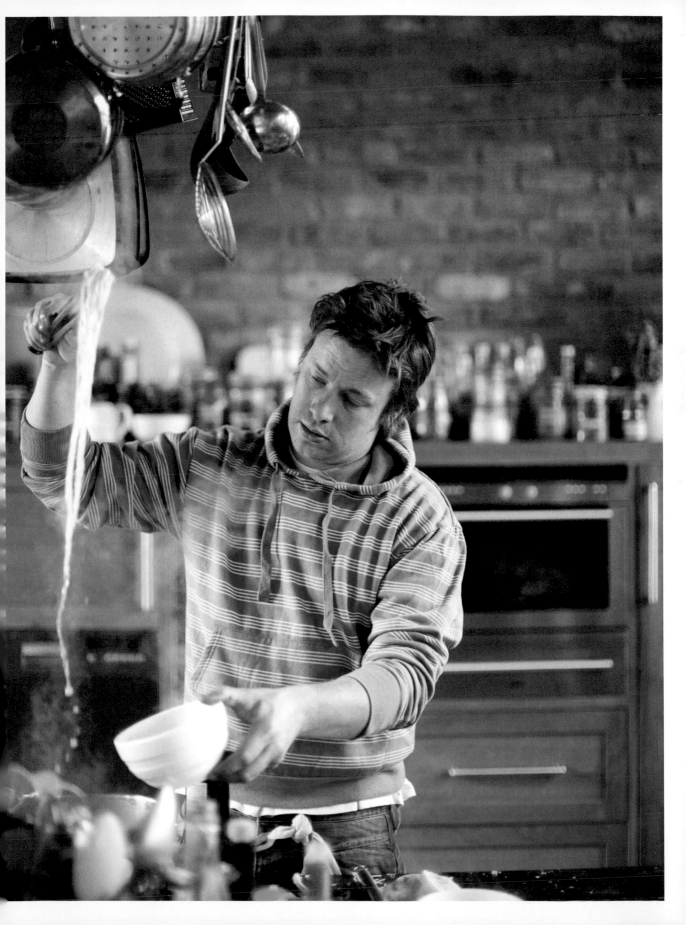

SUPER-FAST BEEF HASH

JACKET POTATOES

GODDESS SALAD

LOVELY BUTTER BEANS & BACON

SERVES 4

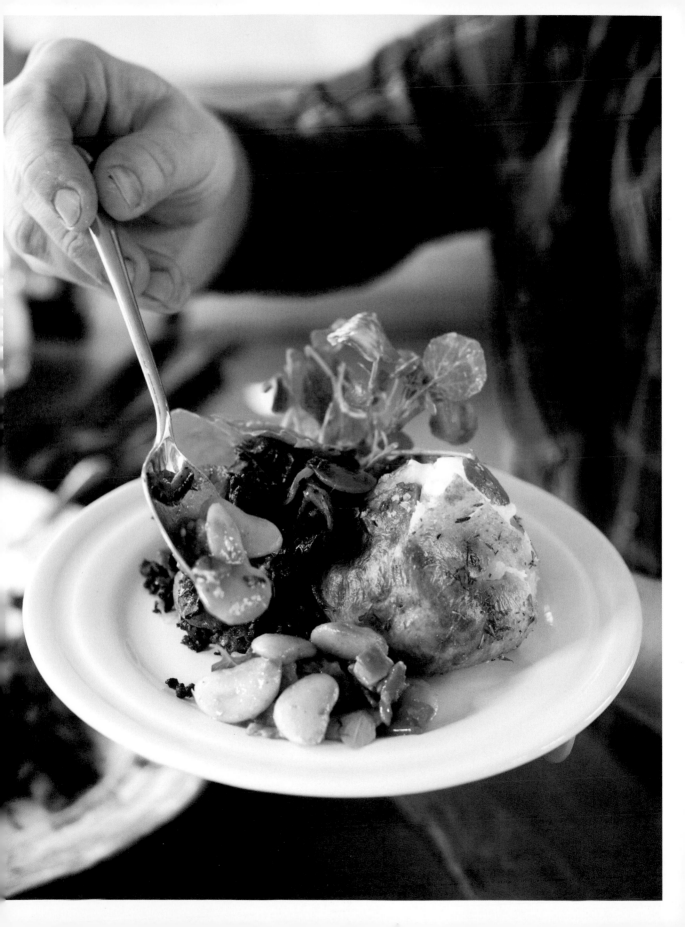

POTATOES
4 large baking potatoes
2 sprigs of fresh rosemary
4 teaspoons soured cream

HASH
500g good-quality minced beef
2 sprigs of fresh thyme
1 red onion
2 carrots
3 sticks of celery
a few sprigs of fresh rosemary

4 cloves of garlic
6 tablespoons Worcestershire sauce
a small bunch of fresh flat-leaf parsley

BEANS
4 rashers of smoked streaky bacon
2 tomatoes
1 x 400g tin of butter beans
red wine vinegar
2 or 3 sprigs of fresh Greek basil or
   basil, leaves picked

SALAD
1 soft round lettuce
a handful of prewashed watercress
1 avocado
1 heaped tablespoon soured cream
1 lemon

SEASONINGS
olive oil
extra virgin olive oil
sea salt & black pepper

TO START Get all your ingredients and equipment ready. Turn the grill on to full whack and put a baking tray underneath it to heat up. Put a large frying pan on a medium-high heat and another on a low heat. Put the thin slicer disc attachment into the food processor.

POTATOES Wash the spuds, trim off any gnarly bits, stab a few times with a knife, then put into a large microwave-safe bowl and cover with a double layer of clingfilm. Put straight into the microwave for around 14 to 16 minutes, or until cooked.

HASH Put the mince into the largest frying pan and break it up with a wooden spoon. Add 1 teaspoon of salt and 1 teaspoon of pepper and drizzle over some olive oil. Pick in the thyme leaves and cook until golden, stirring often.

BEANS Drizzle olive oil into the second frying pan on a low heat. Finely slice the bacon and add to the pan. Toss occasionally and move the pan off the heat once the bacon is golden.

HASH Peel and halve the red onion. Wash and trim the carrots and celery, then slice all of them in the food processor and set aside. When the mince is golden, pick the rosemary leaves into the pan. Crush in the 4 unpeeled cloves of garlic and add 6 tablespoons of Worcestershire sauce. Stir well, cook until nicely glazed, then add the sliced veg and stir again. Reduce the heat to medium and remember to toss often.

POTATOES Put a knife through each potato to check they are cooked through. Pick and finely chop the rosemary leaves, and add them to the bowl with a pinch of salt & pepper and a drizzle of olive oil. Gently toss to coat them in the flavours, then use tongs to transfer the spuds to the hot baking tray and put under the grill to crisp up.

BEANS Now get your pan of bacon on a high heat. Roughly chop the tomatoes and add them to the bacon. Tip in the butter beans and their juices, and simmer gently to cook the liquid down.

SALAD Click the leaves off the lettuce, then wash and spin them dry. Put into a serving bowl with the watercress. Halve and stone the avocado, then use a spoon to scoop slivers from one half into the serving bowl. Whiz the soured cream in a liquidizer with the remaining avocado flesh, the juice of 1 lemon, 4 tablespoons of extra virgin olive oil and a pinch of salt & pepper. If it's too thick, add a splash or two of water until you have a creamy dressing.

HASH Finely slice the parsley. Add most of it to the hash pan, reserving a few leaves. Taste and correct the seasoning, then transfer it to a large serving platter.

POTATOES Take the potatoes out of the oven. Cut a cross on each one and pinch them open. Serve on top of the hash. Top each with 1 teaspoon of soured cream and scatter over the remaining parsley. Take the platter to the table.

BEANS Add a little extra virgin olive oil and a good splash of vinegar, then season. Sprinkle over the Greek basil leaves. Take the pan to the table.

SALAD Toss with the dressing and tuck in!

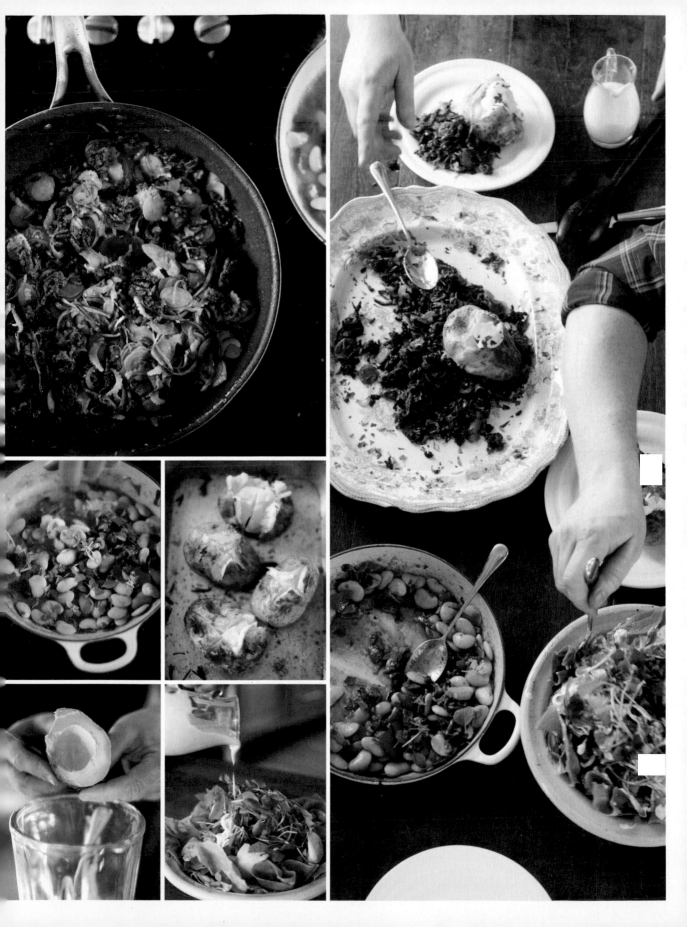

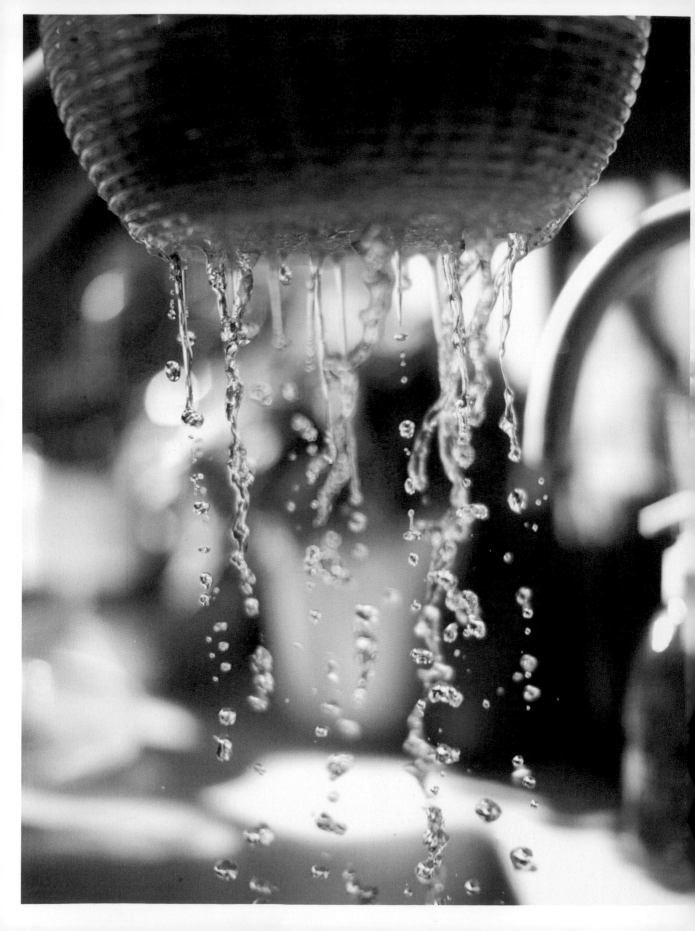

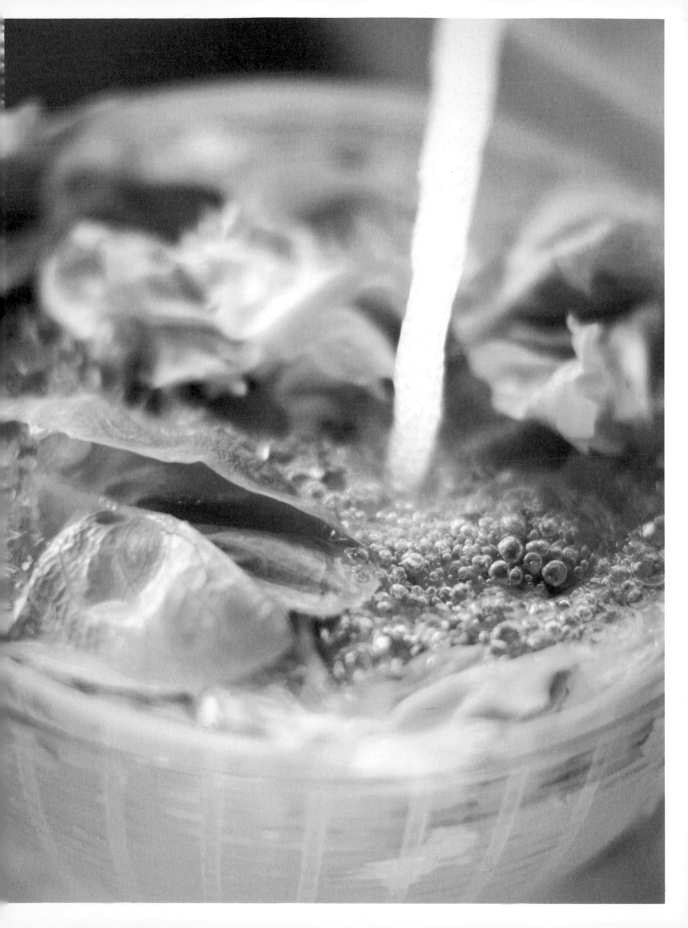

STEAK
INDIAN-STYLE

SPINACH & PANEER SALAD

NAAN BREADS

MANGO DESSERT

SERVES 4

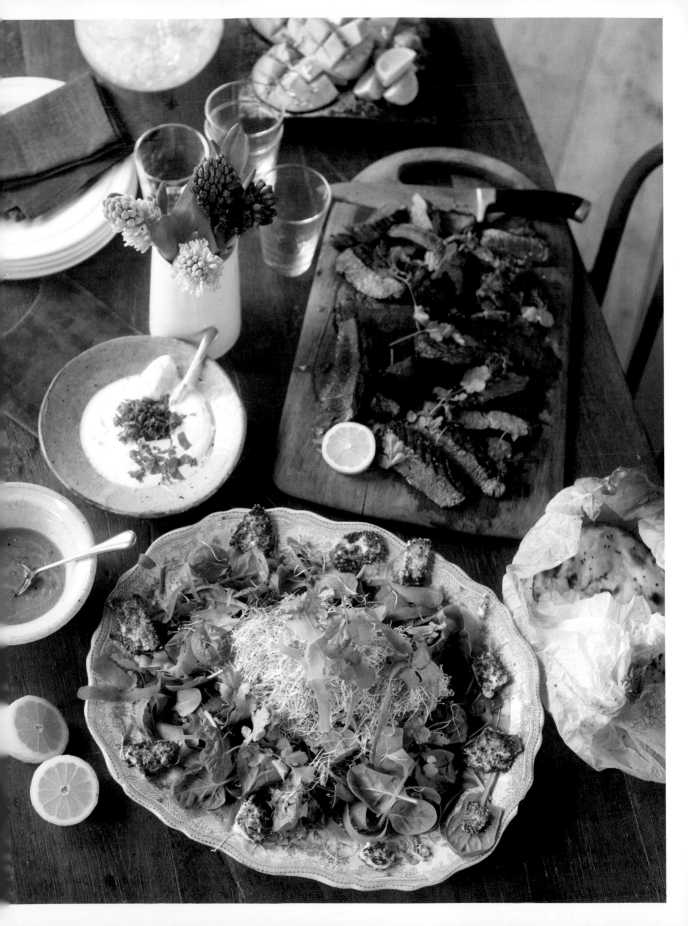

STEAKS
¼ of a 283g jar of Patak's jalfrezi
  paste
½ a lemon
3 x 300g best-quality rump steaks
a few sprigs of fresh coriander

YOGHURT DIP
250g natural yoghurt
a few sprigs of fresh mint
½ a lemon

NAAN BREADS
2 naan breads

PANEER & SPINACH SALAD
200g prewashed baby spinach
a small bunch of fresh coriander
1 packet of alfalfa sprouts
1 punnet of cress
1 large carrot
200g paneer cheese
3 tablespoons sesame seeds
1 lemon

CURRY SAUCE
¼ of a 283g jar of Patak's jalfrezi
  paste
½ a 400ml tin of coconut milk

SEASONINGS
olive oil
extra virgin olive oil
sea salt & black pepper

MANGO DESSERT
2 ripe mangoes
1 heaped teaspoon icing sugar
a few sprigs of fresh mint
1 lime

TO START Get all your ingredients and equipment ready. Put a griddle pan on a high heat. Turn the oven on to 180°C/375°F/gas 4.

STEAKS Dollop ¼ of the jar of jalfrezi paste into a large flat bowl and mix in the juice of ½ a lemon, a few good lugs of olive oil and a good pinch of salt & pepper. Put the steaks on top, rub this marinade all over them, then set aside and wash your hands.

YOGHURT DIP Spoon the yoghurt into a dish. Finely slice the leafy tops of the sprigs of mint, then add to the yoghurt with a drizzle of extra virgin olive oil, the juice of ½ a lemon and a good pinch of salt. Take to the table and stir just before serving.

PANEER & SPINACH SALAD Tip the spinach on to a platter. Tear and scatter over most of the coriander leaves, top with the alfalfa sprouts and snip over the cress. Use a speed-peeler to peel the carrot into ribbons on top.

NAAN BREADS Scrunch up a large piece of greaseproof paper under the tap, then flatten out and drizzle with olive oil. Wrap the naans in the paper and pop into the oven to warm through.

STEAKS Use tongs to transfer the steaks to the screaming hot griddle pan. Cook for about 6 minutes in total, turning every minute, for medium-rare steaks, around 8 minutes in total for medium and about 10 minutes for well done. You know how you like your meat, so use your instincts and move it to a board once cooked to your liking. Put a small frying pan on a medium heat.

CURRY SAUCE Put a small saucepan on a medium heat. Add ¼ of the jar of jalfrezi paste, pour in ½ the tin of coconut milk, mix well, then leave to bubble and thicken.

PANEER & SPINACH SALAD Chop the paneer into bite-sized pieces and add to the hot frying pan with a splash of olive oil. Check on your steaks.

CURRY SAUCE Once the sauce has boiled down to a nice consistency, turn the heat underneath down to low, or turn off. Check your steaks again.

PANEER & SPINACH SALAD Turn the paneer over – it should be nicely golden underneath. Add a good pinch of salt and 3 tablespoons of sesame seeds. Turn the heat down if it looks like it's cooking too fast.

MANGO DESSERT Slice both mangoes down either side of the stone. Take each half and score a crisscross pattern about 2cm down through the flesh, stopping at the skin. Turn the skin inside out so the mango pieces pop up. Trim the skin off the middle bit where the stone is, then either chop chunks of flesh off or eat them as a treat ( )!

Arrange the mango hedgehogs on a board and sieve 1 heaped teaspoon of icing sugar all over, then finely chop a few mint leaves and sprinkle over. Slice the lime into wedges for serving. Take to the table.

STEAKS If you haven't already done so, move the steaks to a board to rest and drizzle over a little extra virgin olive oil.

PANEER & SPINACH SALAD Arrange the paneer around the edge of the salad and cut the lemon into wedges for squeezing over. Take to the table.

TO SERVE Slice up the meat at an angle, toss in the resting juices and oil from the board and scatter over the coriander leaves. Tip the warm curry sauce into a bowl and take to the table with the stack of warm naan breads and the sliced steak.

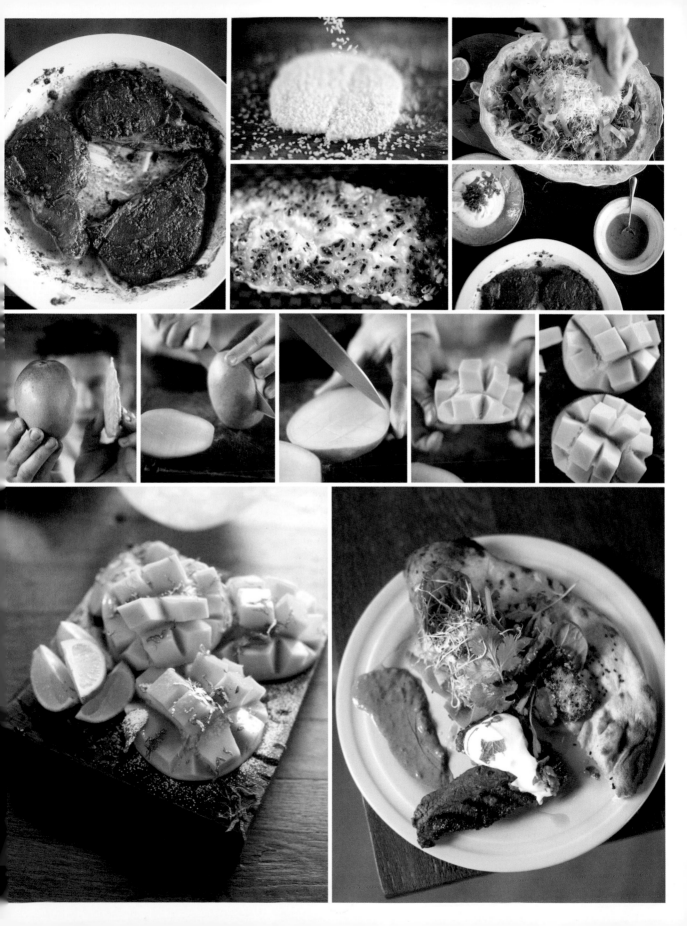

MEATBALL SANDWICH

PICKLED CABBAGE

CHOPPED SALAD

BANANA ICE CREAM

SERVES 4–6

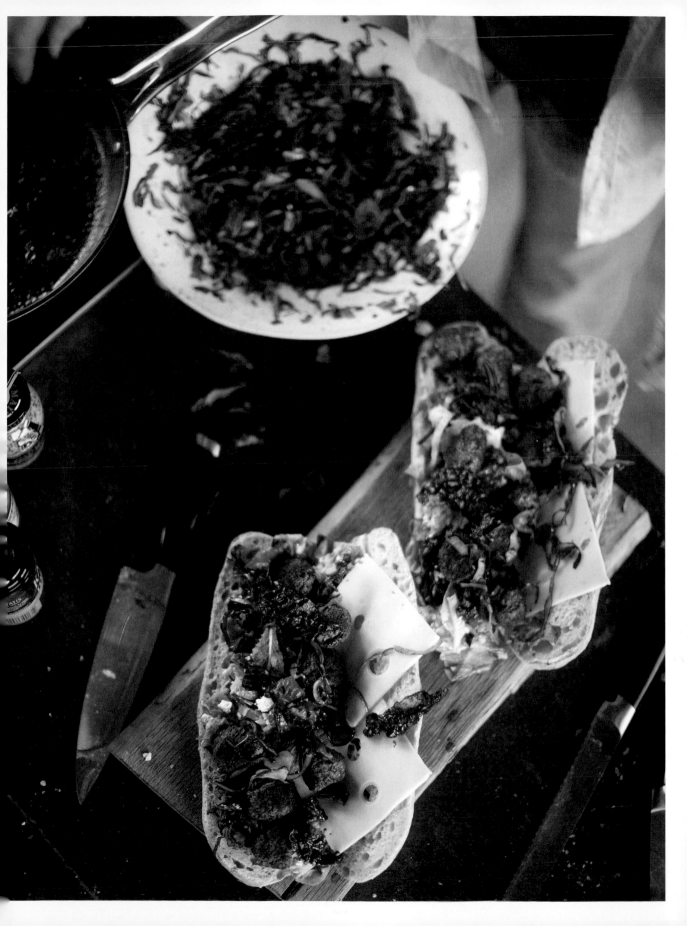

MEATBALL SANDWICH
a small handful of fresh basil
500g good-quality minced beef
1 tablespoon wholegrain mustard
½ a lemon
1 egg
8 slices of smoked pancetta
2 ciabatta loaves
4 slices of Jarlsberg cheese

CABBAGE
½ a small red cabbage
1 red onion
a small bunch of fresh mint
1 fresh red chilli
2 lemons

CHOPPED SALAD
½ a cucumber
2 tomatoes
2 avocados
a handful of fresh basil leaves
1 x 110g bag of prewashed Italian
  leaf salad
1 teaspoon English mustard
1½ tablespoons red wine vinegar
50g feta cheese

SEASONINGS
olive oil
extra virgin olive oil
sea salt & black pepper

ICE CREAM
6 bananas (approx. 900g), peeled,
  sliced and put into the freezer in
  sandwich bags at least 6 hours in
  advance
1 x 250g tub of low-fat natural yoghurt
1 tablespoon runny honey
2–3 handfuls of desiccated coconut
  for coating
8 sweet, crunchy biscuits

TO SERVE
cold beer

NOTE: Make sure your bananas are frozen ahead of time, at least 6 hours before. Peel and slice them, then put in sandwich bags in the freezer. This is a great habit to get into, especially with fruit that is starting to turn.

TO START Get all your ingredients and equipment ready. Turn the oven on to 160°C/320°F/gas 3. Take the bananas out of the freezer. Put a large ovenproof frying pan on a medium heat. Put the thin slicer disc attachment into the food processor. Get 4 tumblers out for dessert, then check your freezer to make sure you have room for them.

MEATBALL SANDWICH Roughly chop the basil and put it into a large mixing bowl with the minced beef, wholegrain mustard, a pinch of salt & pepper and the zest of ½ a lemon. Separate the egg and add the yolk to the bowl with 1 tablespoon of olive oil. Add a drizzle of olive oil to the ovenproof frying pan, then really scrunch and mix up the mince mixture with clean hands. Quickly divide the mince mixture into 4, then divide each portion into 4 again. Work quickly to pat, roll and shape these into meatballs (it helps if you wet your hands as you do this). Place them in the pan as you go, then wash your hands. Shake, toss and cook the meatballs for about 12 to 14 minutes, or until they are golden all over.

CABBAGE Slice off the base of the cabbage half, peel off the outer leaves and cut into 4 wedges. Push them into the food processor to finely slice. Peel and halve the onion, rip the top half off the bunch of mint and add to the processor with the chilli (stalk removed).

MEATBALL SANDWICH Lay the pancetta slices in the frying pan, around the meatballs, and put into the oven with the ciabattas on the shelf underneath.

CABBAGE Tip the shredded veg and chilli into a large bowl and add a good lug of extra virgin olive oil. Squeeze over the lemon juice and add a good pinch of salt. Toss everything together.

CHOPPED SALAD I like to use 2 knives for this, but do whatever feels safe and comfortable. Roughly chop the cucumber and tomatoes together on a really large board. Halve and stone the avocados. Spoon out the avocado flesh, add it to the cucumber and tomatoes and chop again. Add the basil leaves and continue chopping. Tip the Italian leaves on to the board on top of the rest of the salad. Make a well in the centre of the leaves, then add a teaspoon of English mustard, a pinch of salt, 5 tablespoons of extra virgin olive oil and 1½ tablespoons of red wine vinegar. Chop and toss again to dress. Add more olive oil if needed, then crumble over the feta.

ICE CREAM Quickly wash the food processor bowl with cold water, then swap in the standard blade attachment and whiz the frozen bananas with yoghurt and honey until thick and creamy. Put the desiccated coconut into a large bowl, then take 1 dessertspoon of banana ice cream and roll it in coconut until covered. Do this with each scoop putting them into tumblers as you go. Once you've used up all the ice cream, pop the tumblers into the freezer until you're ready for dessert.

MEATBALL SANDWICH Remove the pan of meatballs and ciabattas from the oven. Open out the hot ciabattas, drizzle over a little extra virgin olive oil, lay 2 slices of Jarlsberg on each loaf, scatter over some cabbage salad, then top with meatballs and a few slices of crispy pancetta.

TO SERVE Take the meatball sandwich to the table with the chopped salad. Squeeze the sandwiches shut, halve them, then dive in. When ready, get the banana ice cream out of the freezer and tuck in with a crunchy biscuit.

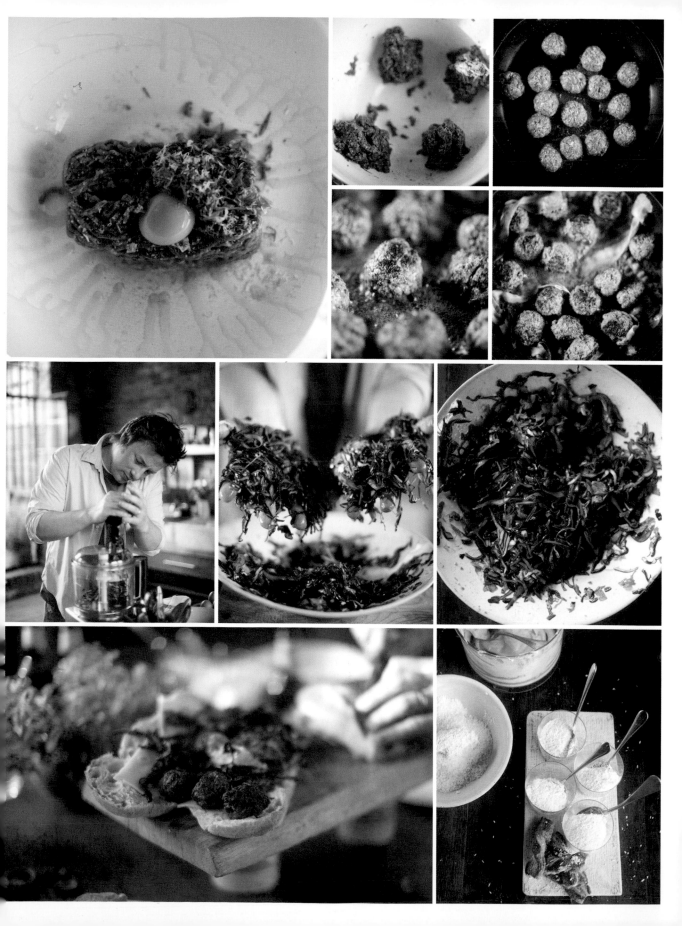

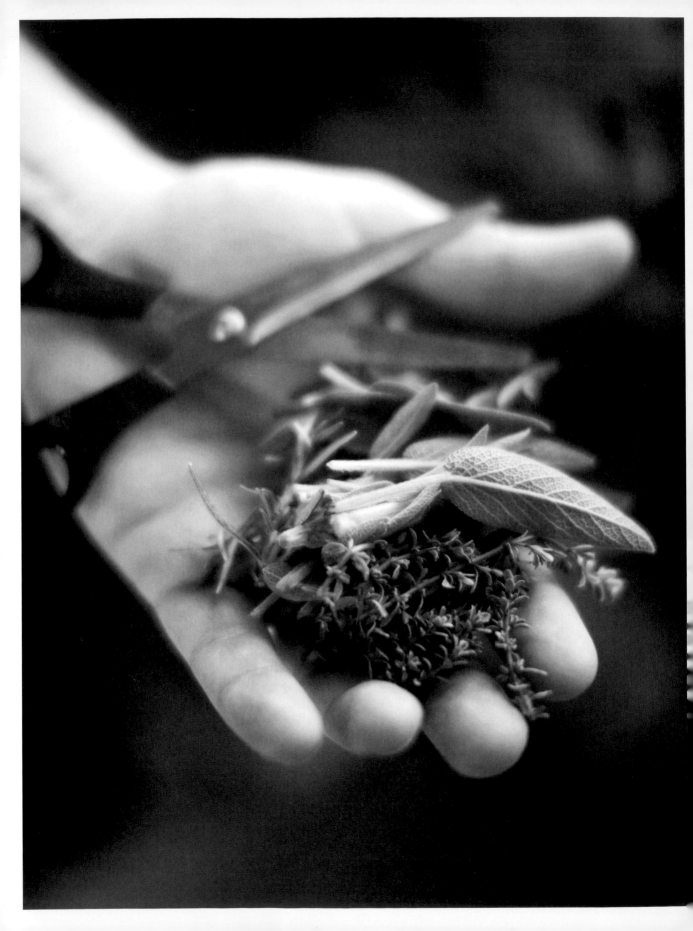

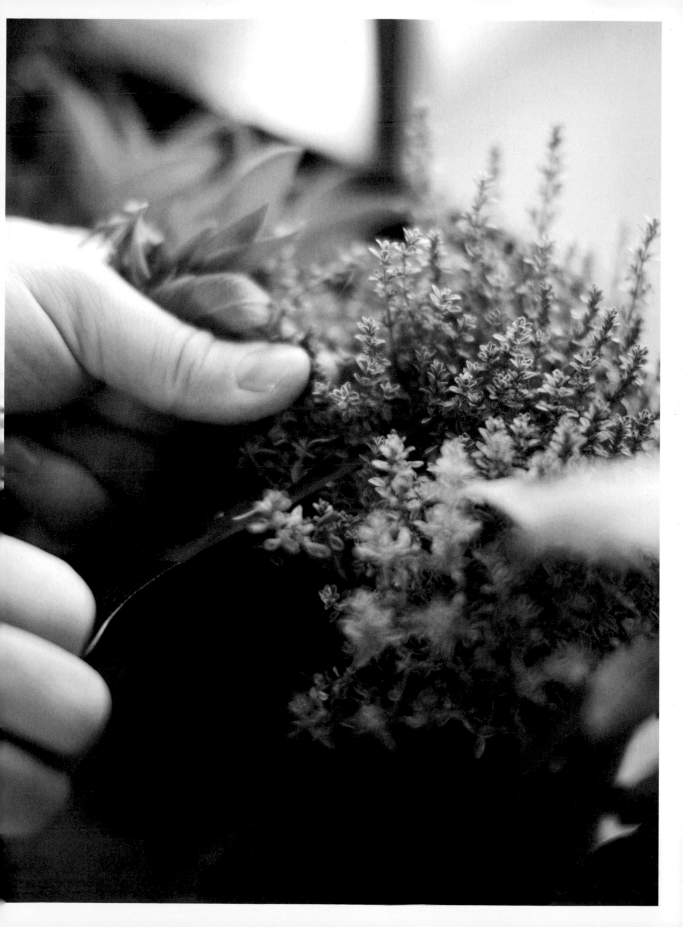

LIVER & BACON

ONION GRAVY

SMASHED POTATO

DRESSED GREENS

MERINGUES

SERVES 4

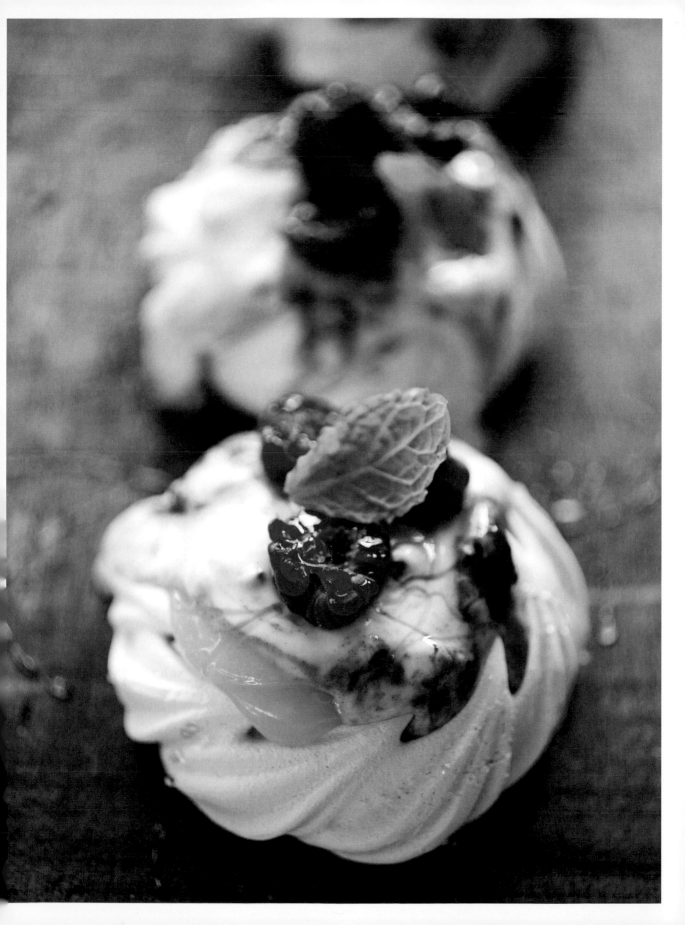

SMASH
500g red-skinned potatoes
1 lemon

GRAVY
2 red onions
a few sprigs of fresh rosemary
1 teaspoon runny honey
2 cloves of garlic
1 heaped tablespoon flour
1 wineglass of red wine
3 tablespoons balsamic vinegar
1 organic beef stock cube

LIVER
8 rashers of smoked streaky bacon
300g calves' liver
plain flour
4 sprigs of fresh rosemary

GREENS
200g of Swiss chard or other seasonal
  greens
½ a lemon

SEASONINGS
olive oil
extra virgin olive oil
sea salt & black pepper

DESSERT
150g raspberries or strawberries
1 tablespoon runny honey, plus a little
  extra
4 tablespoons Greek yoghurt
4 individual meringue nests
4 teaspoons good-quality lemon curd
a few fresh baby mint leaves

TO START Get all your ingredients and equipment ready. Fill and boil the kettle. Put a 3-level steamer pan and 2 large frying pans on a medium heat. Put the thin slicer disc attachment into the food processor.

SMASH Wash the spuds. Leave the skins on but remove any gnarly bits. Cut into 3cm pieces. Fill the steamer pan with boiled water, add a pinch of salt and the potatoes and put the lid on.

GRAVY Peel and halve the red onions and slice up in the food processor. Put into one of the hot frying pans with a splash of olive oil and stir. Pick and finely chop the rosemary leaves and add them to the pan with the teaspoon of honey. Crush in 2 peeled cloves of garlic. Stir occasionally while you crack on with the rest of the meal.

LIVER Put the bacon into the other frying pan with a lug of olive oil. Keep turning it until golden on both sides, then move to a plate and take the pan off the heat.

GREENS Wash the chard well. Finely slice the stalks and add to the lowest pan of the steamer. Roughly chop the larger leaves and add to the top level of the steamer. Stack both above the potatoes and put the lid on. Refill and boil the kettle.

DESSERT Put half the berries in a bowl with 1 tablespoon of honey and mash till soft. Add the Greek yoghurt and gently swirl and marble through, then put into the fridge. Put the meringue nests on a serving board, with 1 teaspoon of lemon curd in the centre of each. Leave them like this

until you're ready to serve them, then dollop a spoonful of your berry yoghurt mixture over each one. Top with a few berries, a drizzle of honey and a few small mint leaves.

GRAVY Stir the heaped tablespoon of flour into the pan of onions. Add the glass of red wine. Cook away, then add the 3 tablespoons of balsamic vinegar and stir again. Add the beef stock cube and 300ml of boiled water. Stir and simmer till it's a good consistency.

LIVER Put the bacon pan back on the heat. Lay the liver on greaseproof paper. Season with salt & pepper and dust both sides with an even coating of flour. Turn the heat up under the pan and add the liver and a splash more olive oil. Don't be tempted to turn it. Leave to cook for 3 minutes.

SMASH Check the potatoes are cooked through, then drain them and mash with a really good drizzle of extra virgin olive oil, a good pinch of salt & pepper and a few gratings of lemon zest. Spoon on to a large serving platter.

LIVER Turn the liver over, add the rosemary sprigs and return the bacon to the pan. Cook for 2 more minutes, then lay it on top of the smash and take the platter to the table.

GREENS Put the chard on a serving plate, drizzle over some extra virgin olive oil and squeeze over the juice of ½ a lemon. Add a pinch of salt & pepper and take to the table.

TO SERVE Pour the gravy into a jug and you're ready to tuck in.

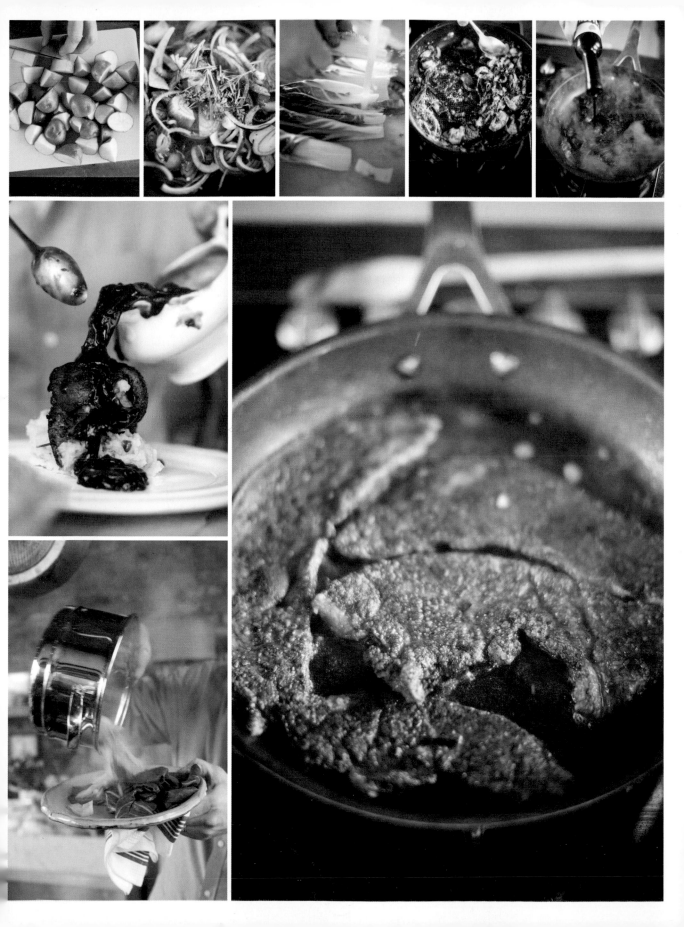

STUFFED FOCACCIA

PROSCIUTTO

CELERIAC REMOULADE

DRESSED MOZZARELLA

FRESH LEMON & LIME GRANITA

SERVES 4–6

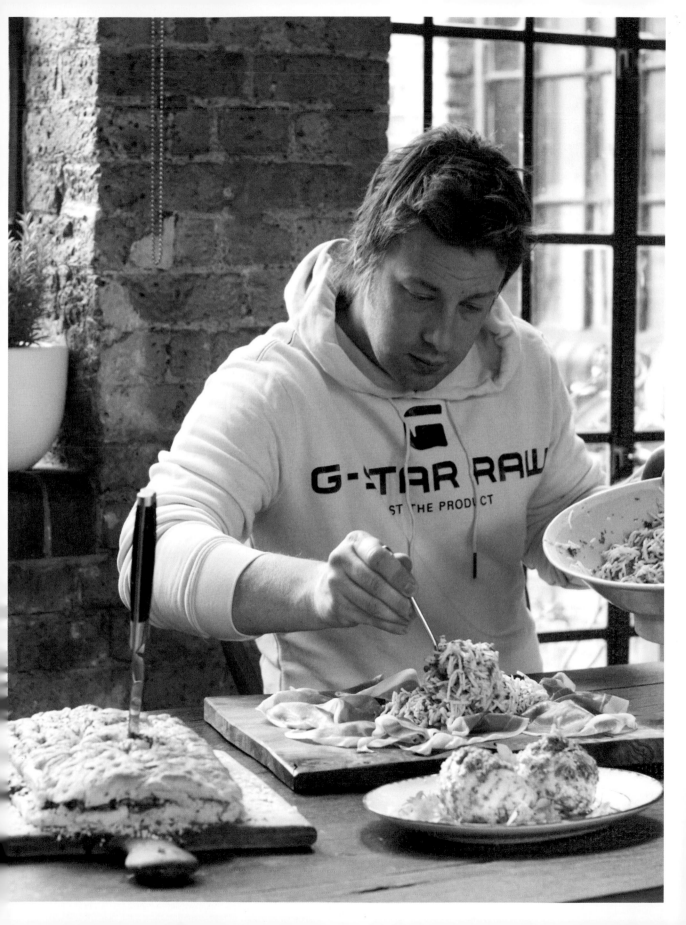

FOCACCIA
1 x 400g focaccia loaf
1 x 450g jar of peppers
1 teaspoon capers, drained
6 sun-dried tomatoes in oil
a large handful of good-quality mixed
  marinated olives
1 fresh red chilli
a large handful of cherry tomatoes
3 or 4 cornichons
a small bunch of fresh mint
½ a lemon
Parmesan cheese, for grating

REMOULADE & PROSCIUTTO
600g celeriac
½ a fresh red chilli
1 pear
a bunch of fresh flat-leaf parsley

1 teaspoon French mustard
1 teaspoon wholegrain mustard
2 tablespoons white wine vinegar
2 x 125g packs of good-quality
  prosciutto

PESTO & MOZZARELLA
2 x 125g balls of mozzarella
100g pinenuts
½ a clove of garlic
75g Parmesan cheese
a large bunch of fresh basil
optional: a few sprigs of fresh Greek
  basil
½ a lemon
½ a dried chilli

SEASONINGS
extra virgin olive oil
sea salt & black pepper

GRANITA
1 bag of ice cubes
3 or 4 sprigs of fresh mint
1 lemon
1 lime
1 teaspoon vanilla paste or extract
3 heaped tablespoons caster sugar
1 pink grapefruit
natural yoghurt, to serve
a small punnet of raspberries, to
  serve

TO SERVE
1 bottle of chilled rosé wine

TO START Get all your ingredients and equipment ready. Turn the oven on to 150°C/300°F/gas 2 and put the standard blade attachment into the food processor. Check you have room in your freezer for a platter.

GRANITA Half-fill the food processor with ice cubes. Add the leaves from 3 or 4 sprigs of mint. Finely grate in the zest of the lemon and the lime and add a teaspoon of vanilla paste or extract, then leave to blitz to a sort of snow. While blitzing, add 3 heaped tablespoons of caster sugar and squeeze in the juice of the lemon and lime. Once the mixture is like snow, spread it over a serving platter and put it straight into the freezer.

REMOULADE & PROSCIUTTO Quickly rinse the food processor, then swap the standard blade for the coarse grater attachment. Halve and peel the celeriac, then cut it into wedges. Deseed ½ a chilli, trim the stalk and base of the pear and halve it lengthways. Grate the celeriac, ½ a chilli, the pear and a bunch of parsley in the processor. Tip everything into a large bowl. Add a teaspoon each of French and wholegrain mustard, 5 tablespoons of extra virgin olive oil, 2 tablespoons of white wine vinegar and a pinch of salt & pepper. Toss together gently with your hands, have a taste to check the flavours, and set aside.

FOCACCIA Put the focaccia into the oven to warm for around 15 minutes. Make your pickle filling: put the jarred peppers, 1 teaspoon of capers, 6 sun-dried tomatoes, a handful of mixed olives, the red chilli, a handful of cherry tomatoes and 3 or 4 cornichons on a chopping board. Pick the leaves from the mint. Remove the stones from the olives. Finely slice the chilli, then chop and slice all the filling ingredients together on the board and sweep into a bowl. Add a lug of extra virgin olive oil, squeeze over the juice of ½ a lemon, then scrunch and mix together with your hands.

Take the focaccia out of the oven. Carefully halve it across the middle with a sharp serrated bread knife and open it like a book. Spread the pickle filling over the bottom half, drizzle over any juices left behind in the bowl, and finely grate over a good layer of Parmesan. Put the top on the sandwich and take it to the table.

REMOULADE & PROSCIUTTO Arrange the prosciutto around a rustic serving board, then place your celeriac remoulade in the centre and take to the table.

PESTO & MOZZARELLA Drain the mozzarella balls and put them into a bowl. Give the food processor a quick rinse then swap the grater attachment for the standard blade. Whiz up 100g of pinenuts, 75g of Parmesan, ½ a peeled clove of garlic and a large bunch of basil with 100ml of extra virgin olive oil. Spoon 2 tablespoons of this pesto over the mozzarella then put the rest in a jam jar for another day. Drizzle over some extra virgin olive oil and a pinch of salt & pepper. Toss and dress the mozzarella in the flavours, then sprinkle over the leaves from a few sprigs of Greek basil if using and drizzle over some more extra virgin olive oil. Squeeze over the juice of ½ a lemon, quickly grate over some Parmesan, crumble over the dried chilli half, then move the mozzarella to a serving dish and take to the table.

TO SERVE Divide the focaccia sandwich and dressed mozzarella up between everyone. Serve with a few slices of prosciutto, some of the crunchy remoulade and a glass of chilled rosé.

GRANITA When you're ready for dessert, take the platter of granita out of the freezer. Use a fork to fluff up the ice and squeeze over the juice of the pink grapefruit. Take to the table with the natural yoghurt and raspberries. Delicious!

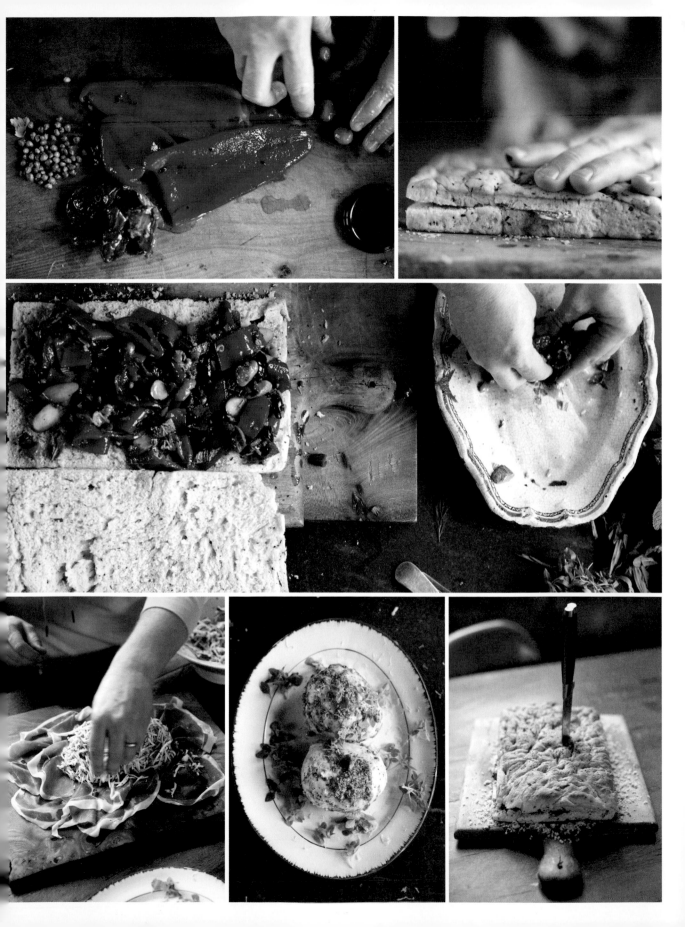

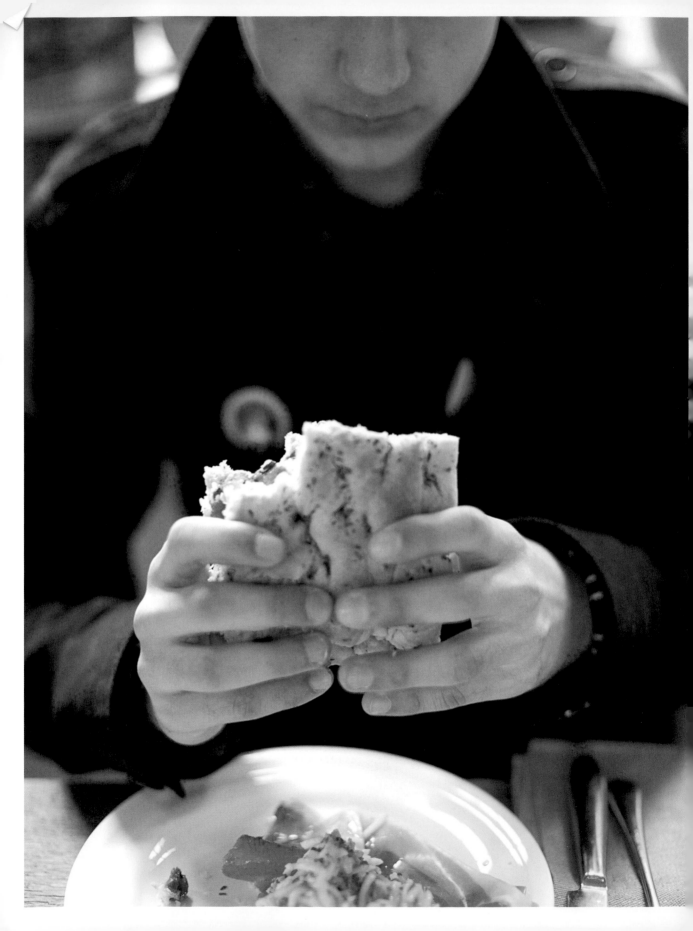

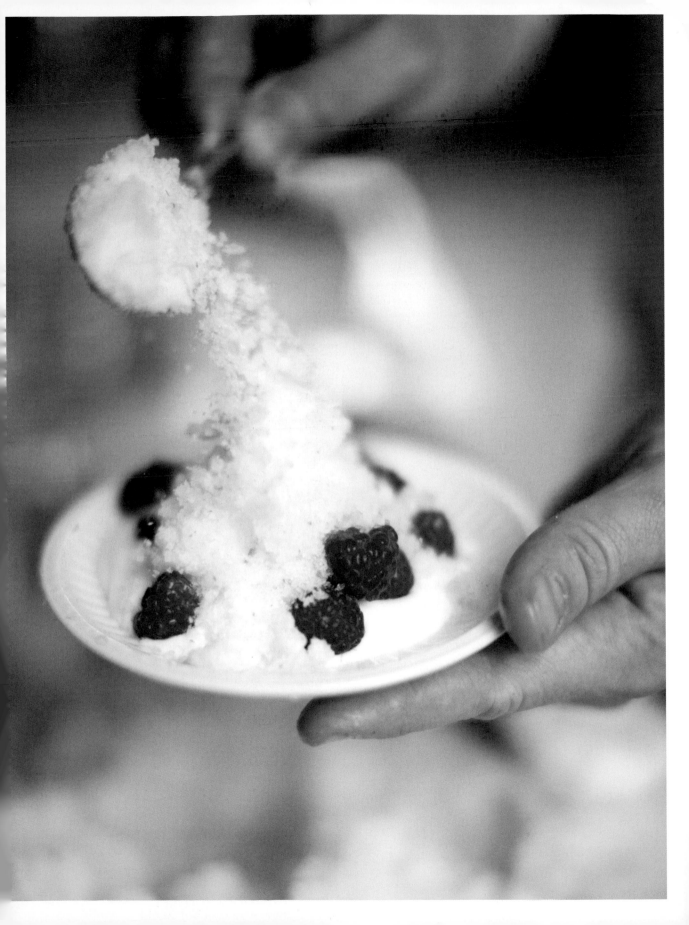

SEARED PORK FILLET & CATHERINE WHEEL SAUSAGE

MEATY MUSHROOM SAUCE

CELERIAC SMASH

GARLICKY BEANS

SERVES 6

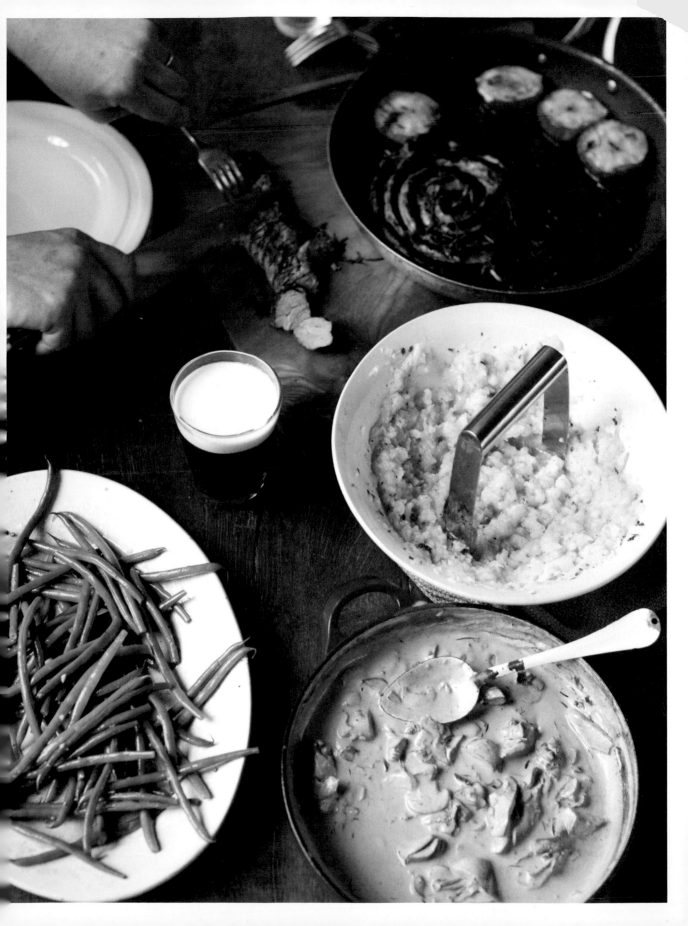

PORK

1 x 500g good-quality pork fillet
1 x 400g string of good-quality pork
  chipolatas
4 sprigs of fresh rosemary
2 small red apples
golden caster sugar

SMASH

1kg celeriac
a few sprigs of fresh thyme
½ a lemon

SAUCE

4 rashers of smoked streaky bacon
a few sprigs of fresh rosemary
200g pork kidney
8 medium white or chestnut
  mushrooms
optional: a swig of Marsala
150ml single cream
1 tablespoon English mustard

BEANS

400g green beans
½ a lemon
1 clove of garlic

SEASONINGS

olive oil
extra virgin olive oil
sea salt & black pepper

TO SERVE

good country ale

TO START Get all your ingredients and equipment ready. Turn the oven on to 220°C/425°F/gas 7. Put your largest ovenproof frying pan on a high heat and a medium frying pan on a medium heat. Fill and boil the kettle.

PORK Butterfly the fillet by halving it lengthways but leaving it joined at the top so it opens out like a book (or ask your butcher to do this for you). Drizzle with olive oil, scatter over a good pinch of salt & pepper, then rub all over so it's well coated. Wash your hands. Put into the large ovenproof frying pan and keep turning it every minute or so for around 5 minutes, while you do other jobs, until golden on all sides.

SMASH Get a clean board, then quickly peel the celeriac with a knife or a speed-peeler and chop into large chunks (🥄). Put into a large microwave-safe serving bowl with a good pinch of salt & pepper. Pick the thyme leaves into the bowl. Squeeze in the juice of ½ a lemon. Add a tiny splash of boiled water and the lemon half, then cover the bowl with a double layer of clingfilm. Microwave on full power for around 12 minutes, or until tender. Wash the board and the knife.

PORK Add a splash of olive oil to the fillet if needed. Turn the heat down a little and keep turning for another couple of minutes.

SAUCE Slice the bacon rashers thinly and put into the empty frying pan with a drizzle of olive oil. Pick in the leaves from a few sprigs of rosemary. Halve the kidney, removing any white bits of sinew. Finely slice the mushrooms and kidney and add to the pan with a really good pinch of pepper. Stir well.

PORK Coil the string of chipolatas around so you end up with a Catherine wheel (just like in the picture) and secure with skewers (🥄). Use tongs to move the fillet to a roasting tray, then put into the oven on the top shelf to cook for 15 minutes, or until golden on both sides. Add a splash of olive oil to the empty frying pan and lay the Catherine wheel in the pan. Brown on both sides, then leave to cook while you

pick some more rosemary leaves into the pan. Turn over the sausage. Halve the apples, then add them to the pan and move them around so they pick up all the juices.

SAUCE Hold the pan carefully and add a good swig of Marsala, if using. Let the alcohol burn off for a minute or light it; after 30 seconds pour in 150ml of single cream and stir in 1 tablespoon of English mustard.

BEANS Put a small saucepan on a high heat, fill it ¾ full with boiled water and add a pinch of salt. Trim the beans by cutting across all their ends at once. Add the beans to the water, put a lid on and cook for 5 minutes, or until tender enough to eat.

PORK Sprinkle a little pinch of sugar over each apple, then put the frying pan on the middle shelf of the oven to continue cooking for 10 minutes while you finish everything off.

SMASH Get the bowl out of the microwave, check the celeriac is cooked, and if so discard the lemon half and any excess water. Add a lug of extra virgin olive oil and season with salt & pepper. Mash until it's a nice consistency. Take to the table.

SAUCE Go back to the creamy mushrooms. Stir in a little cooking water from the beans to loosen if necessary, then taste, adjusting the seasoning if needed and take straight to the table.

BEANS Drain in a colander, then tip on to a platter. Squeeze over the juice of ½ a lemon and crush over an unpeeled clove of garlic. Drizzle over some good-quality extra virgin olive oil, add a pinch of salt & pepper, then toss and take to the table.

TO SERVE Put the sausage wheel and the pork on a wooden board and take to the table with the platter of beans. Let the pork rest for a minute or two while everyone helps themselves, then slice up and serve with some good country ale.

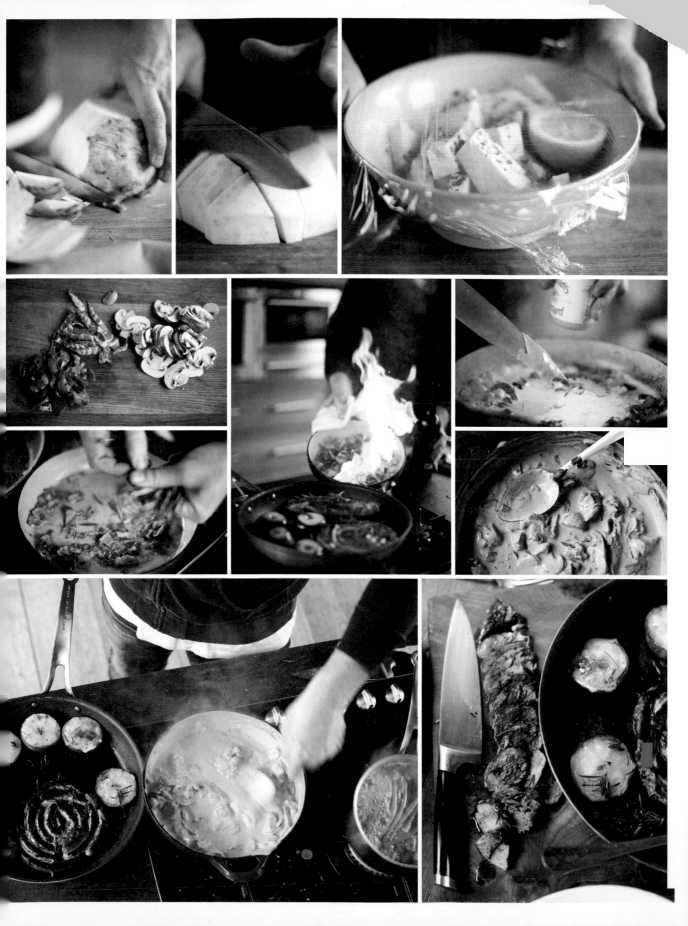

PORK CHOPS & CRISPY CRACKLING

CRUSHED POTATOES

MINTY CABBAGE

PEACHES 'N' CUSTARD

SERVES 4

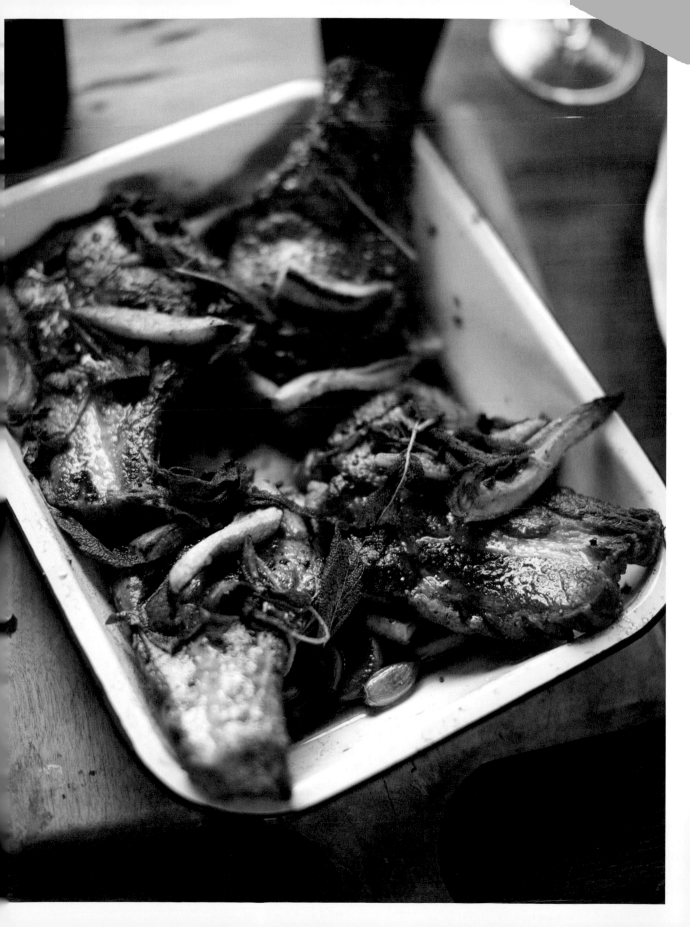

**180g good-quality chops, skin on
8 cloves of garlic
1 teaspoon fennel seeds
a small bunch of fresh sage
runny honey, for drizzling

POTATOES
700g Maris Piper potatoes
½ a lemon
1 heaped teaspoon wholegrain
  mustard
a small bunch of fresh flat-leaf parsley

CABBAGE
1 small Savoy cabbage
2 heaped teaspoons good-quality
  mint sauce

SEASONINGS
olive oil
extra virgin olive oil
sea salt & black pepper

PEACHES 'N' CUSTARD
2 x 415g tins of peach halves in juice
1 cinnamon stick
1 x 425g tin of good-quality custard
4 shortbread biscuits
a couple of sprigs of fresh mint

TO START Get all your ingredients and equipment ready. Turn the oven on to 180°C/350°F/gas 4. Fill and boil the kettle and put a large frying pan on a high heat.

PORK Put the pork chops on a plastic chopping board and trim off the skin and some of the fat. Cut the skin into 1cm slices and put them into the frying pan, fat side down, to make crackling.

POTATOES Wash the potatoes and get rid of any gnarly bits. Cut any large ones in half, quickly stab any whole ones and put into a large microwave-safe serving bowl. Add ½ a lemon and a good pinch of salt & pepper. Cover with a double layer of clingfilm and microwave on full power for around 17 minutes, or until cooked through.

PORK Use tongs to flip the crackling over. Score across the fat on the chops all the way along, then season on both sides with a good pinch of salt & pepper. Take the pan off the heat once the crackling is crisp and golden.

CABBAGE Halve the cabbage, trim the base, and remove the outer leaves. Cut into 8 wedges, put into a large saucepan and set aside.

PORK Lightly squash 8 unpeeled cloves of garlic with the heel of your hand and add to the frying pan – put it back on the heat if you've taken it off. Push the crackling and garlic to the sides of the pan, then stand all 4 chops up in the pan with the fat side down (look at the picture to see what I mean). Use the tongs to transfer the pieces of crackling and garlic to a roasting tray. Scatter the fennel seeds into the roasting tray, then put it into the oven on the top shelf. Wash your hands well, then pick the sage leaves.

CABBAGE Pour boiled water into the saucepan and add a good pinch of salt. Put the lid on and turn the heat underneath to high. Cook the cabbage for 6 to 8 minutes, or until tender enough to eat.

PORK Once the chops are golden on the fat edge, use the tongs to lay them flat in the pan. Cook for around 4 minutes, turning until golden. Get the crackling tray out of the oven and add the sage leaves and the pork chops. Mix together then arrange the sage leaves and crackling over the pork chops. Drizzle the chops with a little honey from a height, then return the tray to the oven for around 10 minutes, or until the chops are cooked through and look amazing.

PEACHES 'N' CUSTARD Pour the peaches and their juices into a small saucepan. Add the cinnamon stick and put over a high heat. Leave to tick away.

CABBAGE Drain the cabbage in a colander, then return it to the pan and stir in 2 heaped teaspoons of mint sauce, a pinch of salt & pepper and a splash of extra virgin olive oil. Gently toss with tongs. Pop the lid back on so it stays warm, and take to the table.

POTATOES Get the potatoes out of the microwave. Carefully pierce and remove the clingfilm. Check they are cooked, then discard the lemon half. Add 1 heaped teaspoon of mustard, a few good lugs of extra virgin olive oil and a good pinch of salt & pepper. Finely chop the parsley and add. Break and crush the potatoes with a spoon, mixing all the flavours together. Take to the table.

PEACHES 'N' CUSTARD Drizzle the custard over a platter. Spoon the hot peaches on top, and crumble over the shortbread. Drizzle over a little of the warm cooking juices, discarding the rest, then pick the leaves from the mint sprigs and tear over the top.

PORK Remove the pork from the oven and take it straight to the table. Serve with the lovely minty cabbage and crushed potatoes.

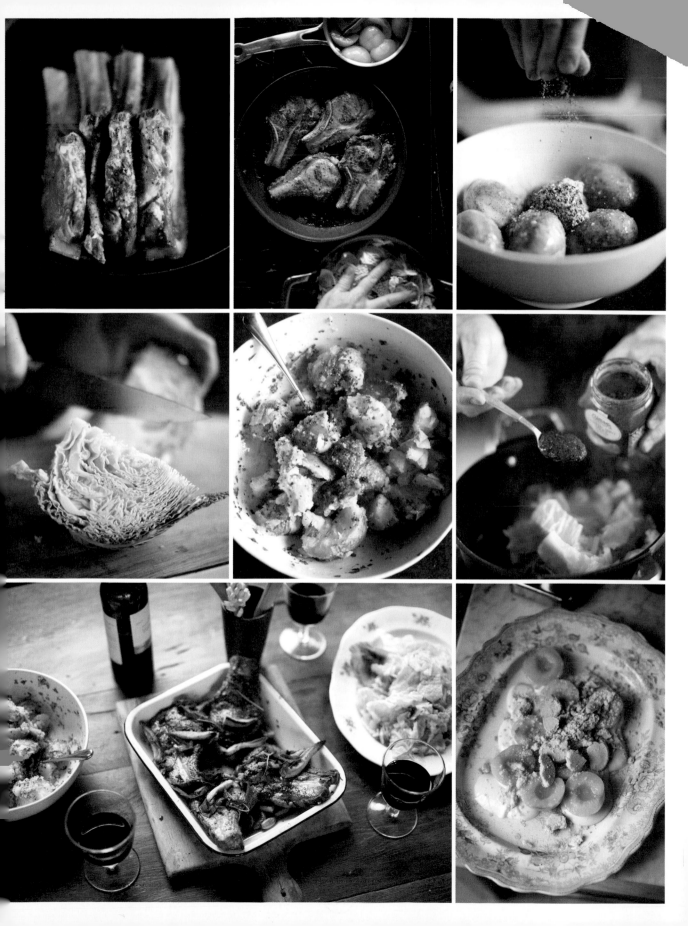

KINDA SAUSAGE CASSOULET

WARM BROCCOLI SALAD

BERRY & CUSTARD RIPPLE

SERVES 4–6

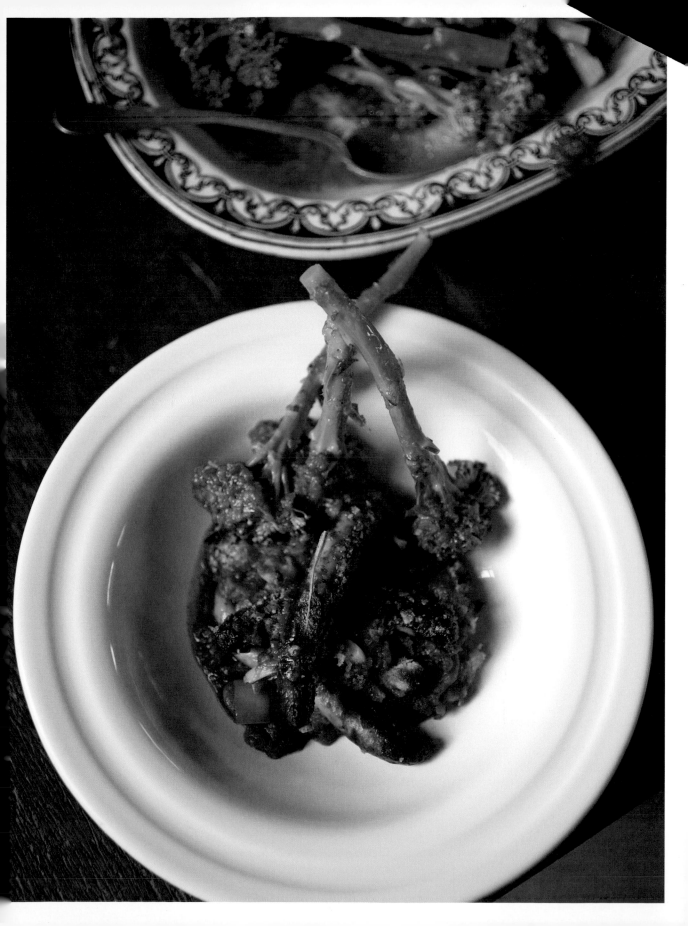

̷OULET

̷shers of smoked streaky bacon
1½ red onions
a few sprigs of fresh rosemary
½ a small bunch of fresh sage
3 fresh bay leaves
2 leeks
400g good-quality chipolata sausages
3–4 thick slices of bread
2 cloves of garlic
1 x 680g jar of passata
1 x 390g carton of butter beans
1 x 390g carton of haricot beans

BROCCOLI

400g tenderstem broccoli
¼ of a small red onion
1 clove of garlic
2 ripe plum tomatoes
1 lemon

SEASONINGS

olive oil
extra virgin olive oil
sea salt & black pepper

BERRY DESSERT

1 x 350g jar or tin of gooseberries,
 peaches or pears in juice
150g blueberries, blackberries or
 other nice berries
3 or 4 tablespoons elderflower cordial
1 x 425g tin of good-quality custard
150g Greek yoghurt
1 teaspoon vanilla paste or
 extract
a few shortbread biscuits, to serve

TO SERVE

a bottle of red wine

TO START Get all your ingredients and equipment ready. Turn the grill to full whack. Fill and boil the kettle. Put the standard blade attachment into the food processor.

CASSOULET Slice 4 rashers of bacon about 1cm thick and add to a sturdy roasting tray with a few lugs of olive oil. Put over a high heat. Halve, peel and slice 1½ red onions. Pick the rosemary and most of the sage leaves and sprinkle into the tray with the bay leaves, keeping a few sage sprigs back for later. Trim the leeks and peel back the outer leaves. Cut down the length of the leeks, then wash away any grit and finely slice. Add the leeks and onions to the tray with a few splashes of boiled water, stir, then leave to soften. Lay the sausages in another roasting tray, drizzle and rub a little olive oil over them, then put under the grill to cook for 8 minutes. Stir your vegetables.

BROCCOLI Put a small saucepan on a high heat. Trim and discard the ends of the broccoli.

BERRY DESSERT Pour the juice from the jar of gooseberries into the empty saucepan on a high heat and bring to the boil.

CASSOULET Tear the slices of bread into large chunks and put into a food processor with a pinch of salt & pepper, ½ of the reserved sprigs of sage, 2 cloves of garlic and a good drizzle of olive oil. Pulse until you have fairly even, coarse breadcrumbs. Stir the passata and the beans and their juices into the tray of vegetables.

BERRY DESSERT Add the gooseberries and fresh berries to the pan and stir occasionally until thick.

BROCCOLI Peel and coarsely grate ¼ of a red onion into a mixing bowl. Crush over 1 clove of garlic. Halve the 2 plum tomatoes, discard the seeds, then carefully grate them, flesh-side down, through the coarse grater. Discard the skins left behind. Add a couple of lugs of extra virgin olive oil, season carefully then squeeze in the juice of 1 lemon and mix.

CASSOULET Take the sausages out of the oven. Sprinkle half the breadcrumbs from the food processor over the veg and beans. Lay the sausages dark side down and sprinkle over the rest of the breadcrumbs. Pick the rest of the sage leaves, drizzle with olive oil and scatter on top. Put the roasting tray into the oven on the middle shelf for around 4 minutes, or until the breadcrumbs are crisp and golden.

BROCCOLI Put the broccoli, stalks down, into a pan of boiling water and put the lid on. Cook for a couple of minutes, or until tender.

BERRY DESSERT This should be lovely and jammy by now, so turn the heat off and stir in 3 or 4 tablespoons of elderflower cordial to taste. Spoon the custard around a platter, then pour the fruit and syrup into the centre. Dollop over the yoghurt, spoon over 1 teaspoon of vanilla paste or extract, then fold and ripple through. Take to the table with a few shortbreads.

TO SERVE The broccoli should be tender by now, so drain it, then scatter on a platter and spoon over the dressing. Toss quickly, and take straight to the table. Remove the cassoulet from the oven and take to the table with a nice bottle of red wine.

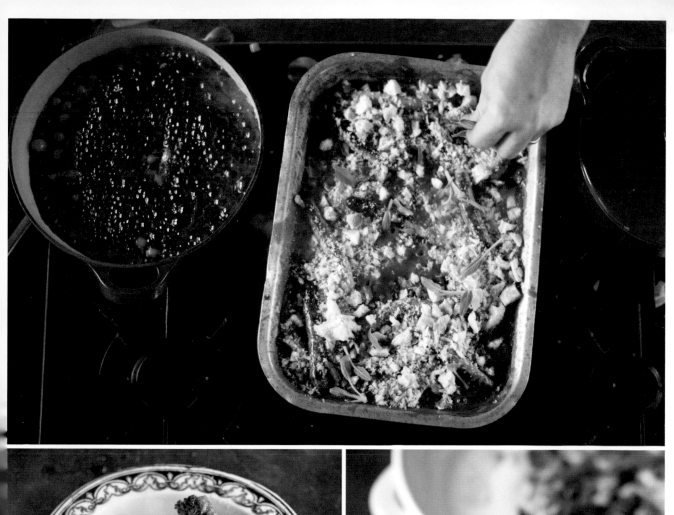

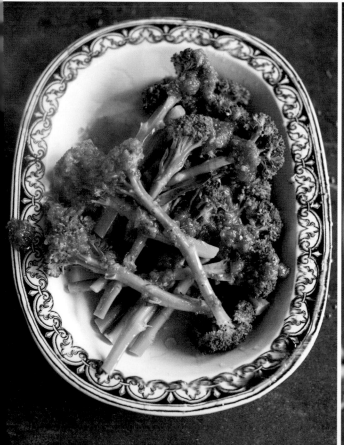

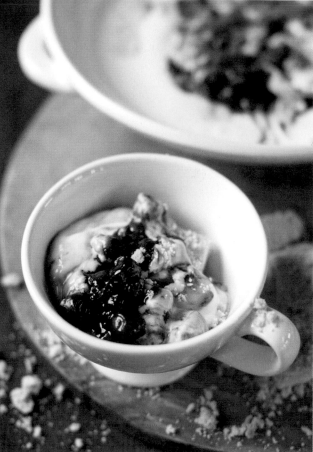

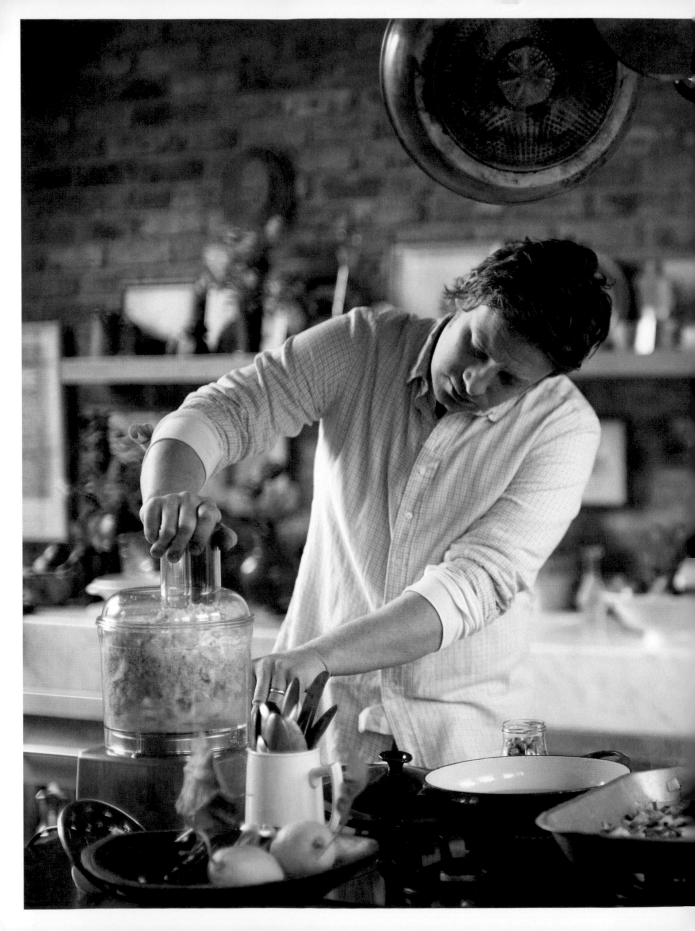

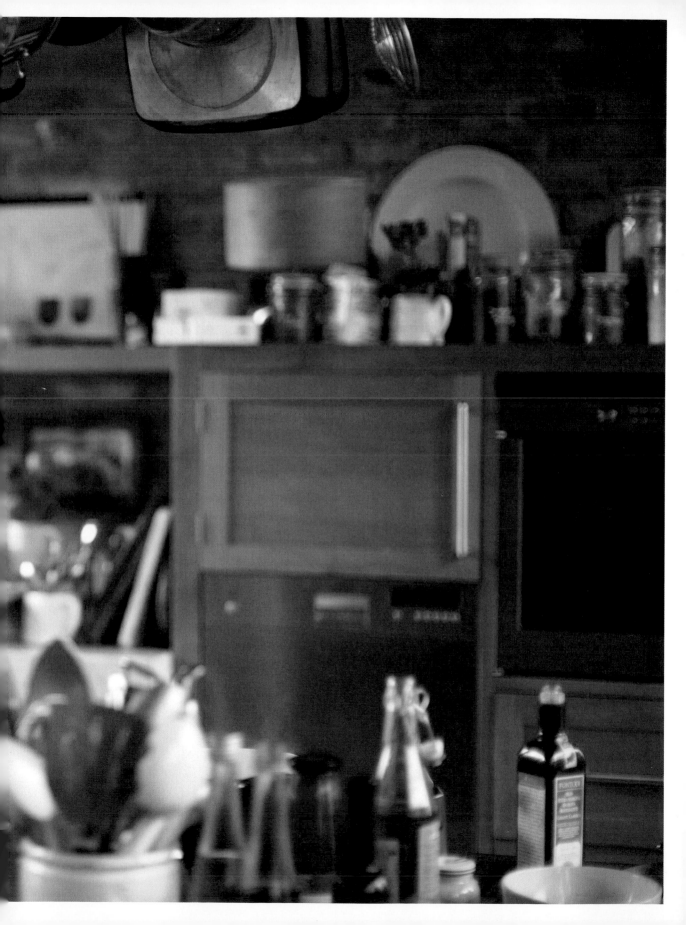

BRITISH PICNIC

SERVES 4 (with great leftovers or 8 as a light lunch)

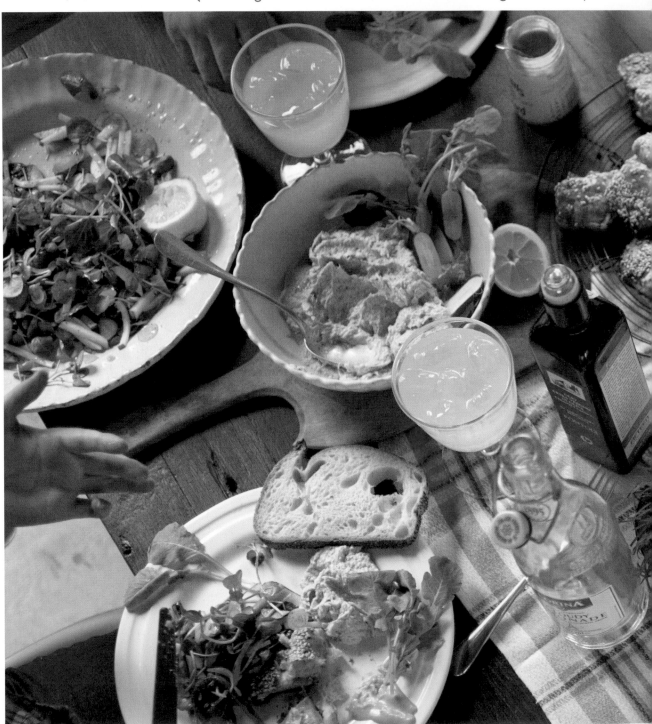

SAUSAGE ROLLS, MACKEREL PÂTÉ, LOVELY ASPARAGUS CRUNCH SALAD, PIMM'S ETON MESS

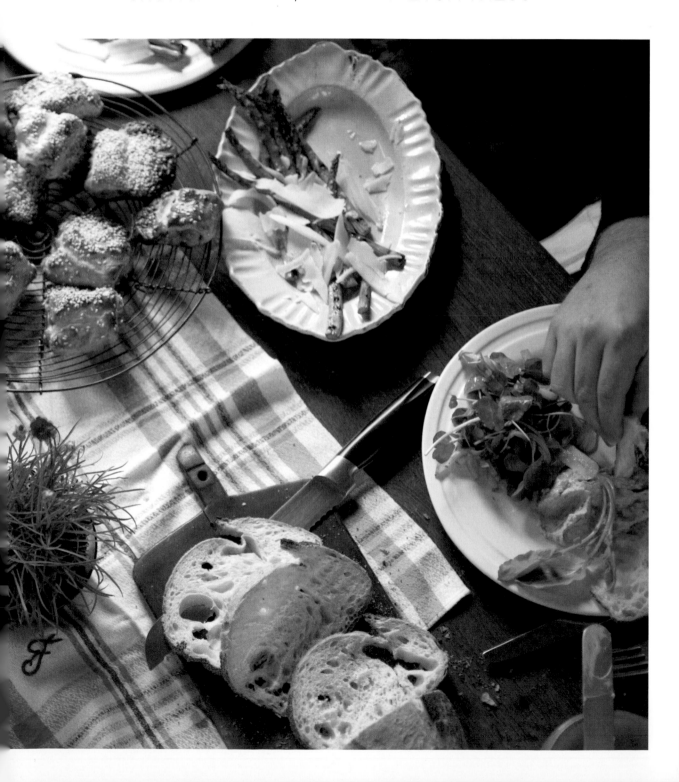

SAUSAGE ROLLS

plain flour, for dusting
1 x 375g ready-rolled puff pastry sheet
1 egg
1 x 12-pack of good-quality lean
  chipolatas (approx. 400g)
1 teaspoon fennel seeds
Parmesan cheese, for grating
1 tablespoon sesame seeds

ASPARAGUS

350g asparagus
½ a lemon
Lancashire cheese, to serve

PÂTÉ

1 heaped dessertspoon creamed
  horseradish
300g smoked mackerel
1 x 200g tub of light cream cheese
a bunch of fresh flat-leaf parsley
2 lemons
1 small bunch of radishes
a loaf of crusty bread

CRUNCH SALAD

1 x 100g bag of prewashed watercress
4 pickled onions
1 pear
½ a lemon

SEASONINGS

olive oil
extra virgin olive oil
sea salt & black pepper

ETON MESS

400g strawberries
1 heaped tablespoon golden caster
  sugar
1 blood orange
2 teaspoons vanilla paste or extract
a splash of Pimm's
250g low-fat yoghurt or
  crème fraîche
1 x 8-pack of meringue nests
a couple of sprigs of fresh mint

TO SERVE

English mustard
a large bottle of traditional lemonade

TO START Get all your ingredients and equipment ready. Turn the oven on to 220°C/425°F/gas 7 and get a griddle pan on a high heat. Put the standard blade attachment into the food processor.

SAUSAGE ROLLS Dust a clean surface with plain flour and unroll the puff pastry. Slice the pastry in half lengthways. Beat the egg in a little bowl, then use a pastry brush to paint the pastry halves. Line the sausages up so you get 6 on each half (just like in the picture). Bash 1 teaspoon of fennel seeds in a pestle & mortar and sprinkle over. Finely grate a layer of Parmesan over the sausages.

Fold the pastry over the sausages, then use a fork to quickly crimp the edges together so you end up with 2 long sausage rolls. Paint these with the rest of the egg wash, then sprinkle over the sesame seeds. Drizzle olive oil over a baking tray, then roughly cut each long roll into 10 smaller rolls. Lay the rolls on the oiled baking tray and put into the oven on the top shelf for around 15 minutes, or until golden and puffed up. Wash your hands, then put the loaf of bread for the pâté into the oven to warm through.

ASPARAGUS Trim off and discard the woody ends of the asparagus, quickly rinse the tips, and lay on the hot dry griddle pan. Turn occasionally and cook until nicely charred on all sides.

PÂTÉ Put 1 heaped dessertspoon of horseradish into the food processor with all of the mackerel and cream cheese, the bunch of parsley and a good pinch of pepper. Finely grate in the zest of a lemon and squeeze in the juice of 1½. Let the processor run for a few minutes while you wash and halve the radishes and arrange them around the edge of a serving bowl. When everything is quite smooth and well mixed, spoon it into the serving bowl. You can put it into the fridge to firm up a bit if you like, but I prefer it a little softer. Drizzle over some good extra virgin olive oil, then take it to the table with the loaf of warm bread and a lemon half for squeezing over.

ASPARAGUS Turn the asparagus.

CRUNCH SALAD Tip the watercress on to a platter. Finely slice 4 large pickled onions and sprinkle all around the watercress. Finely slice the pear into rounds, core and all, then slice the rounds into matchsticks and scatter over. Dress with a good drizzle of extra virgin olive oil and a good pinch of salt & pepper, and take to the table with a lemon half for squeezing over.

ASPARAGUS Drizzle a little extra virgin olive oil over the spears and squeeze over the juice of ½ a lemon. Shake the pan, lightly season, then tip everything on to a serving plate. Take to the table with a wedge of Lancashire for shaving over.

SAUSAGE ROLLS If they are golden brown and cooked through, take them out of the oven. If not, leave in while you make your pudding.

ETON MESS Slice the strawberries and put them into a bowl with 1 heaped tablespoon of sugar. Grate over the orange zest, then squeeze in the juice from ½ the orange. Add 2 teaspoons of vanilla paste or extract, then really mash and mix everything together with a fork. Add a good splash of Pimm's and mix again. Dollop 2 tablespoons of yoghurt or crème fraîche on a platter and spread out, adding the strawberry mixture as you go. Crumble over half the meringue nests, mix again, then rip some mint leaves over and take to the table with the rest of the meringue nests – crumble these over just before you serve dessert.

TO SERVE Remove the sausage rolls from the oven, arrange on a platter and take straight to the table with some English mustard.

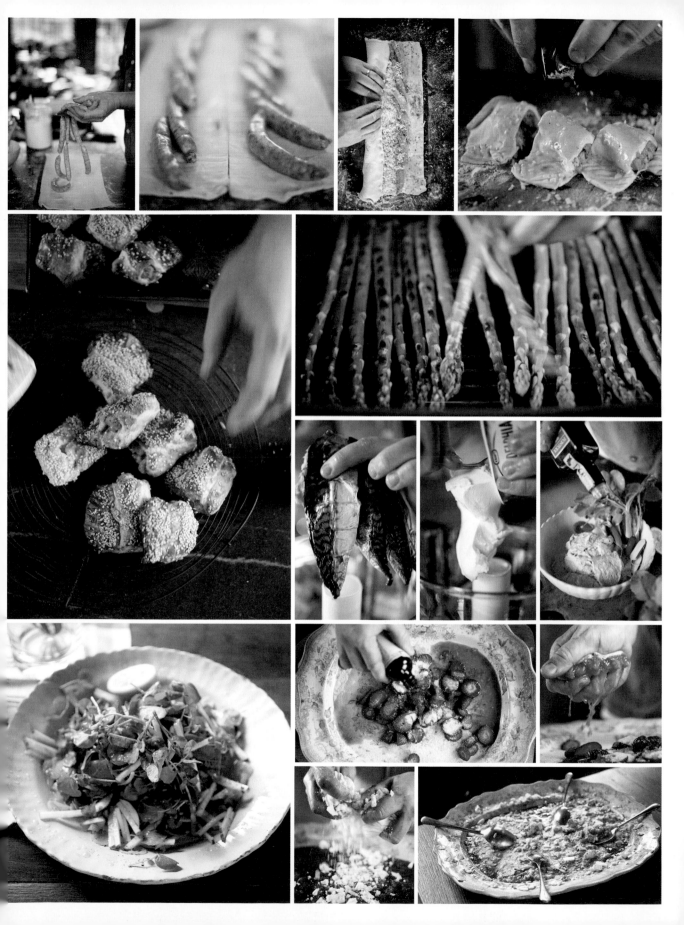

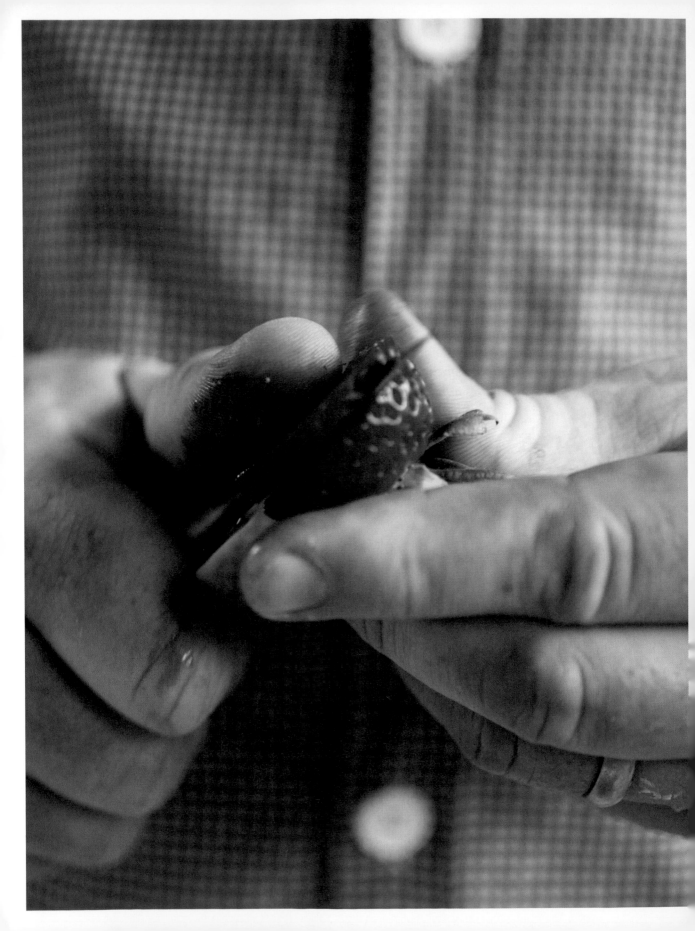

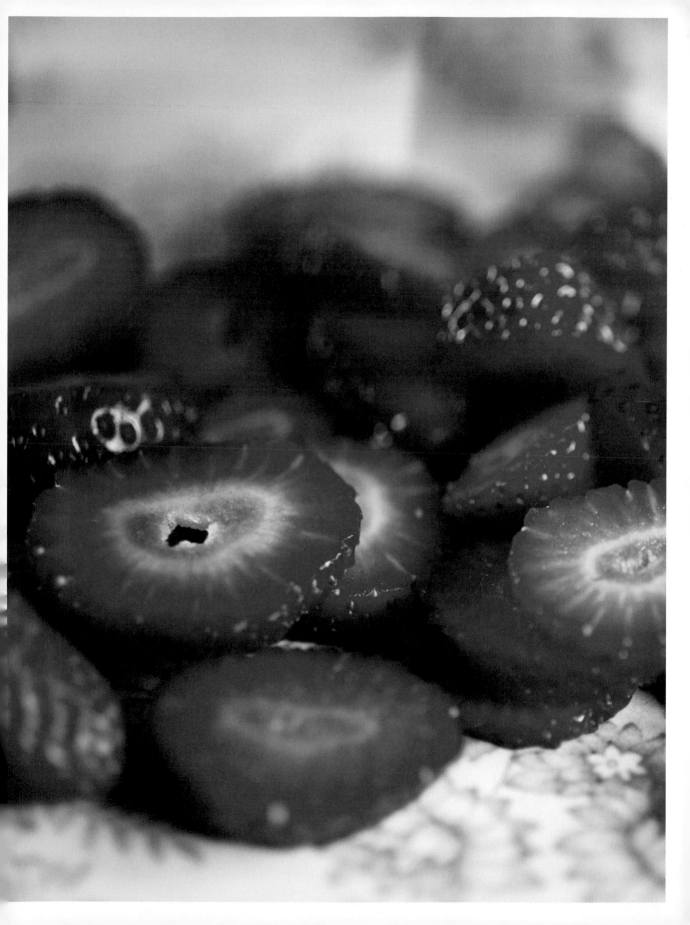

CATHERINE WHEEL SAUSAGE

HORSERADISH MASH

APPLE SALAD

SAGE & LEEK GRAVY

STUFFED APPLES

SERVES 4–6

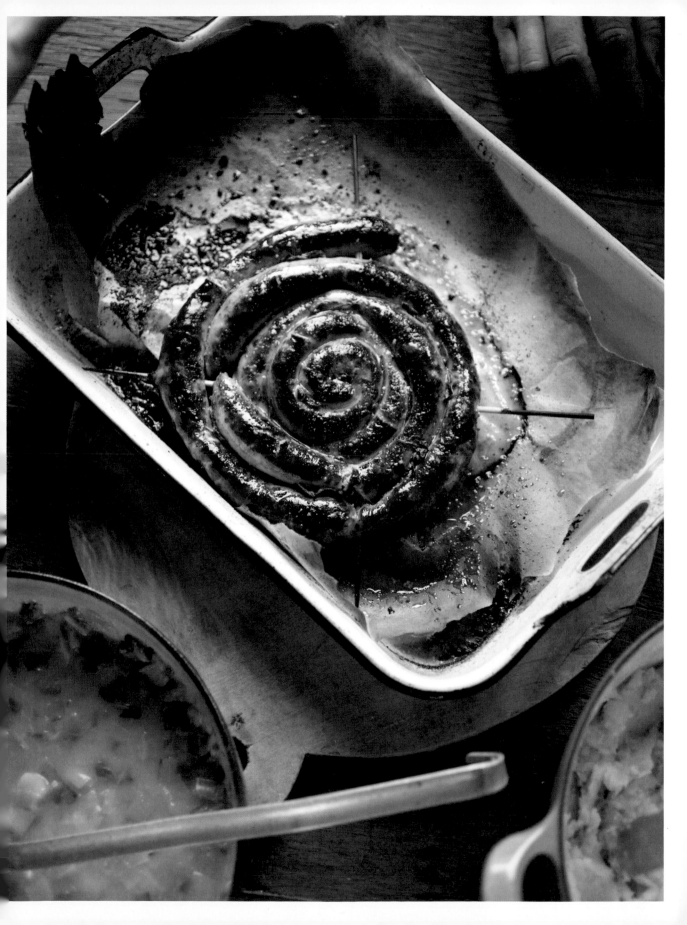

CATHERINE WHEEL SAUSAGE
2 x 6-packs of good-quality
 linked sausages (approx. 400g)
3 sprigs of fresh sage

GRAVY
2 leeks
a few sprigs of fresh sage
1 organic chicken stock cube
1 heaped tablespoon plain flour
200ml good-quality cider

HORSERADISH MASH
800g Maris Piper potatoes
a large knob of butter

2 heaped teaspoons creamed
 horseradish

APPLE SALAD
4 multigrain Ryvita
¼ of a 200g tub of cream cheese
1 lemon
1 small apple
50g prewashed watercress

SEASONINGS
olive oil
extra virgin olive oil
sea salt & black pepper

STUFFED APPLES (makes 4 or 6)
4 small apples (or 6 if making for
 6 people)
1 egg
100g golden caster sugar
100g dried apricots
100g blanched almonds
optional: Cointreau, for drizzling
single cream or natural yoghurt, to
 serve

TO SERVE
a pot of English mustard
cold cider

TO START Get all your ingredients and equipment ready. Turn the grill to full whack. Put a large saucepan on a low heat. Fill and boil the kettle. Put the standard blade attachment into the food processor.

CATHERINE WHEEL SAUSAGE Scrunch a large sheet of greaseproof paper under the tap, then lay it out flat. Untwist the links between the sausages and push the meat together to make 2 long sausages. Roll both into one large Catherine wheel. Stab a couple of wooden skewers through, to hold it all together (🔲). Pick the sage leaves and poke them into the gaps. Drizzle with olive oil and rub in. Lift up the greaseproof paper and transfer the Catherine wheel sausage to a large roasting tray. Tear off any excess paper. Wash your hands. Whack the tray under the grill on the top shelf and cook for 10 minutes, or until the sausage is golden.

STUFFED APPLES Core the apples, then score a line around the middle of each one. Crack the egg into a food processor and add 100g of golden caster sugar, 100g of dried apricots and 100g of blanched almonds (how easy is that ratio?!). Blitz until combined. Use a spoon to stuff the apples with this mixture, pushing it in from either end. Spread any leftover mixture around the base of a snug-fitting earthenware dish (make sure it's microwave-safe). Sit the apples on top, then microwave uncovered for 10 minutes on full power.

GRAVY Put a large frying pan with a lid on a low heat.

HORSERADISH MASH Turn the heat under the large saucepan up to high. Quickly cut the potatoes into 1cm pieces, then put them into the pan and just cover them with boiled water, keeping some water for later. Season with a pinch of salt and put the lid on.

GRAVY Wipe the chopping board. Trim 2 leeks, then halve lengthways and rinse under the tap. Slice into 1cm thick pieces and add to the empty frying pan with a lug of olive oil and a generous splash of boiled water. Pop the lid on and turn the heat up to medium. Stir occasionally.

CATHERINE WHEEL SAUSAGE By now, the 10 minutes should be up. Take the tray out of the oven, flip over the sausage, and return the tray to the top shelf.

APPLE SALAD Snap 4 Ryvitas into bite-sized pieces. Use the back of a teaspoon to smear a little cream cheese over each one. Arrange around a platter. Finely grate over the zest of ½ a lemon and sprinkle over a little black pepper. Slice off the base of the apple so it sits flat, then slice into rounds as finely as you can. Stack the slices up and cut across them into matchsticks. Squeeze over the juice of the zested ½ a lemon to stop the apple discolouring, and toss.

GRAVY Finely slice the sage leaves and add to the leeks. Crumble in a chicken stock cube and add 1 heaped tablespoon of flour. Stir well and add 200ml of cider. Leave to sizzle away, then add 200ml of boiled water. Reduce the heat to low and leave to tick away until you have a good consistency.

APPLE SALAD Put little pinches of watercress among the Ryvita pieces. Scatter over the dressed apple. Put the other lemon half on the side for squeezing over, drizzle over a little extra virgin olive oil, and take to the table.

STUFFED APPLES Take the dish of apples out of the microwave. If their stuffing has come out, use a spoon to push it back in. Move the Catherine wheel to the bottom shelf of the oven and pop the apples on the top shelf to caramelize for the last couple of minutes.

HORSERADISH MASH Drain the potatoes in a colander, then return them to the pan and mash with a large knob of butter and a pinch of salt & pepper. Stir in 2 heaped teaspoons of creamed horseradish and take to the table.

STUFFED APPLES Pour the cream into a small jug to serve. When golden and delicious, remove the apples from the oven. If you want to be dramatic, like me, drizzle over a splash of Cointreau, then quickly and carefully set alight with a match. Once the flame has burned away, serve with the cream.

TO SERVE Put the sausage on a board and take to the table with the gravy pan. Put a pot of English mustard on the side and dish up. Serve with glasses of cold cider.

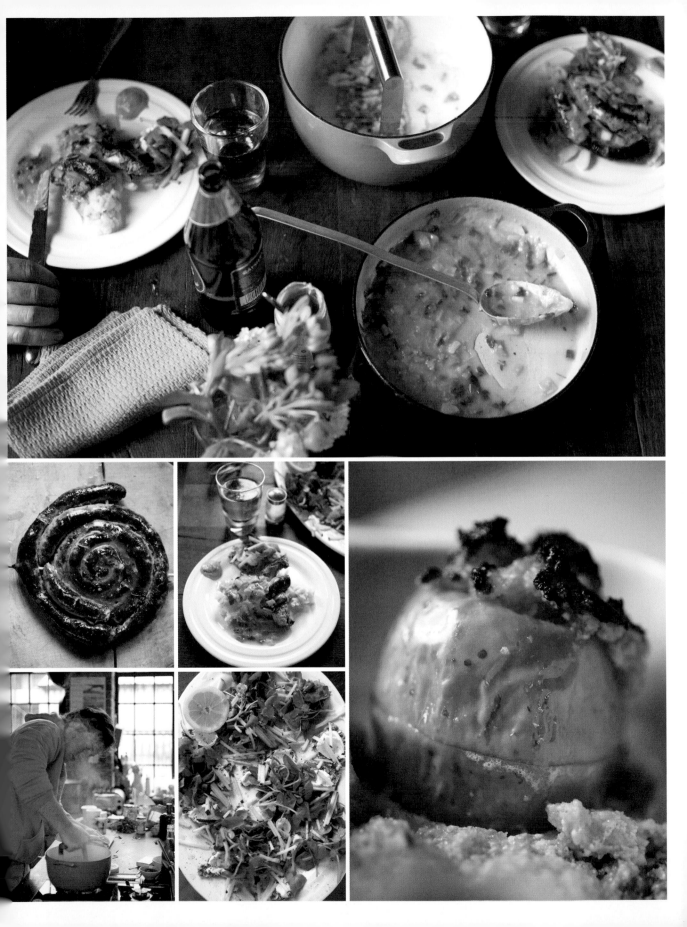

TAPAS FEAST

SERVES 6

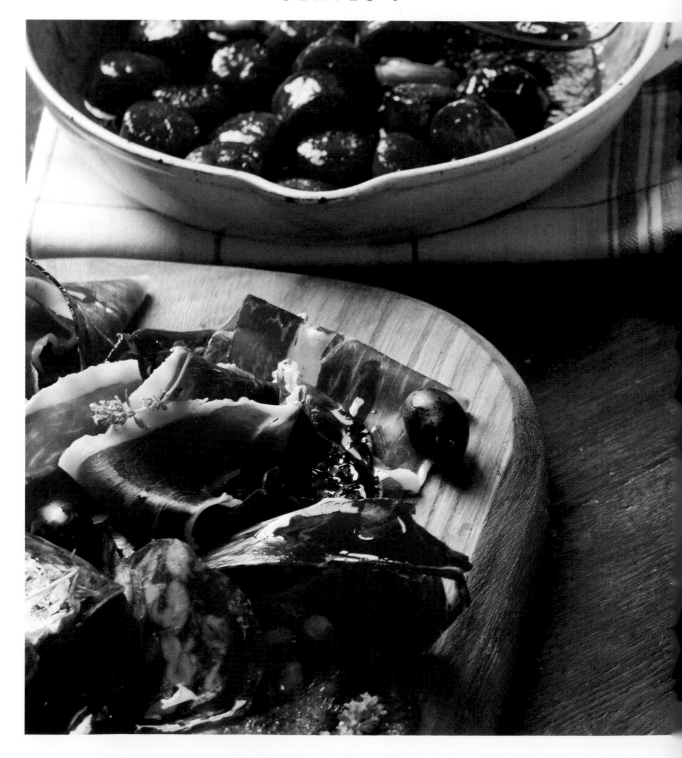

TORTILLA, GLAZED CHORIZO, MANCHEGO CHEESE, CURED MEATS & HONEY, STUFFED PEPPERS, ROLLED ANCHOVIES

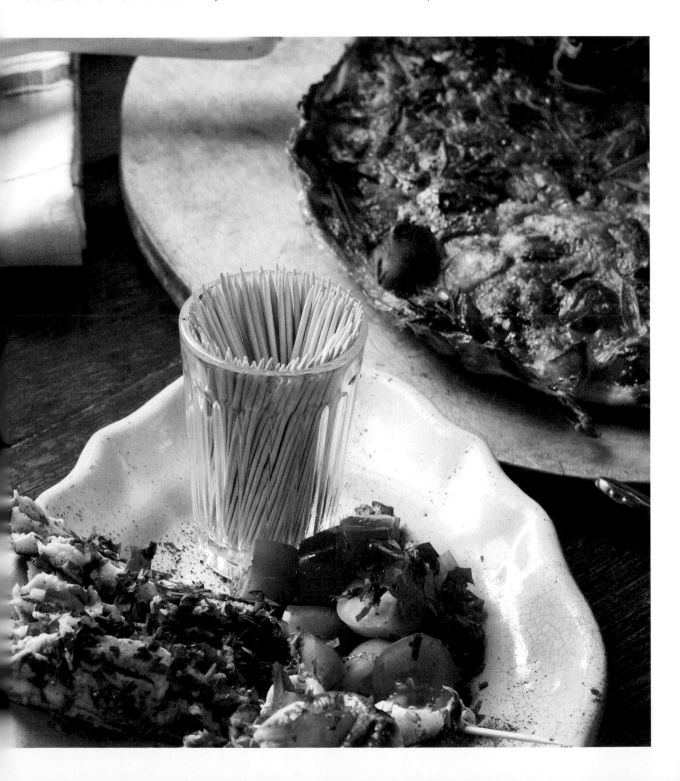

TORTILLA
250g baby new potatoes
1 small red onion
1 teaspoon fennel seeds
2 cloves of garlic
½ a small bunch of fresh rosemary
8 eggs
a large handful of prewashed rocket,
  to serve

CHORIZO
250g good-quality semi-cured whole
  chorizo
2 cloves of garlic
4 tablespoons red wine vinegar
1 tablespoon runny honey

PEPPERS
100g Manchego cheese
1 ciabatta loaf
50g blanched almonds
a small bunch of fresh thyme
red wine vinegar
1 x 450g jar of whole peppers

MANCHEGO
100g Manchego cheese
100g Spanish cured meats, such as
  pata negra
runny honey, for drizzling
instant or quality ground coffee
a handful of black olives
optional: a couple of sprigs of fresh
  thyme or oregano

ANCHOVIES
1 x 100g pack of marinated or dressed
  anchovies, from chilled section
a few sprigs of fresh flat-leaf parsley
1 lemon
150g cherry tomatoes
smoked paprika, for dusting

SEASONINGS
olive oil
extra virgin olive oil
sea salt & black pepper

TO SERVE
a bottle of sparkling water
1 orange
a chilled bottle of dry sherry

TO START Get all your ingredients and equipment ready. Put a medium ovenproof frying pan (approx. 26cm) on a high heat and a small frying pan on a low heat. Turn the grill on to full whack. Put the standard blade attachment into the food processor.

TORTILLA Chop the potatoes into 1cm chunks. Put them into the medium ovenproof frying pan with a lug of olive oil and toss. Halve, peel and roughly chop the red onion. Once the potatoes have a good colour, add the onions to the pan along with the fennel seeds and mix well. Now get on with other jobs but remember to keep tossing the potatoes occasionally.

CHORIZO Slice the chorizo into 2cm rounds. Put into the small frying pan with a splash of olive oil and toss occasionally until golden and crisp.

PEPPERS Trim off the rind from the Manchego, then crumble into the food processor with a handful of torn-up ciabatta, 50g of blanched almonds, the leaves from the bunch of thyme, a good pinch of salt & pepper and a swig of red wine vinegar. Whiz up until fine, then stuff inside the peppers – no need to pack it in. Once full, put them into a baking dish. Scatter any remaining breadcrumbs over the peppers. Top with the remaining thyme sprigs, drizzle with olive oil, then put on the middle shelf, under the grill, for 8 minutes. Rip the remaining ciabatta in half and take to the table.

MANCHEGO Lay the slices of cured meat on a board alongside the large wedge of Manchego. Drizzle a little honey over the cheese, then sprinkle over a pinch of ground coffee. Scatter a handful of black olives and a few leaves of thyme or oregano (if using) over the meat. Drizzle with a tiny bit of extra virgin olive oil, sprinkle lightly with pepper and take to the table.

CHORIZO Lightly bash 2 unpeeled cloves of garlic with the heel of your hand or the bottom of a saucepan and add to the pan.

TORTILLA The potatoes should be lovely and golden by now, so turn the heat down to low. Crush 2 unpeeled cloves of garlic into the pan. Pick most of the rosemary leaves into the pan and stir. Season with a good pinch of salt & pepper.

CHORIZO Carefully drain away most of the fat, leaving about 1 tablespoon of it behind. Add the red wine vinegar and runny honey and leave to reduce down to a really sticky glaze. Keep an eye on it, giving the pan a shake every so often so it doesn't catch.

TORTILLA Taste the potato mixture for seasoning, then crack the eggs directly into the pan and gently stir with a wooden spoon to create a marbled effect. Turn the heat up to medium. Once the eggs start to set around the sides, scatter the rest of the rosemary leaves on top and put under the grill on the top shelf for 3 to 5 minutes, or until set, golden and fluffy.

ANCHOVIES Put the anchovies into a nice serving bowl. Finely chop a few sprigs of parsley and sprinkle over. Finely grate over the zest of ½ the lemon, then drizzle over some extra virgin olive oil. Halve the cherry tomatoes and pile them next to the anchovies with a bunch of cocktail sticks. The idea is to get everyone to make their own skewers. Add a pinch of paprika and take to the table.

TO SERVE Take the tortilla and stuffed peppers to the table. Pop a large handful of rocket next to the tortilla. Take the pan of sticky chorizo to the table. Serve with a jug of iced sparkling water filled with orange slices, and a chilled bottle of dry sherry.

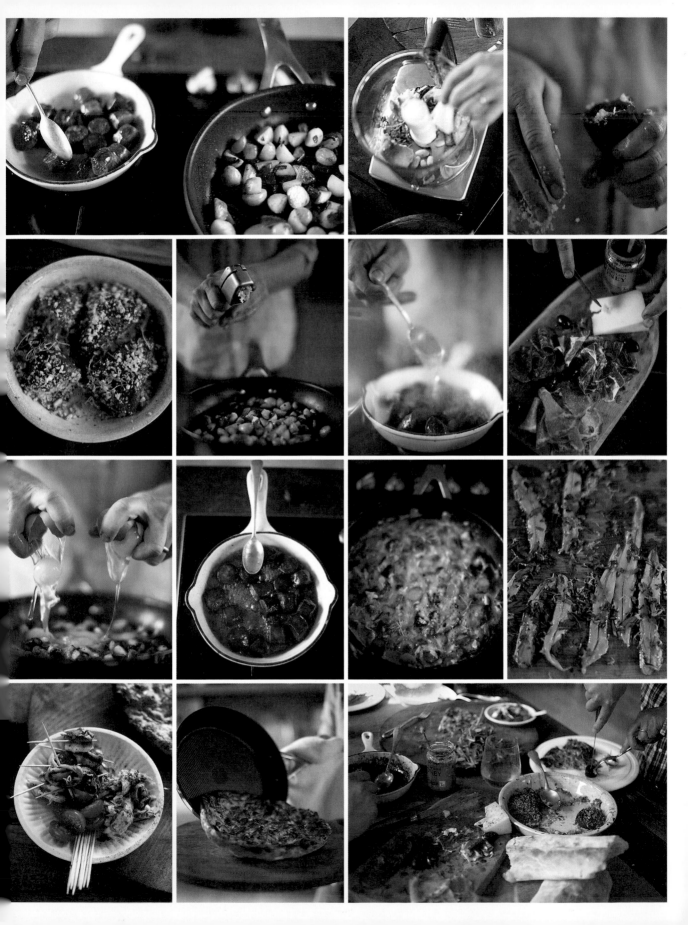

MOROCCAN LAMB CHOPS

SERVES 4–6

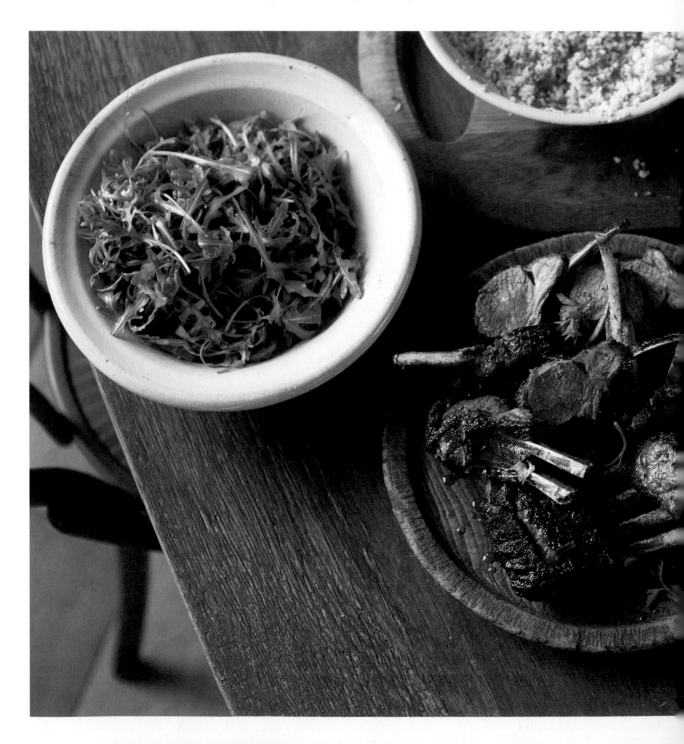

FLATBREADS, HERBY COUSCOUS STUFFED PEPPERS, POMEGRANATE DRINK

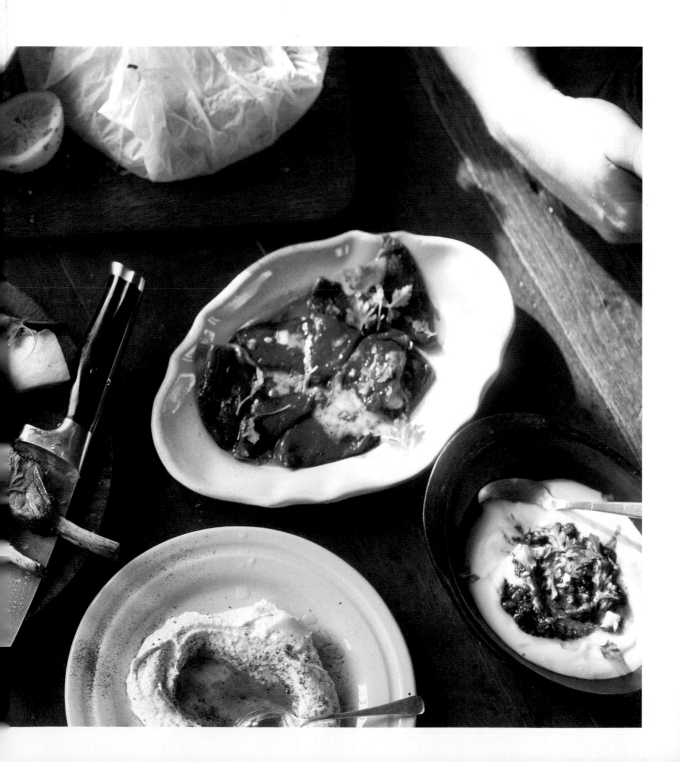

LAMB
2 racks of lamb (8 chops per rack), fat removed
1 whole nutmeg, for grating
1 teaspoon ground cumin
1 teaspoon sweet paprika, plus extra for dusting
1 teaspoon dried thyme
1 lemon

COUSCOUS
200g couscous
1 fresh red chilli
a large bunch of fresh flat-leaf parsley or mint
1 lemon

GARNISHES
1 pack of flatbreads
1 tablespoon dried thyme or oregano
1 x 250g tub of natural yoghurt
1 heaped teaspoon harissa
1 x 200g tub of houmous
½ a lemon

SEASONINGS
olive oil
extra virgin olive oil
sea salt & black pepper

STUFFED PEPPERS
60g good melting cheese, such as Cheddar or fontina
8 small whole jarred red peppers

DRINK
ice cubes
a few sprigs of fresh mint
½ a lemon
1 pomegranate
1 bottle of sparkling water

TO START Get all your ingredients and equipment ready. Fill and boil the kettle. Put a large frying pan on a medium heat. Put a roasting tray in the oven and turn the oven on to 220°C/425°F/gas 7.

LAMB Put the racks of lamb on a sheet of greaseproof paper over a board and cut each rack in half so you have 4 smaller racks. Quickly score the surface area of each rack in a crisscross fashion, then finely grate over ½ the nutmeg, and sprinkle with the cumin, paprika and thyme. Massage the flavours into the meat, then place in the hot frying pan with a splash of olive oil. Discard the greaseproof paper. Turn and colour the meat on all sides for around 5 minutes as you get on with the rest of the meal.

COUSCOUS Tip the couscous into a large bowl with a drizzle of olive oil and add just enough boiling water to cover. Season with a pinch of salt, then cover with a plate and set aside for a few minutes.

GARNISHES Lay the flatbreads on a board. Drizzle with olive oil, then sprinkle with salt and dried thyme or oregano. Scrunch up and wet a large piece of greaseproof paper under the tap and flatten out. Stack up the breads and wrap in the greaseproof paper, then pop on to the lowest oven shelf to warm through.

LAMB Check the lamb. Once brown, transfer to the hot roasting tray, bones facing up, and put on the top shelf of the oven. Set the timer for 14 minutes for blushing to medium meat, slightly less for rare, and more for well done. Halfway through, turn the racks over. Rinse out the lamb pan and wipe clean with kitchen paper. Put on a low heat.

DRINK Half-fill a large jug with ice. Scrunch up a few sprigs of fresh mint and add, squeezing in the juice from ½ a lemon. Place a sieve over the jug, then halve the pomegranate and really squeeze each half so all the capsules break and the juice pours into the jug. Discard

what's left behind in the sieve. Top up with sparkling water, stir with a wooden spoon and take to the table.

STUFFED PEPPERS Divide the cheese into 8 slices and put 1 slice inside each pepper.

LAMB Turn the racks now, gently shake the tray and hit it with a good pinch of salt. Return to the oven.

COUSCOUS Deseed and finely chop the red chilli. Finely chop most of the parsley or mint leaves (reserving a small handful of leaves). Take the plate off the couscous, add the chopped parsley and chilli, a few lugs of extra virgin olive oil and a pinch of salt & pepper. Squeeze in the juice of a lemon. Toss and fluff up with a fork. Taste and tweak until happy, then take to the table.

GARNISHES Put the yoghurt into a bowl and swirl in the harissa. Drizzle over a touch of extra virgin olive oil and add a few reserved parsley leaves. Spoon the houmous on to a plate, make a well in the centre and drizzle with extra virgin olive oil. Add a pinch of salt & pepper, a squeeze of the juice from the lemon half and a pinch of paprika. Take to the table.

STUFFED PEPPERS Drizzle olive oil into the pan you used for the lamb, then add the peppers. Cook for just 1½ to 2 minutes and once the cheese melts, turn the heat off. It's quick and delicious.

LAMB Remove from the oven and transfer to a board to rest for a few minutes.

TO SERVE Tip the peppers on to a plate and scatter over a few parsley or mint leaves. Take the flatbreads out of the oven. Scatter the rest of the parsley over the lamb, cut the lemon into wedges for squeezing over and serve on the side. Take everything to the table and enjoy!

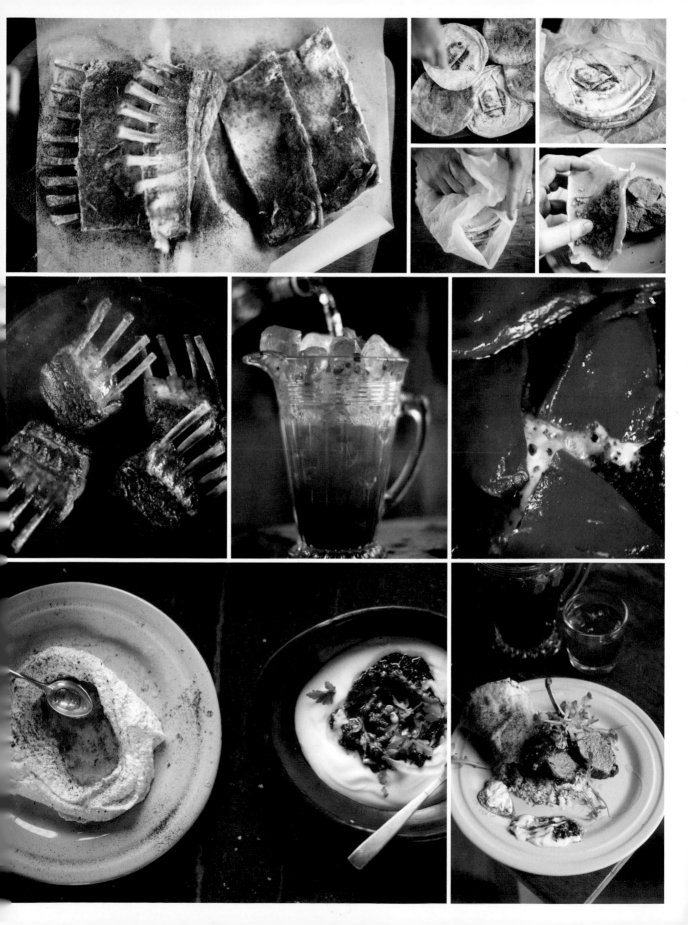

SPRING LAMB

VEGETABLE PLATTER

MINT SAUCE

CHIANTI GRAVY

CHOCOLATE FONDUE

SERVES 4–6

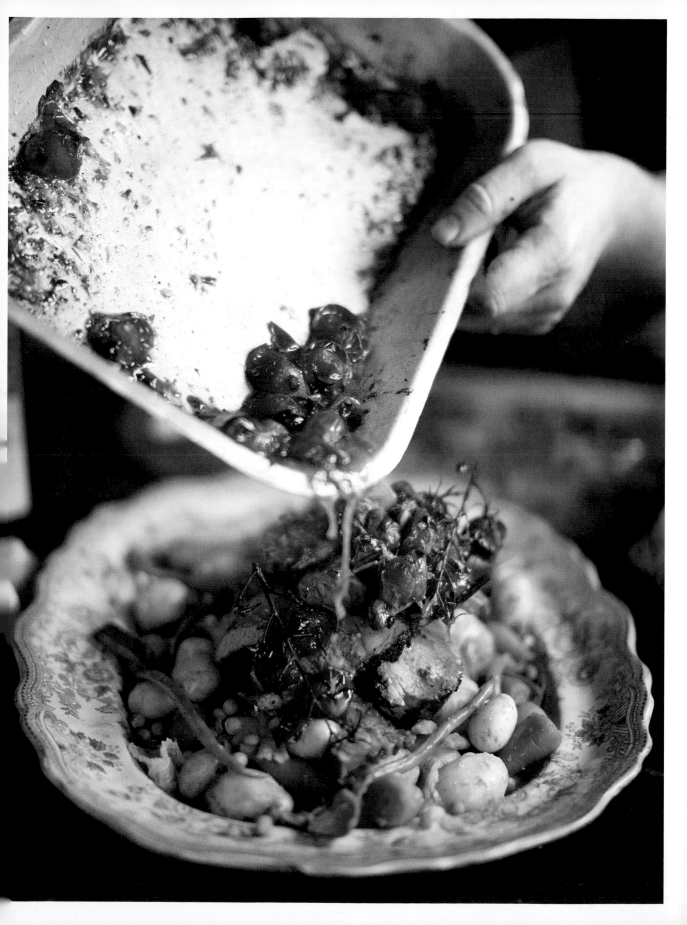

LAMB

1 x 8-bone rack of lamb, fat removed
1 x 2-piece pack of lamb neck fillet
  (approx. 250g)
3 sprigs of fresh rosemary
2 cloves of garlic
1 teaspoon Dijon mustard
white wine vinegar
300g cherry tomatoes on the vine

GRAVY

4 rashers of smoked bacon
2 sprigs of fresh rosemary
1 heaped tablespoon plain flour
½ a glass of red wine

VEGETABLES

500g baby new potatoes
250g baby carrots
stalks from a bunch of fresh mint
1 organic chicken stock cube
200g fine beans
200g runner beans
½ a Savoy cabbage
200g frozen peas
a knob of butter
½ a lemon

MINT SAUCE

leaves from a bunch of fresh mint
4 tablespoons red wine vinegar
1 tablespoon golden caster sugar

SEASONINGS

olive oil
extra virgin olive oil
sea salt & black pepper

FONDUE

1 x 100g bar of good-quality dark
  chocolate (70% cocoa solids)
1 teaspoon vanilla paste or extract
100ml milk
4–6 handfuls of mixed fruit, such as
  mango, strawberries or pineapple

TO START Get all your ingredients and equipment ready. Put a large frying pan and a large saucepan on a high heat. Fill and boil the kettle. Turn the oven on to 220°C/425°F/gas 7.

LAMB Halve the rack of lamb, then season with salt & pepper and add to the frying pan with a lug of olive oil.

VEGETABLES Wash the potatoes and trim the tops of the carrots. Add everything to the large saucepan with a pinch of salt. Rip the leafy tops off the bunch of mint and put aside for the mint sauce. Make sure the band is still around the stalks, then add them to the saucepan. Just cover with boiled water and crumble in the chicken stock cube. Put the lid on.

LAMB Drizzle olive oil straight into the pack of neck fillet and season. Turn the racks of lamb then put the two neck fillets in the pan. Sear the ends of the meat and keep coming back to the pan and turning each piece so they brown all over.

Pull the leaves off 3 sprigs of rosemary and put into a pestle & mortar with a good pinch of salt & pepper. Peel the garlic, add to the mortar, and pound really well. Turn the lamb over. Add Dijon mustard to the mortar with a good couple of lugs of olive oil and a swig of white wine vinegar. Mix well.

Make sure all sides of the lamb are seared, then use tongs to transfer all of it to a roasting tray. Pour away most of the fat in the pan, then put it back on a very low heat for the gravy. Spoon the dressing from the pestle & mortar over the lamb and put the vines of cherry tomatoes on top. Move everything around until well coated in the dressing. Sprinkle with salt, then whack on the top shelf of the oven and set the timer for 14 minutes for blushing to medium meat, slightly less for rare, and more for well done. Turn the racks over halfway through.

GRAVY Finely slice the bacon and put into the frying pan.

MINT SAUCE Finely chop the reserved mint leaves and add to the unwashed pestle & mortar. Pound, then add the red wine vinegar, caster sugar, a pinch of salt and 2 tablespoons of cooking water from the veg pot. Muddle together with the pestle, have a taste to check the balance, and add a tiny splash of extra virgin olive oil. Take to the table with a spoon.

GRAVY Turn the heat under the bacon right up and add the leaves from the rosemary. Stir in the flour, red wine and a few ladles of cooking water.

VEGETABLES Trim all the beans and put the runner beans through a runner bean slicer or slice at an angle, 1cm thick. Cut the Savoy cabbage half in two and click off any tatty outer leaves, then discard the stalk. Cut the cabbage into thin wedges. Add the cabbage, beans and peas to the saucepan, then stir and put the lid back on.

LAMB Turn the lamb over. If your tomatoes are colouring too much, lean the meat on top of them.

GRAVY Stir in a spoonful of cooking water if needed.

FONDUE Smash the bar of chocolate in its wrapping then unwrap and put it into a small microwave-safe bowl with the vanilla paste or extract, a small pinch of salt and the milk. Microwave on full power for 1½ minutes, leave to rest for a few seconds and stir, then microwave for 1 more minute on full power. Meanwhile, chop all your fruit into bite-sized chunks and wedges and pile these on a platter. Take the bowl out of the microwave and stir until all the chocolate has melted, then put the bowl on the platter and take to the table.

LAMB When the 14 minutes are up, take your lamb out of the oven and leave it to rest for a minute.

VEGETABLES Drain the veg in a colander, then return them to the pan. Drizzle well with extra virgin olive oil, and add a good pinch of salt & pepper and a knob of butter. Squeeze over the juice of ½ a lemon and toss well. Tip on to a large serving platter and take to the table.

GRAVY Taste and correct the seasoning, then pour into a gravy boat and take to the table.

TO SERVE Cut the racks into individual chops and slice up the neck fillet. Pile on a platter. Move most of the cherry tomatoes to the platter on top of the lamb, mushing the rest into the cooking juices. Stir in a good lug of extra virgin olive oil, then drizzle over the platter and serve.

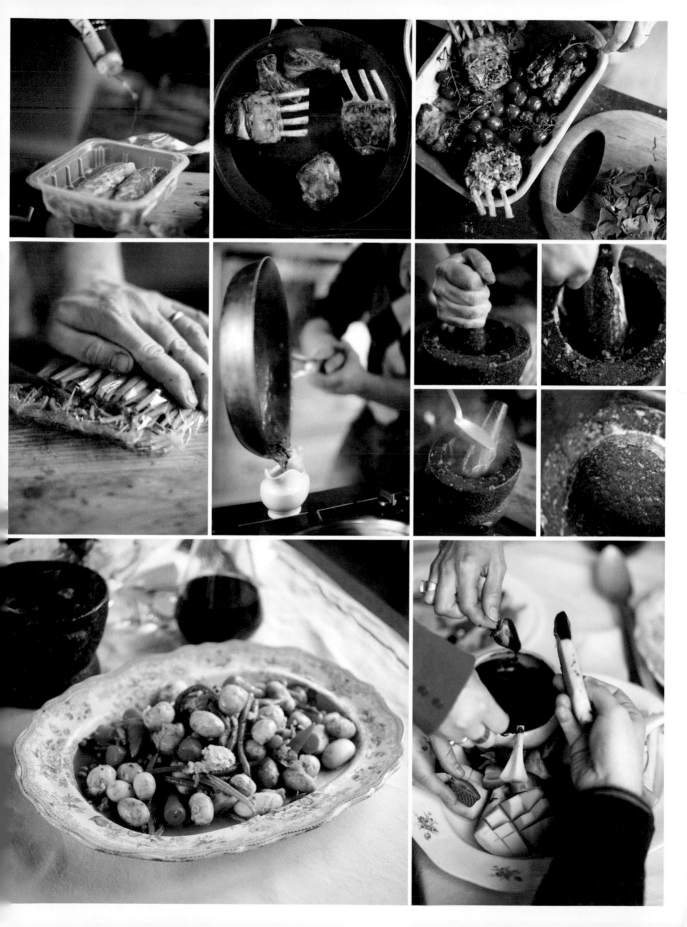

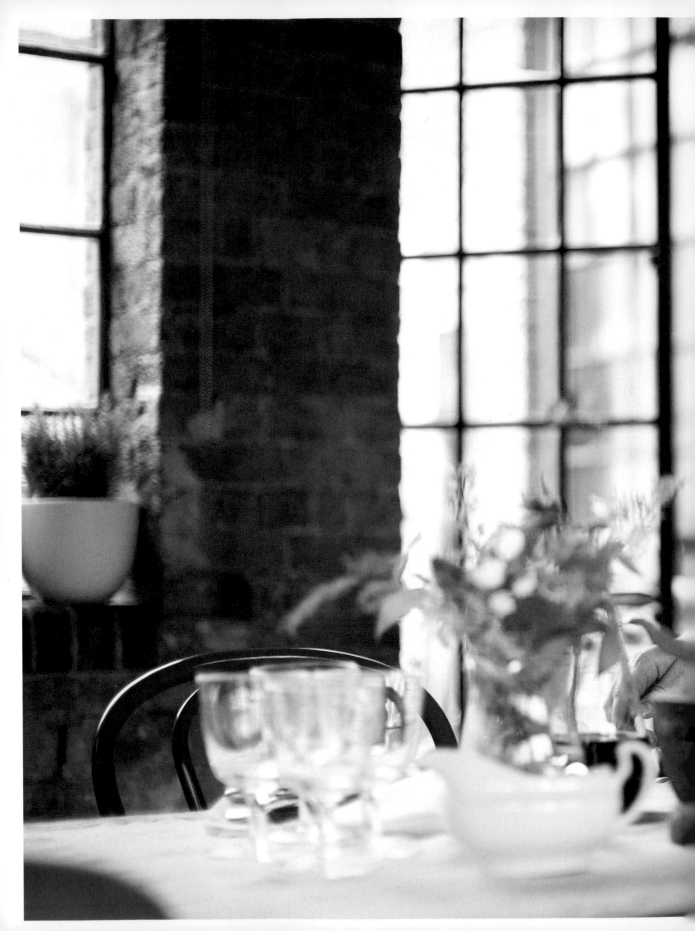

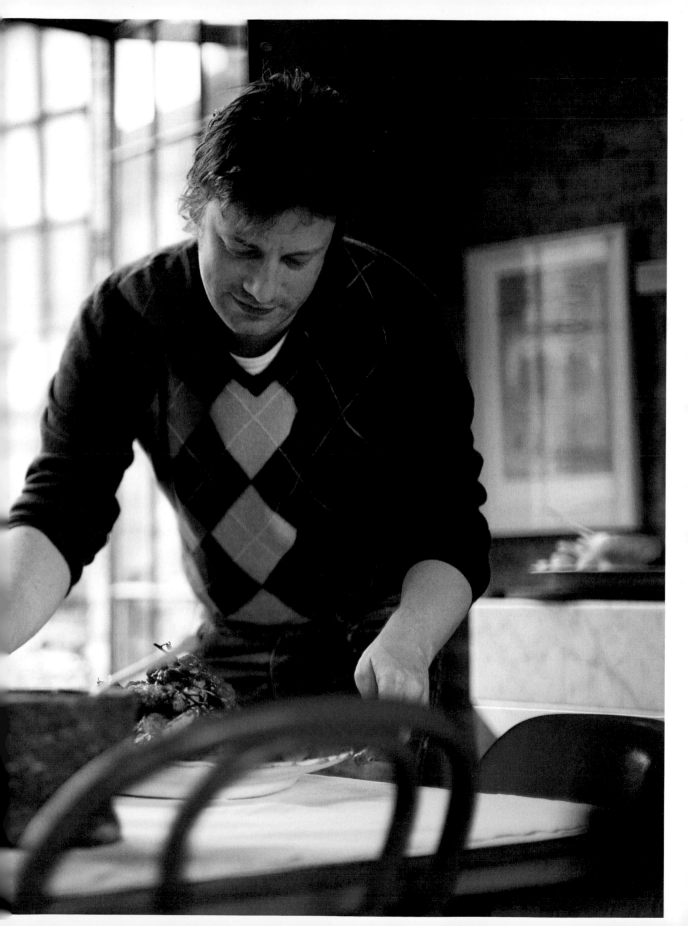

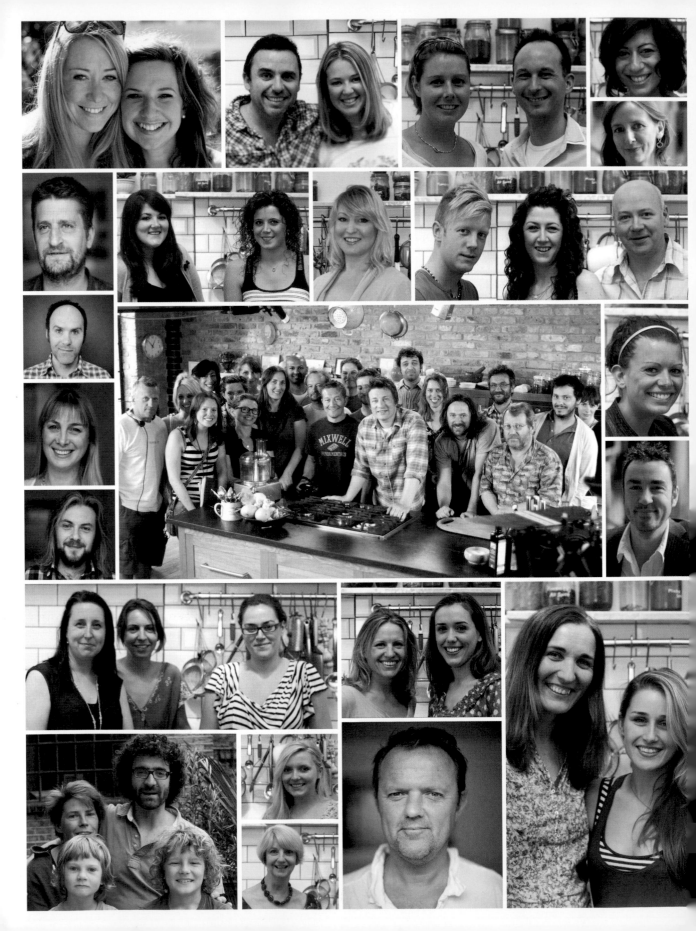

THANKS

This list gets longer and longer every year but, as always, I'm going to do my very best to not leave anyone out. If I do, please forgive me and let me know so I can get you into the reprint! Thanks, first and foremost, to my beautiful and patient wife, Jools, who is still willing to share a meal with me, even when I'm home later than expected. Love you. Thanks to my kids, Poppy, Daisy, Petal and — (I haven't met this one yet!) for being such funny, interesting and generally wonderful little people. Thanks and love as always to Mum and Dad and, of course, to Gennaro Contaldo.

To my dear friend and photographer extraordinaire 'Lord' David Loftus: once again, mate, you've outdone yourself. Choosing between all your beautiful photographs this time around has been a real struggle. Much love.

Huge thanks and love to my wonderfully supportive, creative and energetic food team. You've been excited about this book right alongside me and done an incredible job as usual: to the brilliant style girls Ginny Rolfe, Anna Jones, Sarah Tildesley, Georgie Socratous and little Christina 'Scarabooch' McCloskey. Big love to my main men Pete Begg and Daniel Nowland and, of course, to superb ladies Claire Postans, Bobby Sebire, Joanne Lord, Helen Martin, and to Laura Parr for keeping an eye on nutrition for me! I honestly don't know what I'd do without you guys. Big shout out as well to Abigail 'Scottish' Fawcett, Becca Hetherston and Kelly Bowers for their help on recipe testing.

Love and thanks to my hard-working word girls: my editor, Katie Bosher, and the lovely Rebecca 'Rubs' Walker and Bethan O'Connor.

Big shout out to the Penguin crew, who are always brave enough to get behind my crazy ideas. Especially to my dear friends John Hamilton, Lindsey Evans, Tom Weldon and Louise Moore – it has been a pleasure working on another one of these books together. Thanks, as well, to my new mate, Alistair (Al, Aladdin, Aslan, Alsace) Richardson, for his help designing this book. To the rest of the Penguin team who keep the wheels turning and do such a great job under pressure: Nick Lowndes, Juliette Butler, Janis Barbi, Laura Herring, Airelle Depreux, Clare Pollock, Chantal Noel, Kate Brotherhood, Elizabeth Smith, Jen Doyle, Jeremy Ettinghausen, Anna Rafferty, Ashley Wilks, Naomi Fidler, Thomas Chicken and all the people on their teams – great work, guys. And big thanks, as always, to the very lovely Annie Lee, and to Helen Campbell and Caroline Wilding.

This book also has a digital edition with lots of great bonus content. So big thanks, once again, to David Loftus and also to Paul Gwilliams for the beautiful filming they've done for that. Thanks also to Matt Shaw and Gudren Claire from Fresh One for sorting out all the footage and editing it so beautifully. My marketing exec, the very lovely and clever Eloise Bedwell, worked hard to bring all the digital stuff together, so a big shout out to her.

To my CEO, John Jackson, managing director, Tara Donovan, and manager, Louise Holland ('Yoda', 'M', or my 'Chief of Staff' as she's known in America), and all of their teams – thanks so much for doing what you do so brilliantly. Same goes for my personal team, who do the most incredible job of looking out for me and keeping my life on track: Liz McMullan, Holly Adams, Beth Richardson, Paul Rutherford, Saffron Greening and Susie Blythe – thanks, guys. The rest of my wonderful office work so hard every day and make coming into work an absolute pleasure. Lots of them got stuck in and tested the recipes in this book for me (a few pictures of them are opposite) so a big round of applause to them for giving me such great feedback. You guys are brilliant!

And big, big love and thanks to the wonderful television team pictured with me on the opposite page. You guys helped me turn this book into a brilliant series and we had a great time doing it. To my lovely Fresh One team: Zoe Collins and Jo Ralling, Roy Ackerman, Martha Delap, Emily Taylor, Kirsten Rogers, Gudren Claire, Lou Dew, Esub Miah and Alex Gardiner. The brilliant crew: Luke Cardiff, Dave Miller, Olly Wiggins, Paul Gwilliams (cheers for the extra pics), Mike Sarah, Godfrey Kirby, Daryl Higgins, Andy Young, Pete Bateson, Jeff Brown and Chris Stevens – you guys really are the best. Shout out again to my incredible food girls who helped make the filming go so smoothly. Big thanks as well to Kate McCullough, Almir Santos and also to the edit team, Jen Cockburn, Jackie Witts, Barbara Graham, Steve Flatt and Mike Kerr.

And, of course, a big thanks to the Forster family. The last thing Jools needed while pregnant with our fourth child was me shooting a whole book in our kitchen. So I was very lucky that these guys were willing to let me invade their beautiful home to cook for days on end. Crispin, who's been my favourite carpenter for a few years now, made the table in this book especially for me. Thanks so much, mate, and big hugs to Gemma and your two boys, Jago and Felix. I enjoyed every minute.

INDEX

Page references in **bold** indicate an illustration
v indicates a vegetarian recipe

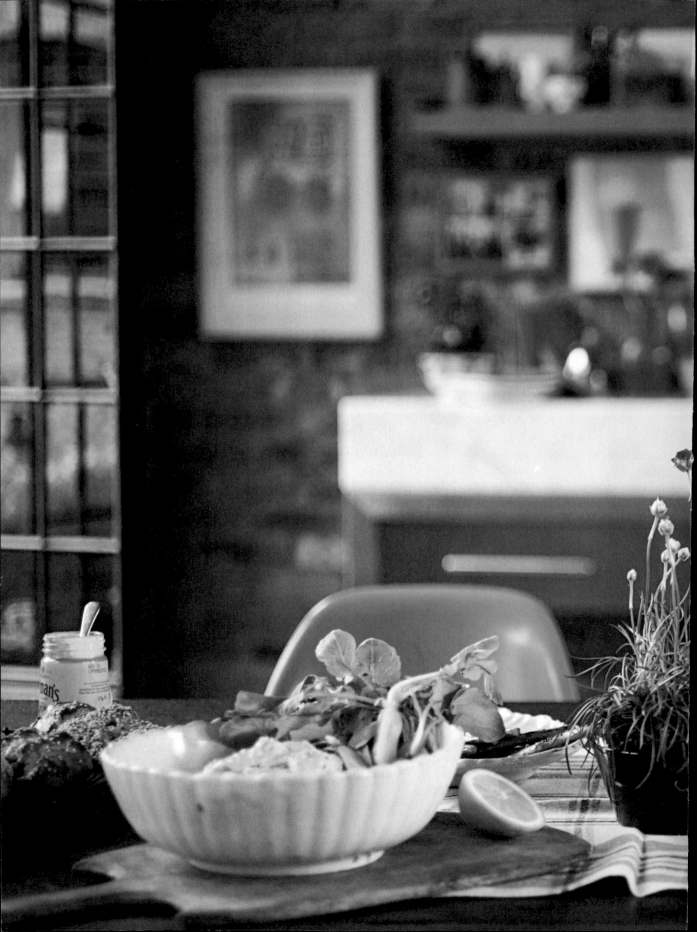

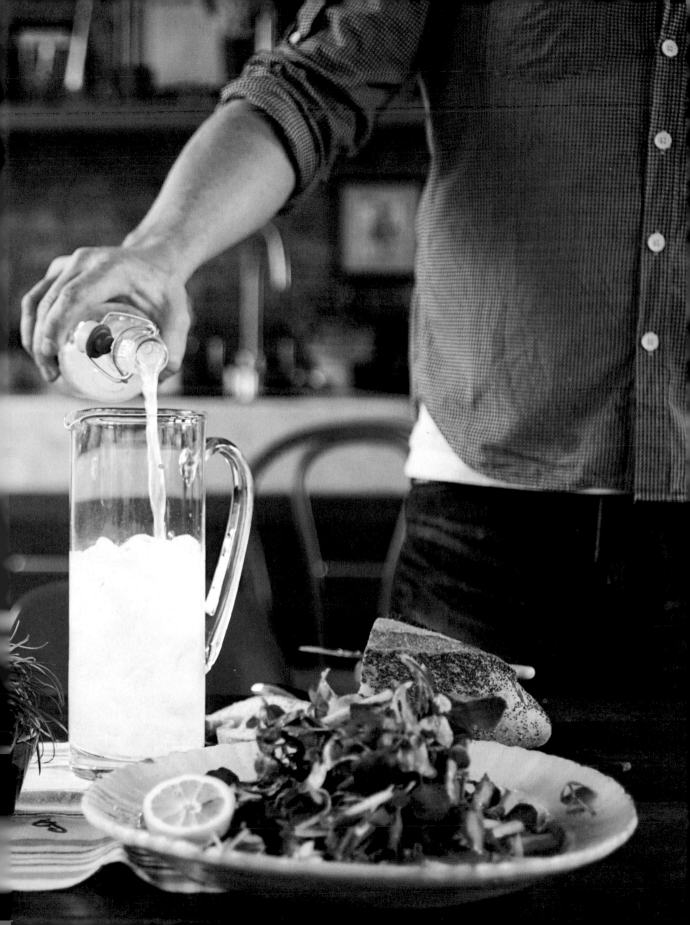

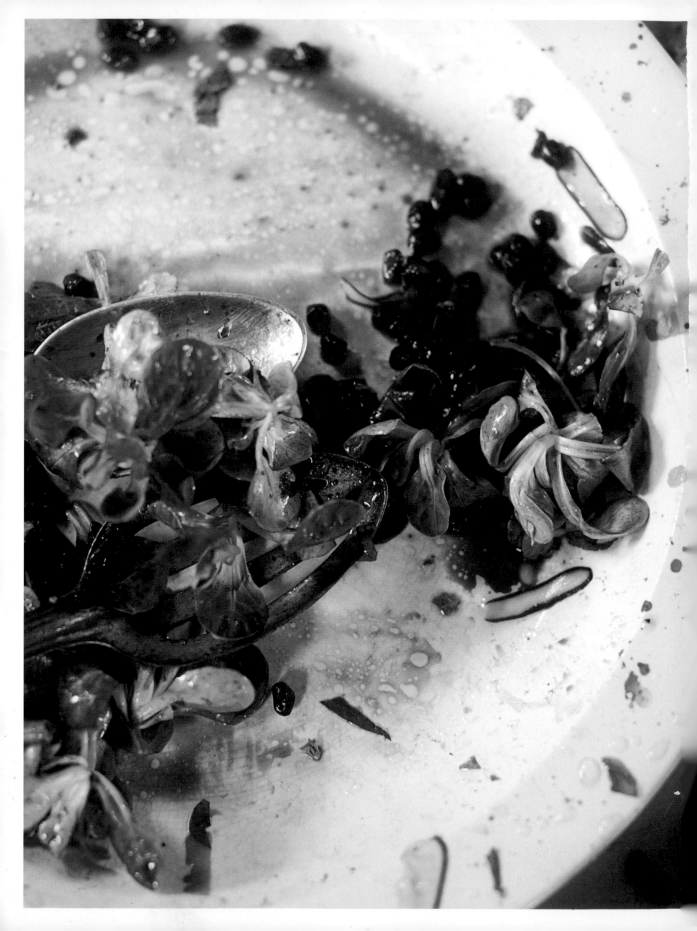